Respiratory Diseases in Cattle

Current Topics in Veterinary Medicine

Volume 3

Respiratory Diseases in Cattle

A Seminar in the EEC Programme of Coordination of Research on Beef Production held at Edinburgh, November 8-10, 1977

Sponsored by the Commission of the European Communities, Directorate-General for Agriculture, Coordination of Agricultural Research

Edited by

W. B. Martin

Animal Diseases Research Association,
Moredun Institute,
Edinburgh

Martinus Nijhoff - The Hague/Boston/London   1978
for
The Commission of the European Communities

Publication arranged by

Commission of the European Communities,
Directorate-General Scientific and Technical Information
and Information Management, Luxembourg.

EUR 6010 EN

ISBN-13:978-94-009-9752-3   e-ISBN-13:978-94-009-9750-9
DOI: 10.1007/978-94-009-9750-9

Table of contents

PREFACE

Not so many years ago little attention was paid to non-parasitic
respiratory diseases of cattle because they seemed of minor importance.
However, in the past twenty years, as the number of cattle kept on any farm
unit increased under economic pressures, there has been a concomitant rise
in the prevalence of respiratory illness.

Investigations into cattle respiratory diseases have become a significant
part of the research effort in most countries of Europe. Initially much work
went into finding, like the alchemist's stone, the organism responsible for
causing cattle respiratory disease. Many viruses were isolated and over the
years a long list of those recovered from the respiratory tract of cattle
has been prepared. Unfortunately, few of these viruses on their own are
recognised as proven pathogens and no single virus provides the complete
aetiological answer to bovine respiratory disease.

More recently, perhaps in despair, greater attention has been directed
to the role of mycoplasma and, additionally, a revival of interest has taken
place in the significant part played by bacteria in the later stages of respiratory disease. Now, phrases such as "multifactorial disease" are being
commonly used to describe the complex situation with respiratory disease.

The respiratory infections of cattle do not respect international
boundaries. All countries involved in intensive beef or dairy production
are afflicted with the problem and the movement of large numbers of cattle
within, and between, countries disseminates infection and encourages outbreaks
of disease. Changes in agricultural methods as the result of economic pressures must be accepted. Consequently, veterinary surgeons and others engaged
in combating livestock diseases must perforce be involved in finding effective
ways to reduce or eliminate the deaths and performance losses which follow in
the wake of intensive animal production.

It is with this aim in mind that this Seminar has been organised on
behalf of the Directorate General of Agriculture of the Commission of the
European Communities and the participants collected together for three days
of intensive discussion. By such exchange of information and ideas it is
hoped that all those involved in the problem of respiratory disease in cattle

will be brought up to date with the situation in each country and with the current research findings throughout Europe.

Answers to the problems of respiratory disease must and will be found, and it is through the stimulation of seminars such as this one that progress will be hastened.

OPENING REMARKS

P. L'Hermite *(EEC)*

I would like to welcome you all to the Moredun Institute, and to this seminar on respiratory diseases of cattle. I will only say a few words about the problems and objectives of this kind of seminar.

You know that we have a research programme at the Commission on improvement in beef production. A certain part of this programme is set aside to deal specifically with enteric diseases in calves and respiratory diseases.

In 1975 we organised the first seminar on perinatal health in calves, under the chairmanship of Dr. Rotin, and this represents the second seminar in the field of bovine pathology. We are planning another seminar in France, in Thiverval Grignon in April 1978, about the use and quality of colostrum. In Dublin in November 1977 we are having another research workshop, organised by Professor Kelly, on the problems of animals and human health hazards caused by livestock effluents. It is the purpose of the Commission to maintain the free exchange of animals between the member States, and to avoid the communication of diseases to humans.

For this purpose we are in permanent communication with veterinarians within the Commission who are responsible for the establishment of the Veterinary Code, and who are already setting up four eradication programmes, one on bovine tuberculosis, one on bovine cysticercosis, one on bovine brucellosis, and one on classical swine fever.

I hope that we will obtain a better knowledge of some of the problems connected with respiratory disease from this seminar, in order to track down the origins of the diseases for the betterment of relations within the Commission.

I would like to take this opportunity to thank Dr. Martin
for his co-operation in organising this seminar, both scientific-
ally and administratively, and I would also like to thank his
co-ordinators who have participated in the organisation of this
seminar.

SESSION I

INCIDENCE

Chairman and Co-ordinator:

W.B. Martin

VARIATION IN THE RESPIRATORY VIRUS STATUS OF LARGE BOVINE UNITS IN BELGIUM

F. Lomba

Université de Liège, Faculté de Médecine Vétérinaire,
Rue des Vétérinaires 45, 1070 Bruxelles, Belgium.

ABSTRACT

Cattle in six large bovine units in Belgium were studied for five years. Blood and colostrum samples from cows near parturition, as well as blood samples from the calves before colostrum feeding and at different ages, were checked for the commonest viruses. Paired sera were also examined when respiratory infections occurred.

Results of this study were as follows:

1. Clinically and economically, the incidence of viral respiratory disease was important only in the beef units. Dairy units suffered only mild outbreaks of pneumo-enteritis caused by adenovirus.

2. Of the autumn respiratory infections, by far the most important identified viruses were RSV, reo. 1 and 2, PI3 and IBR.

3. Before feeding colostrum no calf had antibodies against adeno, reo. 1 and 2, IBR or RSV viruses but 10% of these calves had antibodies against BVD virus.

4. Antibody titres in colostrum were not related to the circulating antibodies of the cows, except for PI3. There was also no relationship between the antibody titres in colostrum and in the blood of calves two days old.

5. Variations, in the serum antibodies, with age were considerable but apparently unrelated to the clinical history on the farms.

INTRODUCTION

For several years, the marked improvement in the conform-
ation of certain of our herds of cattle, especially the Belgian
Blue White, has been accompanied by an increase in respiratory
infections (Wellemans et al., 1977). As Tapia-Yanez and Rough
(1976) have observed in France, we also noticed that under our
conditions, enzootic infectious bronchopneumonia of young
cattle is more serious than locomotor and digestive problems
so that it constitutes, at present, a serious limiting factor
to the intensive production of meat.

To contribute to the study of respiratory pathology, we
have tried to pinpoint, in the large cattle enterprises that
we follow regularly, certain characteristics of the respiratory
diseases: notably the casual agents, using diagnostic methods,
the incidence of respiratory diseases and their development.

MATERIAL AND METHODS

For the past six years five cattle enterprises have been
followed. Four were comprised of the Frisonne Pie-Noire breed
and the fifth of the primary beef producing Belgian Blue White
breed. Each farm contained approximately sixty cows. We
determined the presence of antibodies directed against infectious
bovine rhinotracheitis (IBR), parainfluenza 3 (PI3), adeno
type A and B, bovine virus diarrhoea (BVD), reovirus I and II
and respiratory syncytial bovis (RSB) viruses in the following:

blood samples from cows at three periods of the year and
at calving time

colostrum

blood samples from calves, before (O hour) and after (48
hours) the ingestion of colostrum

paired sera, collected at the time of each attack involving
more than one animal.

The tests used were those currently used at the Institut National de Recherches Vétérinaires and described by Wellemans et al. (1977). The results were considered positive or negative according to the following plan:

	PI3 FC IHA	Adeno PG FC	IBR FC	BVD PG FC	RSB PG FC	Reo I, II IHA
Positive	8 8	+ 8	8	+ 8	+ 8	8
Negative	4 4	- 4	4	- 4	- 4	4

FC = fluorescein-conjugate   IHA = indirect haemagglutination
PG = gel precipitin.

All of the usual zootechnical information was recorded as well as all illnesses with their development and treatment.

RESULTS

1. Incidence and clinical importance

1.1 Viral infections occurred on all the farms whether dairy or meat producing, but the consequences were clearly different from one farm to another. The farm raising beef cattle was the one that suffered most for the following reasons:

a) A very high morbidity rate: each year all the young cattle on the farm, with the occasional exception of a group of heifers living under exceptionally favourable conditions, were affected by the 'bovine grippe'.

b) Production losses caused by respiratory disease alone were particularly high due to long and expensive medical treatment, weight loss due to anorexia and frequent forced slaughter. These losses were caused, for the most part, by incurable lesions of pulmonary emphysema.

c) A high frequency of involvement of sites other than the respiratory tract, such as encephalitis and, especially, metritis due to the IBR virus which we have recently described (Lomba et al., 1976).

On the dairy farms, despite a hyperthermia of 41.5°C, the clinical signs in the cattle were generally difficult to detect, sometimes even passing unnoticed. Only once, in the winter of 1974, a pneumoenteritis accompanied by a positive sero-conversion to adenovirus type B, struck all the cows on two dairy farms almost simultaneously. This was characterised during a five day period by a strong hyperthermia (41.5°C), profuse diarrhoea, anorexia and by an almost complete, but temporary, halt in milk production.

At one of the four dairy farms, however, (farm 4) the mortality rate for calves from 15 days to 6 months old was high, but the respiratory lesions, regardless of their importance and gravity, were far from being the only ones which could be blamed. Insufficient living space, poor management practice, salmonella infections and parasite infestations also played a role which could not be overlooked.

1.2 The vast majority of respiratory infections occurred in the fourth trimester of the year, from September to December. One case of rhinotracheitis, clinically very similar to IBR but accompanied by a positive sero-conversion to reo I, was observed in April in a group of 10 heifers 9 - 10 months old, of the Belgian Blue White breed. They were transported and held in an area which was too small and where, when at liberty, they displayed incessant and excessive movement.

2. Antiviral antibodies in the blood of newborn calves before colostrum feeding

By examination of the precolostral blood from 215 calves to detect antibodies to adeno, BVD, IBR, PI3, reo I and II and RSB we tried to see if some calves had become infected *in utero*. None of the calves had antibodies against adeno, IBR, reo I and II, RSB, but two calves had antibodies against PI3 and 10 had antibodies against BVD (farm 5). Since they had at the same time higher Ig serum levels than the others, it was concluded that these calves had been infected *in utero* before parturition.

3. Passive transfer of maternal antibodies by colostrum
3.1 Composition of colostrum

Two hundred and eighty samples of colostrum were analysed for their quantity of antiviral antibodies. The results obtained are summarised in Table 1.

TABLE 1

ANTIVIRAL ANTIBODIES IN COLOSTRUM

Virus	N	Total number of positive colostrum	Per cent
Adeno B	280	205	73
BVD	280	152	64
IBR	280	32 (+ 108 AC*)	-
PI3	280	223 (+ 43 AC*)	79 (+ AC)
Reo I	83	76	91
Reo II	83	45	54
RSB	280	205	73

* Anticomplementary

Except for IBR which could not be fully checked, the majority of colostrums contained many antiviral antibodies.

3.1.1 Annual variations in the quantity of antibodies in colostrum

The annual variation in the quantity of antiviral antibodies present in colostrum can be quite substantial for certain viruses. In effect, while the percentages of 'positive' colostrum samples stay relatively constant for BVD (55 - 60%), PI3 ($\approx$ 100%) and for reo I (90%), they varied from 60 to 100% for RSB, from 3 to 35% for IBR and from 3 to 98% for adenovirus B.

The years which gave the highest percentage of positive colostrum samples were:

```
Adeno:  1974 (98%)
BVD:    1972 (60%) and 1974 (65%)
IBR:    1975 (30%) and 1976 (35%)
RSB:    1970 (75%) and 1975 (100%)
PI3 and reo I and reo  II: always very frequent.
```

3.1.2 Variations according to farm enterprises

Particularly when comparing one farm with another, and from one year to the next, colostrum samples appeared extremely useful. This is demonstrated very well in the results presented below as an example. They give the variations of percentages of positive colostrum samples from two farms and at different times.

Farm 5		Adeno B	BVD	IBR	PI3	RSB
Belgian Blue White	1971	0	0	0	100	76
	1972	4	48	8	100	76
	1974	100	100	–	100	100
	1975	80	80	50	100	100
	1976	86	48	57	100	57
Farm 2						
Frisonne Pie-Noire	1972	0	61	0	100	61
	1975	100	0	0	100	100

The increase in the number of colostrum samples positive for IBR on farm 5 might be due to the systematic vaccination of all cattle with a monovalent IBR vaccine. On the other hand it is clear that the farm had problems with BVD after 1971, with adenovirus after 1972, and that 1974 was a difficult year (BVD, RSB, adeno), with a return to a more acceptable situation in 1976. Farm 2 never had a problem with IBR, nor in 1975 with BVD. One notes, however, that since 1972 there was a remarkable increase in the number of colostrum samples positive for RSB and 100% for adenovirus. Looking at the results from farms 1, 3 and 4, we see that they had trouble, with adenovirus, BVD, and with RSB viruses. Antibodies against IBR were rare but not absent. In the four farms where they were systematically examined

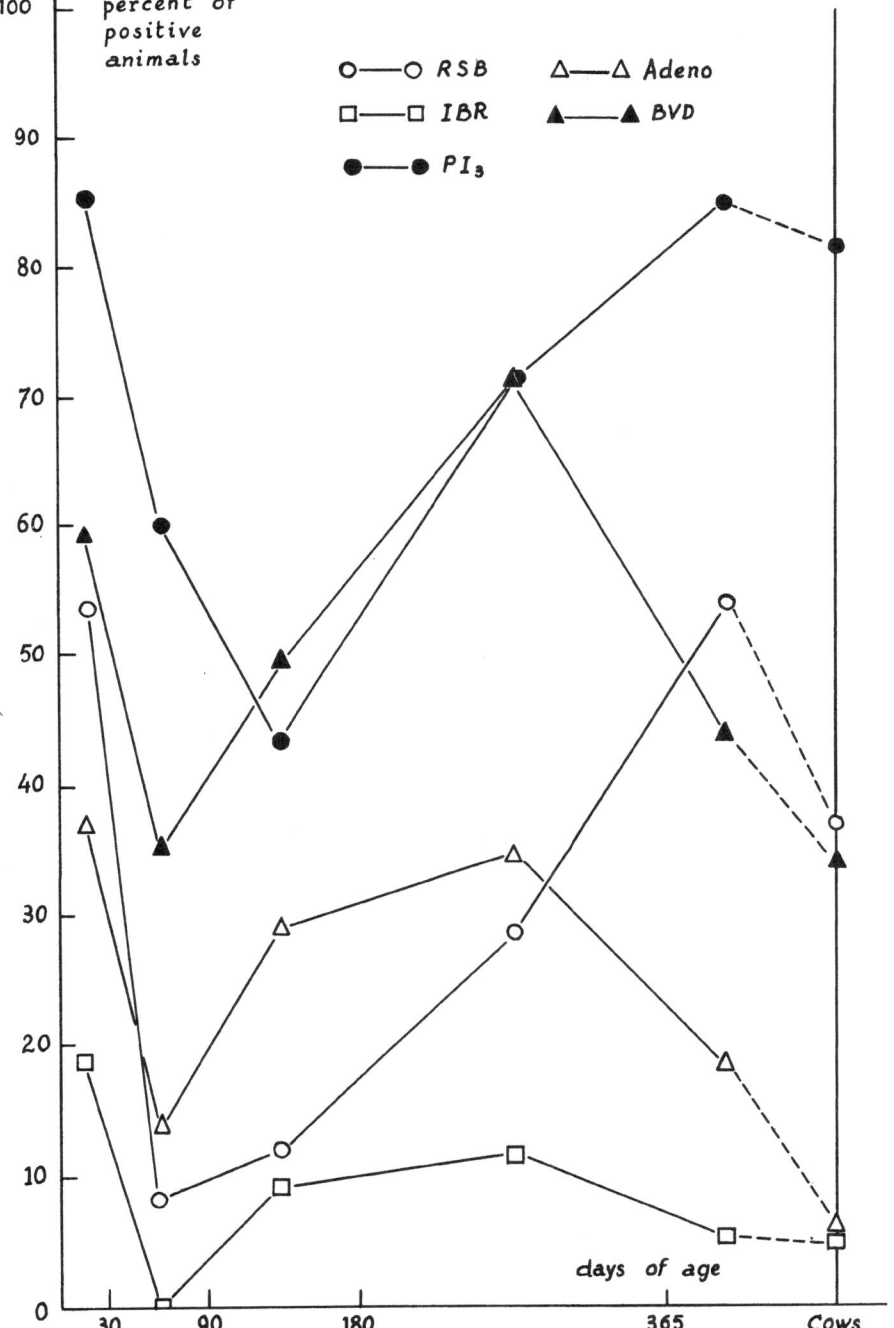

Fig. 1 Variations in antiviral antibodies with age

for, from 1974, antibodies against reo I and II were found with a frequency matching that of PI3.

3.2 Relationship: mother - colostrum - calf

In 106 cases where we had a sample of blood from the mother at parturition, a sample of colostrum, and a sample of blood from the calf at 48 h, it was possible to compare serological titres of the calves at 48 h with the corresponding titres of the colostrum and with the blood of the mothers. The results given in Table 2 show that :

Except for PI3 antibodies which were practically always present in the blood at high titre, the number of positives was much higher in the colostrum sample than in the blood of the cows that produced colostrum.

Even more remarkable was the number of cows which were serologically negative but showed a significant content of viral antibodies in the colostrum.

Except for PI3 virus, a significant number of calves had not acquired a sufficient number of antiviral antibodies at 48 h. For BVD virus, the number of calves serologically positive was higher than the number of positive colostrum samples. As seen earlier, this could be explained partly by the existence of already 'positive' calves before any administration of colostrum.

To evaluate the virological history of an enterprise, as shown in the preceding paragraph, the best method could be to analyse the colostrum rather than the blood of adults or that of the calves.

4. Variations in the serum antibodies with age

The antiviral antibody content was measured in the blood of the same animals at different ages. Figure 1 gives, according to virus group, the number of positive animals in relation to the total number of subjects examined. We notice again, and we will come back to this point later on, that as far as the young are concerned, many animals do not have

TABLE 2

PASSIVE TRANSMISSION OF COLOSTRAL ANTIBODIES

Virus	Number of calvings	Number of positive samples in		
		Serum from dams	Colostrum	Serum from calves (at 48 hours)
Adeno B	106	9	67 (60)	42
BVD	106	25	55 (38)	70
IBR	106	2	22*(21)	30
PI3	106	98	71*(7)	88
Reo I	78	48	71 (27)	56
Reo II	78	51	43 (14)	56
RSB	106	30	79 (59)	61

( ) number of positive colostrums produced by cows which were
serologically negative.

* not including 32 anticomplementary colostrums.

sufficient circulating immunity except for PI3. Nevertheless
many more animals were positive for reo I and II, RSB, and BVD
than for adeno and IBR. One can see a clear difference between,
on the one hand BVD and PI3 and on the other RSB, IBR and adenovirus. For all viruses there was a drop in antibody titres of
the same extent, as animals went from 0 - 30 days to 30 - 90
days. While a high percentage of animals maintained a significant
level of antibodies to BVD and PI3 viruses at 30 - 90 days of
age, this is not the case for the other viruses for which the
antibodies diminish considerably at this same stage to the
point that calves 1 - 3 months of age no longer had circulating
immunity against IBR. In older calves there was an increase in
antibody titre to all the viruses but it was difficult to
ascribe this rise to natural infection or vaccination (IBR for
example).

5. Characteristics of each enterprise

Farm 1.

This farm is both a dairy farm (cows of the Pie-Noire
breed), and a meat-producing farm (fattening resulting from

crossing the cows with Charolais or Blue White Belgian bulls).
Our observations lasted three years. We did not find any
problem there with BVD and, even though 12% of the mothers and
70% of the colostrums were positive for this virus, all of the
animals under 2 years old stayed serologically negative, with
one or two exceptions. IBR was never a threat though the
numbers of animals which were serologically positive increased
after the introduction of 3 Holstein heifers bought in France.

The RSB virus was found in abundance at all times. Each
year, in the fall, young animals could be observed suffering
from the 'grippe'. Only once, out of three episodes, could an
etiological diagnosis be made. In October 1971, calves less
than 3 months old showed a significant sero-conversion and PI3
was shown to be the causal agent. On the other hand, at the
same time calves 3 months to 1 year old, held in another section
of the farm, showed a sero-conversion just as significant but
this time for adenovirus B.

It is interesting to look at the rise of antibodies against
these two viruses both before and after October 1971 for
animals of different age groups

	1970		1971		1972
PI3	spring	autumn	spring	autumn	spring
48 h - 1 month	0/4	1/8	0/12	-	4/4
1 - 3 months	0/6	0/6	-	6/6	2/2
3 - 12 months	6/35	8/37	-	-	13/13
12 - 24 months	3/5	3/5	1/3	-	3/3
adults	41/60	23/60	25/60	-	15/15
Adeno B					
48 h - 1 month	0/4	0/8	0/12	-	-
1 - 3 months	1/15	0/15	0/4	-	-
3 - 12 months	0/9	5/37	-	-	6/6+++
12 - 24 months	0/5	0/2	0/2	-	0/3
adults	7/60	0/60	0/60	-	0/60

It can be seen that the outbreak caused by PI3 was
followed by a spectacular rise in the percentage of positive
animals to this virus while the 'grippe' caused by adeno B had
no effect other than to cause a temporary rise in antibodies
against this virus in affected animals.

In addition, it is surprising to note that in spite of an
average-to-abundant presence of antibodies to adeno B and PI3
in the colostrum (respectively 51% and 91% positive) the young
calves were totally deficient in them. Perhaps this was the
reason for their susceptibility to those viruses as ubiquitous
as PI3. It is difficult to incriminate the distribution of
colostrum because these same calves at 48 h to 1 month of age
had acquired elevated titres against RSB.

Farm 2
One is struck by the fact that practically all the calves
stayed serologically negative (except for PI3) until the age
of 6 months. From 6 months to 1 year but, even more so, from
1 year to 2 years, they became positive for RSB and BVD as
well as other viruses. The cows never encountered IBR virus.
On the other hand they all had antibodies against PI3, reo I
and reo II, and since 1974, against adeno B and BVD. The only
viral episode worth mentioning was pneumo-enteritis with seroconversion to adeno B that struck all the cows simultaneously
in December 1974.

Farm 3
On this farm they experienced no viral diseases other than
a pneumo-enteritis similar to that on farm 2, which occurred
during the same period. However, on this farm antibodies against
all of the viruses studied in the report were present in the
colostrum, in the blood of the mothers, and also in the blood
of the calves with the same frequency during the four year
period.

Farm 4
The same remarks can be made as for farm 3 concerning the

number of antibodies in the different mediums studied. This
farm differed from the other in that there were numerous
fatalities amongst the young. These fatalities, however, could
not be attributed solely to respiratory diseases.

Farm 5

Each fall this farm is troubled by cases of bovine 'grippe'.
Only once in 4 years could a correlation be made with a
positive seroconversion (in 1976 for reo I). RSB virus and
PI3 virus have always been abundant here. Adenoviruses have
shown a marked increase beginning in 1974.

However, it is BVD virus which appears to be most typical.
There were no antibodies against BVD until 1971. During the
second trimester of 1971 the colostrums became positive but
significant titres appeared in the blood of the animals only
after a period of several months. Since this time practically
all of the colostrums and the bloods of the calves at 48 h of
age have proved to be positive for BVD. Three calves of 4 -
6 months of age died of an acute form of BVD in August 1973.

CONCLUSIONS

1.   It is possible to characterise the dynamics of viral
infections on a farm by relying on the presence of antiviral
antibodies in the blood of animals, such as new born calves,
young and adult cattle, and in paired sera of diseased animals.
The anlaysis of colostrum has also proved useful. This
information permits the identification of virus infections
that appear on a farm. It also allows the pinpointing of the
beginning and duration of the virus infection, even after the
blood of the animals, both young and old, no longer contains
the corresponding antibodies.

2.   The passive transmission of maternal antibodies by colostrum
feeding has not yet proved to be totally successful, at least
in the farm enterprises that we followed regularly. In effect,

a very high number of calves of 48 h of age had not acquired significant titres of circulating antibodies.

3.   Only rarely can the development of the titre of antiviral antibodies in the blood of young bovines be connected with a well identified outbreak of the 'grippe'. On the other hand, one must note that at all times, except for such viruses as PI3 and reoviruses, a high number of animals do not have a sufficient circulating immunity.

4.   In the farms we surveyed, those exploiting milk cattle were less affected by viral disease than those rearing beef cattle. Antibodies against RSB, PI3 and the reoviruses are abundantly present. BVD virus is also well represented, and given the complexity of the troubles that it can provoke, even before birth, the situation is an unsettling one.

ACKNOWLEDGEMENT

We wish to thank Mr Herring for the English translation of our manuscript.

REFERENCES

Lomba, F., Bienfet, V. and Wellemans, G. 1976. Br. Vet. J. 132, p.178
Tapia-Yanez, Rough, E. 1976. 9th International Congress of Buiatrics, Paris, p.695
Wellemans, G., Van Opdenbosch, E. and Strobbe, R. 1977. CEC Seminar on Respiratory Diseases of Cattle, Edinburgh.

RESPIRATORY DISEASES IN CALVES - INCIDENCE AND EPIDEMIOLOGY IN DENMARK*

O. Aalund

Royal Veterinary and Agricultural University, Rolighesdsvej 23,
Copenhagen, Denmark.

ABSTRACT

*In a Danish dairy herd of 350 milking cows the respiratory disease
(rd) situation among calves up to the age of 6 months was analysed. During
a 3 year period a total of 1 010 single calves were born. The rd
mortality rate in the herd was 9%. Approximately 85 - 90% of the fatal
cases of rd occurred after the third week of life. Rd accounted for
approximately 50% of the economic loss per calf.*

* This investigation was carried out in cooperation with Claus M. Willadsen,
Royal Veterinary and Agricultural University, Copenhagen, Denmark, and
L. Gjøl Christensen, National Cattle Research Institute, Copenhagen,
Denmark.

INTRODUCTION

This account of the situation in Denmark has been restricted to calves between birth and the end of the sixth month of life. It is during this age interval that respiratory disease constitutes a substantial health hazard. Information collected nationally on causal infectious agents and on associated epidemiology is scarce. Hence, this paper has concentrated on the analysis of the situation in a single Danish dairy herd of approximately 350 milking cows where the situation was comparable to that prevailing in most Danish dairy operations. The investigation (Willadsen et al., 1977) was carried out in an attempt to evaluate the economic aspects of respiratory diseases in calves.

MATERIALS

During a 3 year period a total of 1 010 single calves were born. The fate of these calves was analysed on the basis of detailed health records. The time interval from birth to the end of the sixth month was subdivided in 6 periods (Table 1) and the economic impact associated with mortality and morbidity was calculated for each of the 5 periods (Willadsen et al., 1977).

RESULTS

The mortality rate up to the first few hours after birth was 10%. The overall respiratory disease (rd) attack rate among the calves from birth up to the end of the sixth month was 23% with a case fatality rate of 40%. Hence the rd mortality rate in the herd was 23 x 40/100 = 9%. The mortality rate due to ailments other than rd was 12%, and the overall mortality rate during the first six months of life was 21% (Table 1). The overall mortality rate was higher for male than for female calves, 25% and 17% respectively. This difference was found by Chi-square analysis to be statistically significant (P >0.001).

TABLE 1

MORTALITY: ABSOLUTE PROBABILITIES (PER CENT) BY TIME PERIODS, CAUSES AND SEXES

Time period	Male and female combined				Male				Female			
	Rd.*	G.**	O***	Total	Rd.*	G**	O***	Total	Rd.*	G.**	O**	Total
1st week after birth	0.5	5.7	1.2	7.4	0.6	7.4	1.9	9.9	0.4	4.0	0.6	5.0
2nd week after birth	0.2	0.8	0.3	1.3	0.2	0.4	0.4	1.0	0.2	1.1	0.2	1.5
3rd week after birth	0.4	0.9	0.3	1.6	0.7	1.0	0.5	2.2	0.2	0.9	0.2	1.3
4th week after birth	0.8	0.5	0.1	1.4	1.2	0.7	0.2	2.1	0.4	0.4	0.0	0.8
2nd month after birth	3.2	1.6	0.0	4.8	4.2	1.3	0.0	5.5	2.2	1.8	0.0	4.0
3rd to 6th month after birth	3.8	0.3	0.3	4.4	3.5	0.5	0.5	4.5	4.0	0.2	0.2	4.4
Total	8.9	9.8	2.2	20.9	10.4	11.3	3.5	25.2	7.4	8.4	1.2	17.0

* Respiratory disease   ** Gastroenteritis   *** Other diseases

   Mortality among male calves was significantly associated
with parity of the mother (Table 2). Thus, the mortality rate
for male calves born to heifers was 32% as compared to 29% and
19% for male calves born at parity 2 and parity ⩾ 3 respectively.
The same trend prevailed for male and female calves combined,
whereas for female calves the lowest mortality rate was
observed at parity 2.

   From Table 1 it may be seen that gastroenteritis was the
prime cause of death during the first week of life while
approximately 85 - 90% of fatal cases of rd occurred after the
third week of life.

DISCUSSION

   The mortality figures reported here are not unusual for
the average Danish dairy herd. However, in order to revaluate
the total economic impact of diseases the statistics of non
fatal morbidity will also have to be analysed. The influence
of rd on the economic net return per calf has been shown to be
very substantial (Aalund et al., 1977; Willadsen et al., 1977).
At the current cost and price level, the net return per calf
of the dairy herd studied here was extremely close to zero, and
approximately 50% of the economic loss per calf was associated
with calves dying from rd. These investigations also showed
that the net return per calf would be improved by 40.14 Danish
crowns if the mortality among the calves treated for rd could
be reduced to about half of its present level. If 100% profit
on all extra investments was required and the money had to be
borrowed at an interest rate of 15% p.a. up to 19.32 Danish
crowns could be invested per calf to try to accomplish the above
goal.

TABLE 2

CALF MORTALITY RATES (PER CENT) FOR THE PERIOD BETWEEN BIRTH AND THE END
OF THE 6TH MONTH IN RELATION TO PARITY OF THE MOTHER

Parity	Male and female combined	Male	Female
1	22.5	32.0	17.3
2	23.8	29.0	15.2
$\geq$ 3	19.2	18.9	19.9
Chi-square	6.5	43.52	7.00
2 degrees of freedom	$P < 0.05$	$P < 0.001$	$P < 0.005$

REFERENCES

Aalund, O., Willadsen, C.M. and Christensen, L.G. 1977. CEC Seminar,
     Freising, May.
Willadsen, C.M. Aalund, O. and Christensen, L.G. 1977. Nord Vet Med.
     (in press)

EPIDEMIOLOGICAL SURVEY OF INFECTIOUS BOVINE RHINOTRACHEITIS IN FRANCE

G. Dannacher and M. Fedida

Laboratoire de Virologie Animale, 250 rue Marcel Merieux,
69342 Lyon, France.

ABSTRACT

Epidemiological surveys and diagnostic examinations show that IBR exists in France but that its frequency is still relatively low (2 to 5% of reactors) and certainly much less important than was first suggested. Serological positivity is more frequent in dairy farms of more than 50 head which include imported Holstein cattle. This result should caution breeders wishing to import cattle which are likely to be positive.

Most of the time, imported animals can be held responsible for infection with IBR but, in some cases, such an origin cannot be incriminated. Serological testings repeated at an interval of 6 to 8 months suggest that infection is rather stationary. However, actual outbreaks of IBR infection have been observed in several cases. The incidence of the disease in French cattle does not appear to have changed radically since 1974; IBR virus can be recognised as cause of clinical disease in 5 to 7% of investigated respiratory outbreaks.

Epidemiological features of infection result in necessary control measures. Imported cattle should be serologically tested in order to prevent further spread of infection and the introduction of possibly virulent virus strains. Bulls have to be examined for antibodies before entrance to artificial insemination stations. In herds known to run the risk of being infected, the losses caused by the disease can be reduced by an inactivated IBR vaccine which is now available commercially in France.

Infection with IBR virus has been described frequently in North America. For some years, in France, evidence of infection was obtained by the isolation of virus. However, only a few papers were devoted to this subject (Faye et al., 1967; Charton et al., 1970 and 1973). Severe outbreaks of the disease (Espinasse, et al., 1974; Gilbert et al., 1976; Martel et al., 1976) were correlated with new conditions of management and feeding in large units of dairy cattle or beef cattle and with the introduction of infected animals from other countries.

To answer questions concerning the importance, distribution and epidemiology of infection, the IBR situation in France was followed from 1974 by a series of inquiries initiated by the Director of Veterinary Services with the help of veterinary practitioners.

Virological and serological examinations of respiratory disease outbreaks, supported by laboratory diagnosis, provide further information on the IBR situation.

1. Sero-epidemiological surveys

Extensive serological examinations were carried out in our laboratory on different cattle populations:

Two surveys covering the whole territory.

Two others on a regional basis.

In addition, precise inquiries were started in two sectors:

Calf-fattening farms.

Large dairy-cow farms.

Estimation of serum antibodies was made by the serum neutralisation test and/or by a passive haemagglutination test according to the technique developed in our laboratory (Perrin et al. 1977).

A.   National surveys

   1) First national survey

   The first national survey (Dannacher et al., 1975)
concerned 15 departments which furnished 718 serum samples
from 134 different herds. Sera were collected from animals
without attention to the age, sex, breed or origin. The
percentage of antibody positive animals was found to be less
than 2% (1.95%) and 5.22% of farms showed one or more
positive animals.

   It should be noted that this percentage is similar to that
obtained on the sera from exported cattle (Dhennin, personal
communication). On the whole, the disease seemed not to be as
widespread as was initially thought.

   2) Second national survey

   This survey was conducted on farms where animals were
presumed to run the risk of being infected. Samples were
collected from large farms (50 head or more) essentially
comprising dairy cows of the Holstein breed. Furthermore, most
animals were imported or in contact with imported cows, or with
the progeny of imported cows.

   The laboratory received 2 700 sera collected from 230
farms in 24 departments. Information obtained from the owners
allowed the following conclusions to be drawn (Martel et al.,
1976):

   The total percentage of positive animals was 11.16%.

   The percentage of farms yielding one or more positive
animals was 36.95%.

   The percentages of animals positive according to the breed
were:

   - Holstein: 50%

   - Francaise Frisonne Pie-Noire (FFPN): 10.11%

The percentage of positive animals was found to be close to 5%, which is higher than that of the first survey. Animal concentration and intensive production result in a greater probability of positive reactors.

Serological investigations were carried out twice on the same animals at an interval of 6 to 8 months and eventually allowed a widespread outbreak of IBR infection to be monitored.

The even results obtained from 90% of the sera received periodically should be noted. Initially negative animals remain negative, and initially positive animals remain positive even with some variation in the antibody titre. Concerning the remaining 10% of cattle it appeared that:

- negative titres were obtained from animals with low levels of antibodies.

- increasing antibody titres or seroconversions. Initially negative animals which became positive were generally situated on farms where positive animals were found at the time of the first sample. This point illustrates virus persistence in the herds without clinical manifestation of infection.

Seroconversions in animals on farms where no positive was detected initially suggested two eventualities:

- the initial samples may have omitted some positive animals.

- an IBR virus had recently infected a previously negative herd.

-other and undetermined breeds; 7.50%

- all breeds other than Holstein: 8.49%

The percentages of positive animals, according to their origin, were:

- born in France: 6.46%

- descended from imported animals: 11.34%

- imported from all countries: 34.30%

- imported from North America: 48.80%

The influence of contact with imported animals gave the following percentage of animals positive:

- without contact with imported animals: 7.70%

- in-contact with imported animals: 22.04%

The influence of farm size on the percentage of positive animals:

- herds with 1 to 50 animals: 8.93%

- herds with more than 100 animals: 15.34%.

In fact, this point cannot be clearly demonstrated because the imported Holstein dairy cows were most frequently introduced in large herds. The result of this serological survey indicated that large dairy farms were infected much more than the mean cattle population. IBR positive sera originated principally from Holstein dairy cows and particularly from animals imported from North America.

B.   Regional survey

1) Brittany survey

The investigation concerned dairy cattle in farms devoid of imported cows but of a minimal size of 50 head. About 1 000 sera were tested for the presence of IBR antibodies.

2) Charolais survey

Sera were submitted for examination from beef cattle of the Charolais breed with respiratory symptoms of unknown etiology during the preceding months. Two hundred such sera from 25 herds of more than 50 head were examined for IBR antibodies.

On most farms the animals were found to be negative. Some positive sera were detected on 3 farms without any connection between the positive sera and the respiratory form of the disease being found.

C.   Precise investigations

Serum samples were obtained from calves on fattening farms and these were tested for the presence of antibodies to the respiratory viruses. Out of 415 calves which originated from about 30 farms, no positive serum was detected.

Further investigations were carried out on 2 large dairy farms with Holstein cows. The percentage of positive animals was 85% on one farm and 98% on the other.

2.   Diagnostic examinations

During the 3 preceding years, the laboratory received about 1,000 diagnostic requests for clinically suspected viral respiratory disease. Out of every 10 examinations, 9 consisted of serological tests and 1 virus isolation attempt on nasal fluid from live animals or material from dead animals (Martel et al., 1977). IBR infection was the most frequently suspected infection.

An outbreak was considered to be IBR if the following conditions applied:

a) viral infection was clinically suspected.

b) laboratory examination was positive, either by sero-conversion and/or a significant rise of antibodies on paired sera.

c) and/or recovery of virus from nasal swabs or from pathological material.

Detection of antibody in a single serum sample cannot serve as diagnostic evidence of IBR infection.

Out of 937 cases of bovine respiratory diseases considered as possible IBR infections, only 45 (4.8%) outbreaks could be authenticated.

Infected animals were essentially dairy cows but sometimes they were fattening baby beef. Infection was prevalent in indigenous bovines placed in contact with imported animals as if a persisting virus encountered optimal conditions for developing its pathological potential in the sensitive herd. It should be borne in mind that IBR outbreaks may occur on farms where no imported cattle were introduced. Lastly, another characteristic of outbreaks is their almost exclusive localisation in large animal units.

CONCLUSIONS

Epidemiological surveys and diagnostic examinations show that IBR exists in France but that its frequency is still relatively low (2 to 5%) and certainly much less important than it was first suggested. Serologically positive animals are more widespread in dairy farms of more than 50 head which include imported Holstein cattle. This result should caution breeders who wish to import cattle that there is a high probability that they may be positive.

Most of the time, imported animals can be held responsible for IBR infection but, in some cases, such an origin cannot be incriminated. Serological tests repeated at an interval of 6 to 8 months indicate that infection is rather stationary. However, true outbreaks of IBR infection have been observed several times. The incidence of the disease in French cattle does not appear to have changed radically since 1974; IBR virus can be recognised as a cause of clinical disease in 5 to 7% of respiratory outbreaks investigated.

Epidemiological features of infection necessitate control measures. Imported cattle should be serologically tested in order to prevent further spread of infection and the introduction of possibly virulent virus strains. Bulls should be examined for antibodies before introduction to artificial insemination stations.

In herds known to run the risk of infection, the losses caused by the disease can be reduced by an inactivated IBR vaccine which is now available commercially in France.

REFERENCES

Charton, A., Berkaloff, A., Faye, P., Lecoanet, J., Le Layec, Cl. and
    Bernard, C. 1970. Bull Acad. Vet., 43, pp. 123.

Charton, A., Faye, P., Le Layec, Cl., Mage, C. and Bernard, C. 1973. Bull
    Acad. Vet., 46, p. 225.

Dannacher, G., Fedida, M., Coudert, M. and Peillon, M. 1975. Bull. Off.
    inter. Epiz., report number 110.

Espinasse, J., Gilbert, Y. and Saurat, P. 1974. Rev. Med. Vet., 37, p. 1441.

Faye, P., Berkaloff, A., Charton, Z. and Le Layec, Cl. 1967. Bull. Acad.
    Vet. 40, p. 227.

Gilbert, Y., Espinasse, J., Saurat, P. and Vaissaire, J. 1976. Rec. Med.
    Vet. 127, p. 383.

Martel, J.L., Dannacher, G., Perrin, M., Fedida, M. and Coudert, M. 1976.
    Rec. Med. Vet. 152, p. 829.

Martel, J.L., Dannacher, G., Perrin, M., Fedida, M. and Coudert, M. 1977.
    Bull. Off. intern. Epiz. (In press).

Perrin, M., Dannacher, G., Fedida, M., Martel, J.L. and Coudert, M. (In
    press).

RESPIRATORY DISEASES IN CATTLE
DISEASE INCIDENCE AND EPIDEMIOLOGY - THE SITUATION IN GERMANY

H. Frerking

Klinik für Geburtshilfe und Gynäkologie des Rindes
Tierärztliche Hochschule, 3 000 Hannover, Germany.

ABSTRACT

Respiratory disease in cattle, particularly in young cattle and calves, is getting more and more important in Germany. During the past years, in addition to seasonal bronchopneumonia enzootica on several farms, permanent respiratory problems were observed during the whole year. These problems appeared mostly on farms which fatten calves.

In the spring of 1975 there was a contagious form of bronchopneumonia in Bavaria in the southern part of Germany. Nearly 60 - 70% of all the cattle in affected herds suffered from this sickness. The mortality on average was about 5 - 6% (Wizigmann et al., 1976).

With transport of cattle this infectious disease came to the northern part of Germany, mainly to Schleswig-Holstein (Straub, 1977). The outbreak occurred mainly on farms with bad exogenic and endogenic factors for cattle. Under these poor conditions microbes (viruses and bacteria) cause the diseases.

These respiratory diseases generally became evident after the stress of very long transportation. On the other hand cattle without antibodies, which were brought into districts with a high rate of respiratory disease, became sick in almost every case.

In the past few years, in addition to virus infection, a secondary organism, Pasteurella haemolytica has been found in the lungs of dead animals.

Another problem, mainly in the northern parts of Germany where there are wet pastures, is infection with lung worms (Dictyocaulus viviparus.) In contrast to the bronchopneumonia caused by microbes, this disease has no tendency to spread.

Sporadic cases of respiratory diseases are mostly caused by bacteria and, endemic or epidemic cases, by viruses or lung-worms. In the following paper virus infections will mainly be discussed because sporadic disease and the problems caused by lung-worms are not so important economically.

DISEASE INCIDENCE

It is very difficult to give a report on the true situation in Western Germany about respiratory diseases in cattle. The registration of disease in several counties is not perfect. Only in Bavaria (south east part) and Baden-Würtemberg (south west part) is there accurate information.

Of the animals with the so-called 'Rindergrippe', 75% which died or had to be slaughtered came from farms which fatten calves or young cattle and 25% of all losses occurred in breeding and milk farms. This statement is very important epidemiologically.

In Bavaria, in 1973, about 2 500 head of cattle died or had to be slaughtered. In 1974 the figures were 3 500 head from 2 700 farms; in 1975 6 300 animals from 4 700 farms, and in 1976 8 200 cattle from 6 300 farms. According to these figures respiratory disease, the so-called 'Rindergrippe', has a tendency to spread. Bavaria has its frontiers with Eastern Germany, Czechoslovakia, Austria and Switzerland, but there were no indications that enzootic disease was also a problem in these countries. In Baden-Würtemberg in 1974 there were about 1 200 animals, in 1975 about 1 800 cattle and in 1976 nearly 3 000 head of cattle which had to be slaughtered or which died. In farms which vaccinated prophylactically the total losses decreased to 20%.

Baden Würtemberg has its frontiers with France, Switzerland and Bavaria. Nothing is known about any connection with disease in the two foreign countries.

As a result of this tendency for the disease to spread, the number of young cattle which have been prophylactically vaccinated against 'Rindergrippe' is increasing. The figures were in Baden-Würtemberg in 1974 - 20 000, 1975 - 43 000 and 1976 - 180 000 animals.

In the most northern part of Western Germany - Schleswig-Holstein - there was an epidemic outbreak of respiratory disease in the winter of 1975/76. This occurred in two districts only - Kreis Schleswig and Kreis Flensburg. These two districts have their frontiers with Denmark but the disease did not spread to Denmark.

I am sure that, in the other nine counties of Western Germany, there are also sporadic problems with respiratory diseases mainly in young cattle, but as there is no complete registration, I am unable to give representative figures.

EPIDEMIOLOGY

The outbreak of respiratory disease in young cattle mostly occurs when many factors work together. These are non-microbiological (endogenic and exogenic) factors and microbiological causes (microbes and viruses). Generally an outbreak on a farm happens when a lot of cattle are introduced as a new batch, weakened and stressed by long transportation. Very often they are introduced into a housed environment, with new holding conditions and are fed new food.

In addition to viruses, in more and more cases, *Pasturellae* are found in the lungs.

INFECTION BY LUNG-WORMS

Respiratory diseases caused by lung-worms occur mainly in the northern pasture district of Germany. True figures about the extent of this disease could not be found. In 1969 from 4 040 000 slaughtered head of cattle, 13 631 lungs were confiscated because of *Dictyocaulus viviparus* infestation, that is 0.3% of all slaughtered head of cattle (Burger, 1973).

REFERENCE

Burger, H.J. 1973. In 'Helminthological diseases of cattle, sheep and horses in Europe'. Ed. Urquhart and Armour, Publ. MacLehose & Co. Ltd., University Press, Glasgow, p. 173.

RESPIRATORY DISEASES IN CATTLE IN THE REPUBLIC OF IRELAND

H. Thornberry

Department of Agriculture, Veterinary Research Laboratory,
Abbotstown, Castleknock, Co. Dublin, Republic of Ireland

ABSTRACT

Infections of the respiratory tract constitute one of the major causes of mortality and ill-thrift on many Irish farms. The greatest losses occur during early calfhood.

The viruses involved are parainfluenza type 3 (PI3), bovine adenovirus type 3 (BAV 3), infectious bovine rhinotracheitis (IBR), reovirus type 1 (R1) and bovine viral diarrhoea - mucosal disease (BVD-MD) virus.

Serological surveys for antibodies to each of the abovementioned viruses have been undertaken in several counties.

A field trial of two inactivated adjuvant-incorporated viral respiratory vaccines demonstrated that there was noticeably lower clinical respiratory disease in the vaccinated calves as compared with control animals.

Parasitic pneumonia ('hoose' or 'husk') is fairly widespread amongst calves in the autumn and early winter. Control is obtained by vaccination or by regular medication against gastro-intestinal nematodes.

A growing tendency to intensive rearing of young cattle particularly will, no doubt, lead to increased incidences of viral and bacterial respiratory problems.

Acute pulmonary emphysema ('fog fever') is fairly frequently encountered in autumn.

Infections of the respiratory tract constitute one of the major causes of mortality and ill-thrift in cattle on many Irish farms. While cattle of all ages may be affected the greatest losses occur during early calfhood. On many farms, especially in areas of intensive dairying, the annual occurrence of respiratory disease in housed calves is a source of considerable economic loss arising from the variable mortality associated with the condition, together with the subsequent unthriftiness in many recovered animals.

Parainfluenza type 3 (PI3), bovine adenovirus type 3 (BAV3) infectious bovine rhinotracheitis (IBR), reovirus type 1 (R1) and bovine viral diarrhoea-mucosal disease (BVD-MD) virus, have a widespread geographic distribution in the cattle population of Ireland.

The prevalence of infections with PI3, R1 and BVD-MD viruses is especially high. It is probable that PI3 virus, and to a lesser extent BAV3 and R1 viruses, are primarily pathogens of the young animal, and are involved in many outbreaks of respiratory illness in calves. In contrast, infection with IBR virus would appear to occur sporadically and to be confined to older animals.

Although BVD-MD virus has been associated with many outbreaks of respiratory illness and viral diarrhoea or mucosal disease, its importance as a pathogen of the bovine respiratory tract has not been determined.

Serological surveys for antibodies to each of the above-mentioned viruses have been undertaken several years ago. Samples were so selected as to be representative of as many counties as possible of which there are 26 in the Republic of Ireland.

PI3. Of 2 147 sera examined, 91.4% had haemagglutination inhibition (HI) antibody titres of $\geq 1/32$ to this virus. The percentage for calves and adult cattle were similar.

IBR. The prevalance of serum neutralising (SN) antibodies to IBR virus was 13.2% in over 2 000 bovine sera tested. The average positive rate for adult bovine sera was 17.1% as compared with 7.2% in calf sera.

BAV3. Adenovirus precipitating antibodies were demonstrated in 6.7% of 2 378 bovine sera. No significant difference was noted between the prevalence rate for calf sera of 4.5% and that for adult bovine sera of 5.0%.

R1. Of 966 sera tested for antibodies to R1 virus, 82.7% had titres ≥1/32 although the number of calf sera tested was small, there was no evidence of an increase of reovirus infection with age.

BVD-MD. A total of 75.4% of 1982 bovine serum samples examined contained SN antibodies against BVD-MD virus. The positive rates for calf and adult bovine sera were 71% and 77.3% respectively.

A field trial of two inactivated adjuvant-incorporated viral respiratory vaccines was conducted over a period of two years in a number of selected calf herds. With one exception, respiratory illness of variable extent and severity occurred in all the herds while the trial was in progress. The incidence of clinical respiratory disease was noticeably lower in the vaccinated animals than in the control animals. PI3, BAV3 and R1 viruses were detected in some calves. Under the conditions of the trial the overall response to the PI3 antigen in both vaccines was not significant even though it did confer a dggree of protection in some herds. In contrast, the BAV3 antigen stimulated a significant response in vaccinated calves, and might be considered reasonably successful in protecting calves against natural infection.

It was not possible to evaluate the immunogenicity of the R1

virus component of the trivalent vaccine on the basis of the
antibody response following vaccination. There were indications,
however, that vaccination reduced the number of seroconversions
for R1 virus in the two herds under experiment.

In general the results of the vaccination experiments
showed that inactivated adjuvant incorporated vaccines are of
some value against bovine respiratory disease. However, it
may be that the problem might be more successfully met by the
use of intranasally administered multivalent attenuated viral
vaccines.

Parasitic pneumonia, popularly known as 'hoose' or 'husk',
is fairly widespread amongst calves in the autumn or early
winter, the cause being the nematode *Dictyocaulus vivipara*. Using
questionnaires, the Agricultural Institute collected information
regarding the extent of parasitological problems ('hoose and
'stomach worms'), and the way in which these might be related
to management factors. Sixty-three farms, all with non-suckler
herds, were surveyed in seven counties, and the results published
in the Research Report 1975 on Animal Production by the
Agricultural Institute.

Almost half the farms had between 20 and 40 hectares of
grazing land, and the number of calves reared was between 20
and 50 on about 60% of the farms.

Sixty-five per cent of farmers reckoned that there was a
parasitic bronchitis problem in their calves, about 50% that
there was a problem with parasitic gastro-enteritis, and about
40% that their calves were subject to both these infections.
Twenty-five per cent of farmers considered that they had neither
of these parasitological problems. Twenty-five per cent
vaccinated their calves against parasitic bronchitis, whilst
95% used regular medication to control worms.

On 90% of the farms, most or all of the calves were born
in the spring. The calves were grazed separately from older

stock on about 50% of farms in which set-stocking was practised, and on about 40% of farms where they were rotationally grazed.

Within the past few years the intensive rearing of cattle has been introduced into Ireland, and this system is likely to increase in popularity. As in all situations where numbers of calves and young cattle are brought together from various sources there will, no doubt, be increased incidences of viral and bacterial respiratory problems. In such circumstances, management, hygiene, housing and ventilation will become increasingly important, and expertise in these areas will be essential if disease and mortality are to be kept down to a minimum. The ever-increasing value of cattle should ensure that the necessary attention will be paid to these pre-disposing causes of respiratory conditions.

Acute pulmonary emphysema (so-called 'fog fever') can be quite a problem in the autumn. We have no actual statistics but veterinarians in practice encounter the condition frequently each year. Annually we receive from ten to twelve carcasses of animals which laboratory examination shows to have died of 'fog fever'.

STATISTICAL DATA ON CALF MORTALITY AND DISEASES IN ITALIAN BEEF AND DAIRY HERDS

G. Rognoni and A. Bergamaschi

Instituto di Zootecnia Generale, Facolta di Veterinaria, Università degli Studi di Milano, Italy.

ABSTRACT

In this paper some statistics are given about the mortality in young calves in the following different sorts of Italian herds:

1) Intensive herds of dairy cattle in which young female calves are destined for reproduction and the males for meat production.

2) Intensive herds of veal calves, generally male animals, fed with milk, or milk replacers, which have been imported from various European countries.

3) Intensive herds of baby-beef (400 - 500 kg) animals of 20 - 30 days old, imported from various European countries.

4) Intensive herds for beef production in feed lots systems of imported, weaned calves weighing 150 - 200 kg.

It may be of interest to this audience to report on the rates of mortality and disease prevailing in Italian breeding cattle.

Cattle production in Italy is being carried on along several lines which may be summed up as follows:

1) Dairy cattle production including reproduction.

2) Beef cattle production including reproduction.

3) Rearing of purchased calves for beef production:

    (a) young calves for veal production.

    (b) calves to be weaned or fattened after weaning, or to be sold after weaning.

    (c) weaned calves of 150 - 200 kg live weight to be fattened especially on ensiled maize.

The rate of calf mortality and disease on the various types of cattle production farms obviously varies, usually reaching higher values in purchased calf herds.

DAIRY CATTLE PRODUCTION

This production has undergone marked change during the past two decades, and particularly the last decade. An increase in the number of cattle on the production farms has been recorded, generally with a shift from confined closed housing to free open houses with the cattle gathered in more or less numerous groups.

With this method of rearing the control of the individual calf has become even more difficult and with the group control, which has been consequently adopted for lack of manpower, observation is becoming even more insufficient resulting in an increasing lack of timely attendance in moments of emergency, such as attendance to the calving dam and postpartum attendance to the calf. Breed statistics, particularly in large production

units, revealed during the past five years a considerable
increase in the percentage of stillbirths or perinatal deaths
because of lack of attention (from 3 - 4% to 7 - 9%). This
occurs over the whole year with peak periods in winter, spring
and summer on dairy farms in northern Italy.

I wish to record that during the last decade the spread on
cattle farms of viral agents has caused diseases which increase
the rate of abortion. These viruses, despite the absence of
official statistics, include the virus of infectious rhinotracheitis. Considering that in Italy there are about four
million dairy cows for a production of approximately 2 800 000
calves, the financial loss is very heavy.

Table 1 shows some data on dairy cow production during
1975 - 76.

TABLE 1

Mortality	%	Cause of Mortality	
Precalving or perinatal	7 - 8	Insufficient calving attention	
Precalving or perinatal	3 - 4	Normal calving attention	
During the first month	5 - 8	First 10 days:	
		Digestive diseases	70%
		Respiratory diseases	30%
		After first 10 days:	
		Digestive diseases	30%
		Respiratory diseases	70%
After the first month	1 - 2	Respiratory diseases	50%
		Other	50%

Deaths of new-born calves during the first month amounted
to 5 - 8%, with morbidity reaching double figures.

Disease affecting the digestive tract during the first
month was encountered in 2/3 of cases, with respiratory
disease in about 1/3 of cases. The former occurred during the
first 10 days, the latter after the first 10 days.

Mortality after the first month was rather low (1 - 2%) and usually the most frequent disturbances were ascribed to the respiratory system; 50% of mortality was due to other causes.

BEEF CATTLE PRODUCTION

Production of beef cattle in Italy is carried on along three main lines:

a)   beef cattle kept on ranges throughout the year.

b)   cattle kept on pastures for 8 - 10 months and for the remaining period free in houses.

c)   Cattle living freely in houses for the whole year.

Calf mortality caused by disease is very limited (1.0 - 2.0%) in type a) range herds; also calving deaths are below the rates registered in dairy cattle production farms and vary depending on the breed (2% - 3%).

In type c) herds, even in the case of free housing, the percentage of stillbirths, as well as of deaths during the first month of life, is lower than on dairy cattle production farms (1.0% - 3.0% stillbirths; 4% - 6% of deaths during the first month of life). Pathological disease of the respiratory system is negligible.

Italian zootechnical and economic statistics reveal that consumption of bovine meat amounts to approximately 1 200 000 tons. Of this 320 000 tons are imported as meat. Beef, dairy cows and bulls, at the end of the reproductive life, produce 190 000 tons; young beef cattle of 300 - 600 kg body weight produce 690 000 tons, over half of which come from intensive and semi-intensive production farms which import young cattle from abroad and particularly from EEC countries (France, Germany, Ireland, etc).

Importation of young cattle roughly amounts to 2 300 000

animals which produce, in the various production units, meat
with very different characteristics. About 600 000 of the
calves in 1976 were destined for veal production and slaughtered
at a live weight of 150 - 180 kg; the rest were destined for
the production of heavier animals of 300 - 350 kg live weight.
Sanitary problems, because of their high economic significance,
are particularly important in imported cattle. Among the
diseases affecting this category, respiratory diseases are
assuming, in Italy, a size and gravity unequalled by any other
European country. The reason obviously can be sought in the
peculiar characteristics of intensive production units and
particularly in cattle importation.

Importation of cattle is responsible for a series of
disturbances in the cattle's normal physiological balance:

a) cattle of all ages, breeds and origins are stocked in
the gathering centres of the exporting countries.

b) after a journey, generally long and uncomfortable, the
young calves arrive in Italy where they are sent to
production farms where not one of the original environmental
traits exist, and where they suffer from the stress of
adaptation.

c) intermixing with other cattle with the consequent
spread of pathogenic forms of microbes in the new environment.

d) different feeding and rearing methods, etc.

The cases mentioned above forcibly accumulate to make up
the background for respiratory and digestive disturbances. A
very complex important pathology is thus taking shape, first as
epizootic 'waves' and then as epizootic forms and the threshold
between local and importation pathology is thereafter difficult
to define. Among such disturbances, stress pneumonia (shipping
fever), and the various viral respiratory diseases, are widespread.

In Italy, for instance, during the years 1968 - 1974 there was a wide diffusion of viral infection by parainfluenza 3 followed by infectious rhinotracheitis (IBR). Focuses of respiratory disease attributed to adenovirus and rhinovirus have been detected recently.

Included among imported enteric syndromes are: salmonellosis which penetrated and spread in Italy during 1968 - 1969, the frequent location of focuses of disease of the mucous membranes, very rare if not absent in the past, and viral diarrhoea which spread widely during 1965 - 1970.

Despite the almost total absence of official statistics on the incidence and damage caused by these diseases, it is possible to determine their incidence as a cause of mortality with reasonable approximation.

Given below are the mean mortality values in various types of rearing units.

1. Suckling calves of 60 - 70 kg live weight within 50 days of arrival   4 - 6%

2. Weaned calves of approximately 160 kg   2 - 3%

3. Young bovines of approximately 250 kg within 60 days of arrival   3 - 5%

The above figures can obviously vary depending on the type of rearing unit, the animals themselves, and their origin etc.

There are no complete statistical analyses in this regard. Nevertheless, from research undertaken in large veal rearing units where calves of various origins are fattened, it appears that French calves are more readily affected by respiratory diseases. Mortality caused by such diseases amounts to 2% against 1% in Bavarian calves.

Respiratory diseases are also chiefly responsible for

mortality as shown in Table 2 below.

TABLE 2

CAUSES OF MORTALITY (DURING THE FIRST TWO MONTHS FROM IMPORTATION)

Suckling calves	Respiratory diseases	60%
	Digestive diseases	18%
	Other	22%
Calves over 180 kg	Respiratory diseases	72%
	Digestive diseases	2%
	Metabolic disturbances	9%
	Other	17%

To the financial loss caused by mortality we should add
the cost of medicines: approximately Lire 6 000 are now being
spent *pro capite* (about Lire 15 of meat produced) for respiratory
diseases only.

Other money is being spent on emergency slaughter occurring
roughly in 5% of suckling calves, and 2 - 3% of weaned calves
of over 180 kg live weight. Another heavy loss, almost
impossible to calculate, is the decline in the conversion ratio
and the slowing of weight gains.

POSSIBLE PREVENTATIVE MEASURES

In order to provide a few considerations and to give some
indication of the perspectives for work necessary to cut down
the rate of mortality and disease in calves on rearing units,
it is necessary to define the action to be taken:

a) on the Italian dairy and beef cattle production farms

b) in connection with imported cattle.

In the former case (beef producing enterprises) a decline

in stillbirths and postpartum losses would be possible by
improving our knowledge of rearing techniques and genetic
improvement of our selected bovine herds. Particular attention
should be given to the study of the pregnant cow in an advanced
stage of gestation, calving attention, the genetic testing of
bulls, prenatal mortality and the frequency of calving
difficulties of related cows. Also it is important to improve
our knowledge of the environmental physiology of calf rearing.

In the latter case, the question of a co-ordinated
research programme to prevent, in reared calves, the pathological
syndromes stated above, requires special emphasis. In fact,
both exporting and importing countries must be interested in the
calf overcoming the crisis of adaptation in the best possible
way.

In order to achieve these aims a 'pre-conditioning' is
necessary which should be studied in the light of the
physiological and pathological conditions of rearing - in their
widest sense - both in the country of origin and the country
of destination. Both countries should undertake to improve the
economy of the European Community.

BOVINE RESPIRATORY DISEASES : THE SITUATION IN THE NETHERLANDS

A. van Nieuwstadt, P. Straver and C. Holzhauer
Central Veterinary Institute, Virology Department, Lelystad,
The Netherlands.

ABSTRACT

In the Netherlands studies on the etiology of bovine respiratory diseases have been devoted mainly to Infectious Bovine Rhinotracheitis (IBR) and bovine respiratory syncytial (RS) virus infections. These two agents are regarded as the most important viral causes of respiratory diseases in bovines.

IBR suddenly became a problem in the Netherlands in the spring of 1974. The virus was not enzootic before then and met – in terms of immunology – a virginal population of animals in most herds. Animals of all age groups became infected and the symptoms could be differentiated from those of other respiratory infections. Economic losses were mainly due to a reduced milk yield. The virus rapidly spread over our whole country and the clinical picture has changed with infections sometimes occurring without symptoms. Infections with IBR virus are most numerous in winter and spring.

RS virus infections, on the other hand, cause problems mainly in the autumn. Symptoms become manifest in young animals after they come back from pasture and are housed for some time. Bovine RS virus infections are probably an important cause of respiratory trouble in young cattle in the Netherlands. Systematic research on the role of viruses in the etiology of respiratory diseases has been performed since the autumn of 1972.

Paired serum samples (acute and convalescent) from sick animals are screened by the complement fixation test for antibodies against para-influenza virus type 3 (PI3), bovine RS virus, bovine virus diarrhoea virus (BVD) and adenoviruses of serogroup A and B.

In the autumn of 1973 and 1974 a study of 33 outbreaks of respiratory

*disease involving 925 sick calves of 3 to 11 months old, demonstrated
that 76% of 292 animals serologically investigated had a significant
increase of complement fixing antibodies for bovine RS virus. Bovine RS
virus is considered as the main cause of a fairly typical disease syndrome
for which fever, dyspnoea and symptoms of acute lung emphysema are most
prominent. On a breeding farm that has been under observation since the
autumn of 1972, the characteristic clinical picture of the disease has
appeared every autumn, and the incidence of the disease correlated well
with the serology and isolation of RS virus. In this herd the epidemiology
of bovine PI3 and RS virus was different from that of BVD virus. Infections
with RS and PI3 virus, which are considered typical respiratory viruses,
showed a peak incidence in the autumn and all young animals became
infected at once. On the other hand BVD virus infections occurred the
whole year round, without clinical symptoms.*

*In view of the role of RS virus, more efforts should be made to
develop and evaluate a vaccine.*

In the Netherlands outbreaks of infectious bovine rhinotracheitis (IBR) virus infection with respiratory symptoms
first appeared on a larger scale in the spring of 1974. The
virus met in most herds - in terms of immunology - a virginal
population. Animals of all ages became infected. In most
cases an experienced veterinarian could differentiate the
symptoms from those caused by other respiratory infections. The
disease is located mainly in the anterior part of the
respiratory tract. In typical cases the disease is distinguished
by lesions on the nasal mucosa and blood in nasal secretions.
Economical losses are mainly due to a reduced milk yield.

Initially nasal swabs, samples taken postmortem, and
blood samples, were sent to our institute for virus isolation
and serological investigation. At the beginning the diagnosis
could be confirmed on the grounds of a single positive blood
sample, as the virus was not enzootic in our country. From
January 1974 until June 1977 blood samples were received from
2986 farms with respiratory disease in livestock and from 1145
farms nasal swabs or organs for virus isolation were sent to
us. In 33% of these outbreaks a diagnosis of IBR was confirmed
serologically and in 29% of these outbreaks the virus was
isolated. The monthly outbreaks of respiratory disease from
which we received material, the number of outbreaks for which
the diagnosis of IBR could be confirmed, either by serological
investigation or by virus isolation, are presented in Figures
1 and 2. By both methods a comparable picture was obtained. The
figures give an idea of seasonal influence on the occurrence
of IBR epidemics.

However, the picture which is indicated by the graphs has
certain shortcomings. IBR is not a notifiable disease and the
results, therefore, give only a part of the total number of IBR
outbreaks in the Netherlands. It is certainly not right to
conclude that 1/3 of all bovine respiratory problems in the
Netherlands are caused by IBR virus.

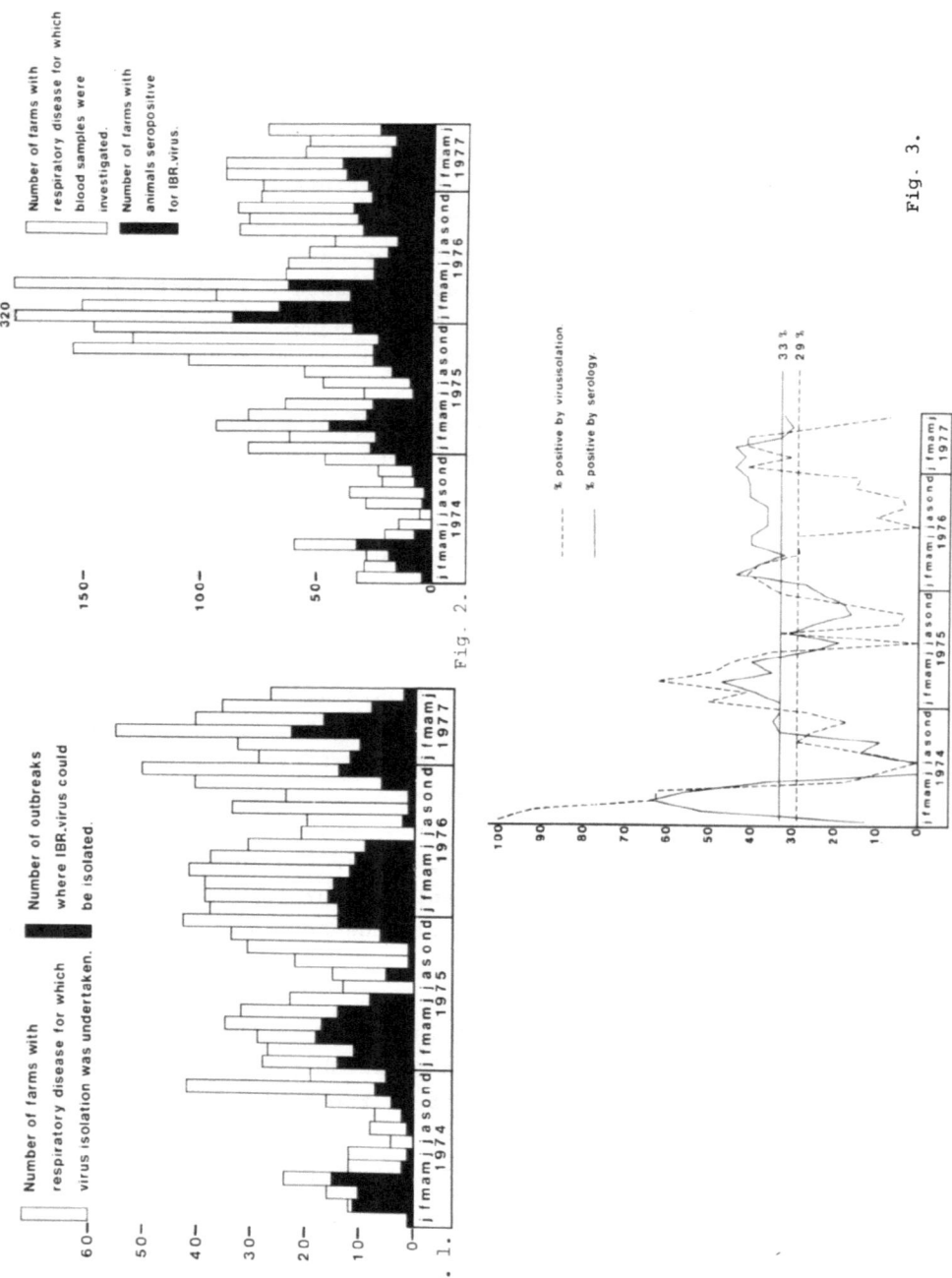

Number of farms with
respiratory disease for which
blood samples were
investigated.

Number of farms with
animals seropositive
for IBR.virus.

Fig. 2.

Number of farms with
respiratory disease for which
virus isolation was undertaken.

Number of outbreaks
where IBR.virus could
be isolated.

Fig. 1.

% positive by virusisolation

% positive by serology

33 %
29 %

Fig. 3.

Undoubtedly there has been a preselection of materials
sent to us for investigation, because IBR was suspected as
the etiological agent on clinical grounds. At the beginning
the clinical picture was new for veterinarians and was not always
differentiated correctly from respiratory diseases caused by
other viruses. The fact that in only 1/3 of cases the diagnosis
could be confirmed as IBR by laboratory investigations indicates
that the disease is not always recognised by its clinical
symptoms. Over the years veterinarians became familiar with
the clinical picture of IBR and material for confirmation of
the diagnosis was sent to us, especially in cases of doubt.
Moreover the clinical picture has somewhat changed as not every
outbreak has typical recognisable IBR symptoms.

The graphs show that IBR infections cause most problems
in the winter and spring, while the virus is less active in
the summer and autumn. Figure 3 depicts the percentage of
outbreaks of respiratory disease investigated every month that
were diagnosed as IBR, either by virus isolation or by positive
serology. It appears that over the whole period an average of
1/3 of all suspected outbreaks could be confirmed by laboratory
investigation. In summer and autumn the percentage of outbreaks of respiratory disease due to IBR is clearly lower. Other
causes must be responsible for the large number of outbreaks,
especially those which occur in the autumn. In general the
curve for the percentage of outbreaks found positive by serological investigation follows that for positive virus isolations.
Only in the summer of 1976 was there a distinct difference and
the serological investigation gives too high a number of positive
results. This may indicate a more widespread dissemination of
the virus among the cattle population. Obviously the diagnosis
can no longer be confirmed by examining one single bood sample,
but should be based on a significant increase of antibodies
between acute and convalescent blood samples.

IBR infections are certainly not as widespread in the
Netherlands as, for instance infections with parainfluenza

virus type 3 (PI3), bovine respiratory syncytial (RS) virus
and bovine virus diarrhoea (BVD) virus, which are enzootic in
practically every large herd.

Problems caused by the IBR virus occur mainly in herds
with an intensive trade in animals and less in more isolated
farms which breed their own calves. Once there has been an
outbreak of IBR in a herd, the risk of infection of young
animals will remain and it will be difficult to eradicate the
virus. In these herds the infection may run a subclinical
course.

In the autumn, especially in large herds, we see a
certain type of respiratory disease in young animals appearing
some time after they have been housed. This is also observed
in beef fattening farms, where animals are kept inside for
their whole lives. We believe the symptoms can be distinguished
from other types of respiratory disease, for instance those of
an IBR infection. (The clinical picture will be dealt with in
detail by Dr. Holzhauer). When an outbreak occurs, symptoms
appear suddenly in all the animals less than one year old.
This is the most critical age for the disease. The animals
cough and there is nasal discharge and conjunctivitis with
lacrymation. After a few days the calves become generally
ill: they are depressed, food uptake and activity are reduced
and respiration rates are increased. The animals become
fevered and dyspnoeic and a number may succumb with symptoms
of acute respiratory distress. The pathological changes are
largely restricted to the respiratory tract. Subpleural
emphysema is visible and sometimes even the pericardium may
be involved; lung tissue may be disrupted extensively. In
acute, fatal, cases bacteriological investigation of the lungs
is negative.

In the autumn of 1973 and 1974 the possible etiological
role of viruses in this disease was investigated. Thirty-
three outbreaks, in which altogether 925 young animals showed
this clinical picture, were examined. Blood samples from 292

animals were collected in the acute and convalescent stage of the disease and tested by complement fixation for antibodies against bovine RS virus, PI3 virus, BVD virus and adenoviruses of serogroups A and B. IBR virus was not suspected on clinical grounds and for some of these outbreaks this was confirmed by a negative virus neutralisation test for IBR virus. There was a significant increase of antibodies to bovine RS virus in 76% of the animals studied. For the other viruses these percentages were 48% for PI3, 13% for BVD, 12% for adenovirus of group A and 11% for group B. In 28 out of 33 outbreaks, half or more of the calves developed antibodies against bovine RS virus. In addition, in 14 of these outbreaks, a significant increase of antibodies was found to PI3 in ⩾ 50% of the animals examined (Table 1). In 12 herds there was no serological indication of a PI3 virus infection during the same period as the respiratory symptoms. In these studies infection with bovine RS virus was diagnosed on the basis of seroconversion as measured by a complement fixation test.

With a virus neutralisation test even higher numbers of RS infections might have been found, as in our experience virus neutralisation is a more sensitive reaction for the demonstration of antibodies against RS virus. Thus we think that an infection by bovine RS virus is the main cause of the disease syndrome.

TABLE 1

SEROLOGICAL INVESTIGATION OF 33 OUTBREAKS OF 'PINKENGRIEP' IN YEARLINGS

Number of outbreaks in 1973 and 1974	Number of animals investigated by serology	Number of calves with a significant CF antibody response to:				
		BRS	PI3	BVD/MD	BAdV1	BAdV4
33	292	223	139	38	35	22
		76%	48%	13%	12%	11%

BRS = bovine respiratory syncytial virus BVD/MD = bovine virus diarrhoea/
PI3 = parainfluenza 3 virus   mucosal disease virus
BAdV4 = bovine adenovirus 4   BAdV1 = bovine adenovirus 1

Since the autumn of 1972 the epidemiology of some virus infections in a breeding farm has been followed. Blood samples were taken regularly from the animals and tested for complement fixing antibodies against IBR, BRS, PI3, BVD/MD and adenoviruses types 1 and 4. This herd receives young female calves from ten dairy farms which are returned to their owner at the age of approximately two years. Nearly every autumn young animals get respiratory symptoms as described above which we attribute to a bovine RS virus infection. Moreover, less serious disease symptoms are observed, but for these we could not demonstrate a clear correlation with a virus infection. In January 1976, IBR virus was introduced on this farm and caused an outbreak with clinical symptoms. In June 1976 there was again an outbreak among animals that had joined the herd since January, but at this time the infection was subclinical.

Between August 1972 and December 1976, 212 animals were involved in our serological investigation. In the survey chart a line is drawn from the moment the animals arrived until the last time a blood sample was collected. The time of sampling is marked by a point on the line. Blood was collected in the acute stage of disease and after recovery. In between, blood samples were also collected and some animals were sampled up to 10 times. Outbreaks of respiratory disease with serious symptoms, as described, started early in December 1972 and ended in April 1973. Symptoms were not observed in the autumn of 1973, but in 1974 symptoms were first reported on the 9th of October and in 1975 on the 15th of November. In 1976 symptoms were observed in August and not in the autumn.

In all cases the time of each outbreak correlates very well with infection by RS virus, as proved by serological investigations. A significant increase in antibodies to bovine RS and PI3 virus is marked on the chart. In some cases, for instance in the autumn of 1974, we found a concurrent increase of antibody titre to PI3 and bovine RS virus. Generally PI3 infection came before the infection with RS virus, as in the autumn of 1972 and 1975, when the increase of antibodies to

PI3 virus occurred before serious clinical symptoms developed. In 1976, PI3 virus infection occurred in the autumn, whereas infection with RS virus, accompanied by disease, was observed in the summer. In the autumn of 1973 infection with RS virus occurred without respiratory symptoms, but minor symptoms were recorded in November. Infection with RS virus does not always cause serious respiratory disease.

In some animals that could be followed for a sufficient length of time, an increase of antibodies against bovine RS virus was found a second time. The first infection was in the spring, followed by another in the autumn. However, the second infection with bovine RS virus does not seem to cause more serious symptoms, as would be expected in the case of an allergic reaction. Symptoms are usually less serious in animals younger than 3 months. Thus maternal antibodies seem to give some protection and are not involved in an allergic reaction as suggested for the pathology of RS infections in children.

The epidemiology of BVD virus infections in this herd was investigated in the same way as described for PI3 and bovine RS virus. All animals become infected with BVD virus sooner or later, but typical symptoms of a BVD virus infection were never observed. It is remarkable that seroconversion for BVD virus occurred throughout the whole year, which is contrary to infections with PI3 and bovine RS virus. The latter two are considered to be agents that specifically infect the respiratory tract, with a seasonal incidence, in which an entire group of young animals is affected more or less simultaneously.

CONCLUSIONS

In the Netherlands IBR virus has been an important cause of respiratory disease in cattle since 1974. However, on clinical grounds the diagnosis is not always made correctly.

There is a seasonal influence on the occurrence of IBR infections; outbreaks are more frequent in winter and spring.

There is a correlation between the occurrence of respiratory symptoms of 'pinkengriep' that have been described, and infection with bovine RS virus.

The relationship between symptoms and infection is clear for infections with PI3 virus.

Infection with bovine RS virus does not always cause the same serious symptoms. Subclinical infection may occur.

DISEASE INCIDENCE AND EPIDEMIOLOGY - THE SITUATION IN THE U.K.

L.H. Thomas

ARC Institute for Research on Animal Diseases
Compton, Nr. Newbury, Berkshire, England.

ABSTRACT

Death rate in beef units recorded by the Meat and Livestock Commission (1970 - 74) averaged 6.2%. The rate in the first 3 months of life was 4.6% and in the period 3 months of age to slaughter was 1.9%.

In the period 1970 - 77 enzootic pneumonia accounted for 50% of 448 deaths recorded on a variety of different farms throughout the UK amongst over 8 000 animals (overall death rate 5.5%). Between 22 and 52% of 5 989 animals were treated for enzootic pneumonia. Treatment for this disease was associated with up to 2.6% reduction in liveweight gain on one farm during 1970 - 72.

Abbatoir returns during 1976 show that 5.5% of 109 449 animals had pneumonic lesions at slaughter. In a survey of 935 animals routinely slaughtered from one farm, 11% were found to have significant lesions at slaughter and the majority of these lesions were a 'cuffing' pneumonia. This lesion was associated with up to 7.2% reduction in liveweight gain. A significant correlation was found between the incidence of enzootic pneumonia during life and 'cuffing' pneumonia at slaughter in these cattle (p < 0.01).

Other respiratory disease syndromes are confined largely to cattle over 3 months of age. Overall death rate in this age range (1970 - 74) is quoted above as 1.9%. No absolute figures are available on the incidence of the individual diseases.

The national cost to beef producers in 1976 of death from enzootic pneumonia may be estimated to be £4.8m.

Both season and age may be seen to influence the incidence of enzootic pneumonia during 7 years on a large beef rearing farm.

INTRODUCTION

Data from beef units recorded in the UK by the Meat and
Livestock Commission (MLC) show that death rate during the
period 1970 - 74 was around 6.2% with small variations depending on the fattening system used (Kilkenny and Rutter, 1975).
The death rate was highest in the first 3 months of life (4.6%)
and in the period 3 months of age to slaughter dropped to 1.9%.
These figures have not altered materially in the succeeding
period 1975 - 77 (Kilkenny, personal communication).

In the UK 6 respiratory disease syndromes of cattle may
be defined by clinical and/or pathological criteria, they are:
enzootic pneumonia, cuffing pneumonia, parasitic bronchitis,
farmer's lung, fog fever and thrombosis of the posterior *vena
cava*.

Enzootic pneumonia

The importance of each respiratory disease syndrome as a
cause of death cannot be determined from the MLC figures above.
However, separately obtained records from 12 different beef
units, in 11 counties, involving some 11 000 animals, during
1970 - 77, indicate that enzootic pneumonia accounted for just
under 50% of 650 deaths (Table 1). Data from some of these
farms also show that 33% of 9 016 animals were treated for non-
fatal enzootic pneumonia. On one of the farms (Berks 1) it was
possible to observe the recurrence of enzootic pneumonia. If
the 449 animals (22%) treated for the disease over 5 years,
8.9% were treated on one or more subsequent occasion and 3.6%,
although treated, had to be culled before reaching slaughter
weight.

The incidence of the non-fatal disease on this farm has
been shown to be associated with up to a 2.6% reduction in
live weight gain during 1970 - 72. (Thomas et al., 1977).
This figure excludes animals that failed to reach slaughter
weight.

TABLE 1

INCIDENCE OF ENZOOTIC PNEUMONIA RECORDED ON 12 BEEF UNITS*

Farm		Number Animals	% deaths		% treated pneumonia
			Total	pneumonia	
Berks 1.	1970-76	3224	5.2	2.8	22
2.	1975-76	250	4.8	4.0	38.4
Oxon	1972-76	951	7.7	5.6	52
Hants	1972-77	552	4.1	0.4	3.4
Somerset	1970-77	712	5.1	2.8	26.9
Hereford	1971-77	416	3.1	1.4	47.8
Cambs	1974-77	436	6.2	1.2	17.2
Warks	1971-75	1200	6.6	1.9	3.1
Notts	1971-76	952	8.9	4.4	18.0
Lancs	1975-76	160	3.8	0	NA
Yorks	NA	1340	6.2	2.5	NA
Leics	1973-75	762	5.8	1.8	14.3
Total		10955	5.9	2.7	32.6

* calves enter units around 10 days old

NA not available

The overall death rate (5.9%) on the 12 farms compares closely with the 6.2% rate recorded nationally on the MLC units and indicates how data collected on a small scale from a representative group of 'sentinel' farms could be reliably used to project national disease losses.

Cuffing pneumonia

Returns from 60 abattoirs in 1976 show that 5.5% of 109 449 animals had pneumonic lesions at slaughter (Animal Disease Reports, MAFF 1977). In a separate survey of 935 animals routinely slaughtered from the Berkshire farm mentioned above, 11% were found to have significant pneumonic lesions at slaughter and the majority of these lesions were 'cuffing' pneumonia. This lesion was associated with up to 7.2% reduction in liveweight gain (Thomas et al., 1977). A significant correlation was found

between the incidence of enzootic pneumonia during life and
cuffing pneumonia at slaughter in these cattle (p < 0.01).

Parasitic Bronchitis and Fog Fever

Data on the incidence of parasitic bronchitis and fog
fever come from a survey of 69 farms in the West Midlands area
during 1974 - 75. Of the 12 029 animals present on the farms
during that year, 303 cases of parasitic bronchitis (2.5%)
were recorded on 11 farms and 10 cases of fog fever (0.08%)
were recorded on 3 farms. Some qualification of these figures
is necessary: the cases do not distinguish between fatal and
non-fatal diseases; cases of parasitic bronchitis may reflect
the number of animals treated for the disease in a group rather
than the number of clinical cases; and the number of animals
involved in the survey excluded adult cows and bulls.

Additional, but fragmentary, data on the prevalance of
parasitic bronchitis may be quoted. This disease accounted for
9.4% of cattle diseases seen in an Ayrshire veterinary practice
during 1967 (Martin, 1973), and 0.5% of cattle diagnoses as
revealed by the Veterinary Investigation Diagnosis Analysis
(VIDA) during 1971 (Hugh-Jones, 1972). More recently (1975
and 1976) VIDA II showed the prevalance to be 0.07% of cattle
diagnoses (G. Davies, personal communication).

Respiratory Disease Syndromes of Adult Cattle

The prevalance of these diseases in 295 cases of adult
respiratory disease examined over 6 years at the Glasgow
Veterinary School was: farmers lung (96 cases), acute and
chronic bacterial pneumonias (enzootic pneumonia) (78 cases),
fog fever (62), thrombosis of posterior vena cava (23), parasitic
bronchitis (23), other disorders (13) (Wiseman et al., 1976).

Some indication of the combined death rate caused by
parasitic bronchitis, fog fever and other respiratory disease
syndromes of cattle over 3 months of age may be derived from
MLC data; overall death rate in this age range (1970 - 74) is
quoted as 1.9%.

Cost of Disease

The national cost of fatal disease (all causes) to the
beef producer may be estimated from the figures calculated
annually by MLC for mortality cost per head of cattle sold and
the national abbatoir returns for the number of steers and
heifers sold/slaughtered for beef in the same year. The MLC
figure gives the cost of mortality as spread over the total
number of cattle sold for slaughter off MLC recorded farms.
The figure varies with the fattening system used but for 18
month, grass/cereal beef, which is the most commonly used
system in the UK, the figure for 1976 was £3.04 per head of
cattle sold (Kilkenny, 1976). If this figure is taken as a
national average and multiplied by the 3.2 million cattle
slaughtered for beef in 1976, the estimate of the national cost
of mortality to the beef producer in 1976 is £9.7 million. If
50% of deaths were due to enzootic pneumonia, as in the sample
of 11,000 cattle above, the cost of fatal enzootic pneumonia
to the beef producer in 1976 was £4.8 million.

Influence of season and age on Enzootic pneumonia

Epidemiological observations over 7 years involving the
3 224 animals on the Berks 1 farm (Table 1) show that both
season and the age of the animal may influence the incidence
of enzootic pneumonia. Calves are collected onto this farm
in even sized batches, at the same age and at regular intervals
through the year so that the influence of season and age on
disease may be examined separately (Figures 1 and 2). With
season, two peaks of disease may be seen in early and late
winter and with age the 3 - 4 month old animal appears the most
susceptible to both fatal and non-fatal enzootic pneumonia.
Enzootic pneumonia may be seen to take over progressively as the
major cause of death after 1 - 2 months of age.

It would appear therefore that the commonly practised
system in this country, of autumn calving, neatly ensures that
calves are at their most susceptible age during the most
disease prone season. From this point of view it might be worth
reverting to the more natural system of calving with the spring
grass.

62

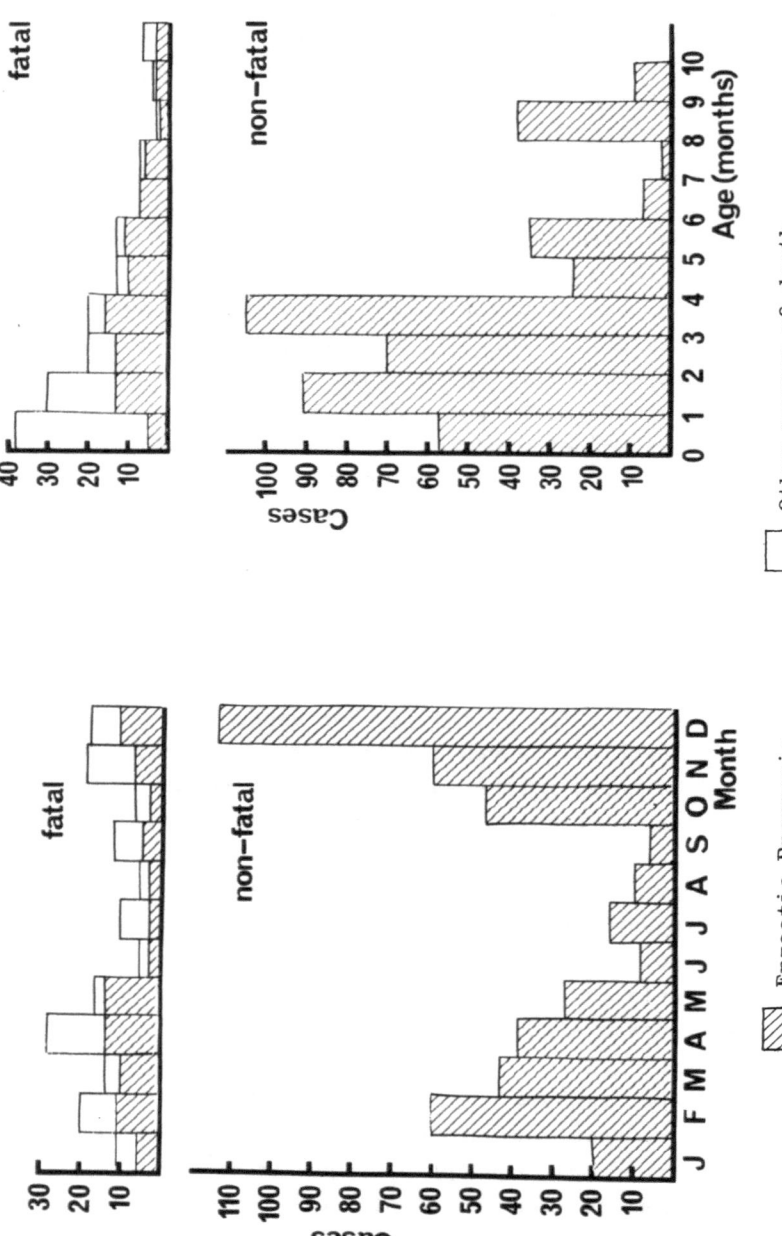

Fig. 1. Incidence of enzootic pneumonia in relation to season.

Fig. 2. Incidence of enzootic pneumonia in relation to age.

Enzootic Pneumonia

Other causes of death

DISCUSSION

None of the data presented in this paper can be claimed to truly represent the UK cattle population and because it comes from a variety of different sources, an overall comparison of incidence for the different disease syndromes is unjustified (even impossible where only prevalence figures exist). More representative data could be obtained, as indicated earlier, from some form of 'sentinel' farm monitoring system but in the absence of this, the present collection of data represents at least a guideline to the situation in the UK.

Some comment should be made on two earlier surveys of cattle disease: Leech et al. (1968) and Hugh-Jones (1972). In the Leech survey 250 carcasses were examined post-mortem and only 11% had lesions of the respiratory tract. In the Hugh-Jones, Veterinary Investigation Diagnosis Analysis only 13% of 6 434 diagnoses involved the respiratory system. Neither of these two surveys would appear to support the thesis that pneumonia accounts for some 50% of calf deaths. However, the populations sampled in these two surveys, differed from the present survey and included also the very young calf of less than ten days of age. In this narrow age range where death rate may be as high or higher than all succeeding periods, lesions of the gastro-intestinal tract, not the respiratory tract, account for the higher proportion of deaths. (The change-over in importance of the two diseases has already been noted in Figure 2 between 1 and 2 months of age). In addition it should be noted that considerable selection is involved in the VIDA sample (Hugh-Jones, 1972), and one may suspect a similar bias towards the smaller and therefore younger carcasses in the 67% of deaths examined postmortem in the Leech survey.

Finally it appears from examination of MLC annual mortality rates, the Leech survey and other surveys discussed by him and from my own rather limited observations over 7 years, that little significant variation occurs from year to year in overall disease patterns.

ACKNOWLEDGEMENTS

I am particularly indebted to Mr. R.D. Caswell, Assistant
Farm Manager, Milk Marketing Board; Mr. G.C. Forth, Veterinary
Officer, MAFF., Kenilworth, Mrs. D.J. Castle, Farmer, Wantage,
Mr. A.H. Andrews, Veterinary Officer, Meat and Livestock
Commission, and Mr. D.C. Ostler and Mr. F.D. Kirby, Veterinary
Officers, MAFF., Reading, for providing disease incidence
data from 12 beef units and to Dr. T.J. Forbes and Mrs. C.
Fenlon at the Grassland Research Institute, Hurley, for
providing disease incidence data from the West Midlands area.

I am grateful also to Mr. Stephen Shaw of the statistics
section at this Institute for the statistical calculation.

REFERENCES

Animal Disease Report MAFF 1977. 1, No. 1, p. 10 and No. 2, p. 10.

Hugh-Jones, M.E. 1972. International Congress of Diseases of Cattle in Great Britain, London, p.1.

Kilkenny, J.B. 1976. Meat and Livestock Commission, Results for Grass/ Cereal systems, p.4.

Kilkenny, J.B. and Rutter, J.M. 1975. Perinatal Ill-Health in Calves CEC. p. 30.

Leech, F.B., Macrae, W.K. and Menzies, D.W. 1968. Animal Disease Surveys Report No. 5, HMSO.

Martin, B. 1973. Vet. Rec. 92, p. 164.

Thomas, L.H., Wood, P.D.P. and Longland, J.M. 1977. Br. vet. J. (In press).

Wiseman, A., Selman, E.I., Pirie, H.M. and Breeze, R.G. 1976. International Congress of Diseases of Cattle, Paris, p. 467.

A SEROSURVEY OF VIRUSES DURING OUTBREAKS OF ACUTE RESPIRATORY/ENTERIC DISEASE IN SWEDISH CATTLE

J. Moreno-Lopez and B. Morein*

The Swedish University of Agricultural Sciences
Uppsala, Sweden.

ABSTRACT

This report presents results on the incidence of serum titres and the increase in titres against viruses and Chlamydia (miagawanella) in Swedish cattle in relation to disease during the period 1973 to 1976. Samples from about 300 animals have been processed. Serological tests with 15 different antigens have been performed including: adenoviruses, parainfluenza-3 virus, virus diarrhoea virus, reoviruses, respiratory syncytial virus and Chlamydia. Serum antibodies were found against all tested antigens and the frequency ranged from 20 to 80%. The frequency of significant increases in titre in connection with disease varied for the different viruses between 2% and 7%.

* Temporary address for next 12 months:

European Molecular Biology Laboratory (EMBL),
69 Heidelberg, Postfach 10,2209, Germany.

A serosurvey of several viruses and a chlamydia
(Miyagawanella) known to occur in cattle was carried out
during outbreaks of acute respiratory and/or enteric disease
on 35 Swedish farms comprising 283 animals. Virus isolation
was also attempted. The age of the animals was between 3
weeks and 6 years. Paired serum samples as well as nasal,
rectal, and conjunctival swabs were collected. For the
serosurvey conventional methods in a microtitre system were
used, ie the HI test for parainfluenza-3 virus (PIV-3) and reoviruses (3 serotypes), the CF test for chlamydia, and the SN
test for bovine virus diarrhoea virus (BVDV), respiratory
syncytial virus (RSV), and adenoviruses (8 serotypes).
Infectious bovine rhinotracheitis (IBR) virus was not included
since antibody to this virus was found only occasionally in
imported cattle. Appropriate pretreatment of the sera was
made with regard to HI tests with PIV-3 and reoviruses. In SN
tests bovine testicle cells (BVDV and adenoviruses 4 through 8),
and bovine kidney cells (RSV and adenoviruses 1 through 3) were
used.

The serosurvey in Table 1 shows the presence of antibodies
to all the agents tested. The number of animals seropositive
to each virus varied considerably. The largest number was
positive to PIV-3 (86%) and reoviruses (70 - 80%) and the
smallest one to RSV (24%). Increases in antibody titre have
also been found to all the agents, but the frequency of increase
per virus was low (Table 1). Groups of animals with antibody
titre increases against one agent often showed similar rises
to two or more other agents (Table 2).

Several virus strains were isolated; some from nasal
swabs (PIV-3) and others from rectal and/or conjunctival swabs.
These latter viruses apparently belong to the entero- and
rhinoviruses, which were not included in the serosurvey.

The results of the serosurvey have not yet been properly
evaluated, ie not related to individual outbreaks. Furthermore,
no data on clinical findings and macro- and micropathology can

be given at present. The frequency of the various viruses and chlamydia in Table 1 is related to the total of 283 sick animals, but pertinent data on the frequency in a representative number of healthy animals are missing. This is true also for the frequencies of antibody titre increases in Table 2 even if these rises indicate infection in association with disease. For all these reasons it is impossible to associate a certain virus or viruses with any disease condition. Virus isolations do not tell us much more.

My report is therefore a preliminary one, ie it shows only the various virus types and the frequency of their occurrence in Swedish cattle do not differ much from those in other countries.

TABLE 1

PRESENCE OF ANTIBODIES AND ANTIBODY-TITRE RISES TO EACH OF 16 AGENTS OF
ACUTE RESPORATROY AND/OR ENTERIC ILLNESS IN DISEASED CATTLE

Agent	Number of cattle tested	Seropositive cattle (%) 1)	Titre rise (%) 2)
PIV-3	283	86	8.8
BVDV	266	41	9.9
RSV	258	24	2.8
Adenovirus			
1	278	54	5.3
2	278	50	3.2
3	280	43	6.4
4	272	45	7.8
5	264	30	4.7
6	259	20	5.8
7	266	50	8.8
8	273	37	6.2
Reovirus			
1	283	81	14.2
2	283	78	7.9
3	283	71	8.0
Chlamydia	283	36	7.3

1) Antibody titre considered as positive in respective test.

2) Four-fold increase of antibody in respective test.

TABLE 2

SIMULTANEOUS RISE OF ANTIBODIES TO DIFFERENT AGENTS IN THE SAME DISEASED CATTLE

Number of cattle with a rise of antibody to respective agent [1]

PIV-3	BVDV	RSV	Adenovirus								Reovirus			Chlamydia
			1	2	3	4	5	6	7	8	1	2	3	
(13)	2	0	2	0	2	2	1	0	0	0	2	2	3	4
2	(11)	0	3	1	1	2	1	1	0	0	3	0	2	3
0	0	(2)	0	0	0	0	0	0	2	0	0	0	1	0
2	3	0	(9)	1	2	1	1	1	1	1	1	1	0	4
0	1	0	1	(3)	1	0	1	1	0	0	0	1	0	2
2	1	0	2	1	(6)	1	0	0	0	0	0	0	0	2
2	2	0	1	0	1	(13)	0	0	8	5	1	2	1	2
1	1	0	1	1	0	0	(8)	2	2	1	3	0	1	1
0	1	0	1	0	0	2	2	(8)	2	1	3	1	0	0
0	0	2	1	0	0	8	5	1	(12)	1	2	1	1	1
0	0	0	1	0	0	5	1	1	6	(9)	1	0	0	1
2	3	0	1	0	0	1	3	3	2	1	(21)	10	8	0
2	2	0	0	1	0	2	0	3	1	1	0	(13)	4	0
3	3	0	1	0	0	0	1	1	0	1	0	8	(11)	2
4	3	0	4	2	2	2	1	0	1	1	0	0	0	(9)

1) Number in brackets: A group of cattle with rise of antibody to a certain agent

(eg PIV-3) was tested for antibody rise to each of the other agents.

DISEASE INCIDENCE AND EPIDEMIOLOGY - THE SITUATION IN THE USA

D.G. McKercher

School of Veterinary Medicine, University of California,
Davis, California.

ABSTRACT

Respiratory infections are most prevalent and severe in feeder cattle enterprises because of stress arising from climatic factors, distant hauling, overcrowding, and rigorous handling, all of which predispose to infection and promote its spread. Shipping fever, in which bacteria such as Pasteurella, Corynebacteria, Mycoplasma, and miscellaneous bacterial species are usually associated with Parainfluenza-3 (PI-3) virus, is the most common and costly infection. Infectious bovine rhinotracheitis (IBR) is a less frequent problem, although it is sometimes complicated by secondary bacterial invasion, with ensuing mortality. Also, because of the latent nature of IBR, problems associated with vaccination against it occasionally occur. Adenoviral infection has not been encountered in feeder cattle, but it appears that these viruses play a role in respiratory-enteric infection in calves. Sporadic outbreaks of respiratory disease attributed to rhinoviruses and bovine respiratory syncytial (BRS) viruses are occasionally reported; but the etiologic significance of these agents, per se, in such infections is unclear. Surprisingly, despite the ubiquity of Chlamydia, the relative scarcity of reports indicates that these agents are rarely involved in respiratory diseases of cattle in the USA. The epidemiology of shipping fever and, to some extent, of IBR, is essentially unresolved.

Respiratory diseases are common in all types of cattle enterprises, but the greatest losses in the USA are incurred by the feeder-cattle industry. Its operations involve large concentrations of closely confined cattle, frequently under adverse physical conditions. Such a situation is incompatible with a healthy environment.

Cattle entering feeder operations come mainly from range pastures, and hence are highly susceptible to infection. On moving into the various commercial channels, they are abruptly exposed to debilitating stresses of a physical and physiologic nature, and to a wide range of infectious agents. As a consequence, losses are extremely high. Calf-rearing establishments for veal production and for dairy cattle replacements, a relatively new development in the USA, also provide conditions favourable for promoting infection and the spread of respiratory diseases.

SHIPPING FEVER

Shipping fever has been, still is, and probably will continue to be, the scourge of the cattle-feeder industry for some time to come, judging by the lack of progress so far in attempts to bring this widespread and costly infection under control. Years ago it was postulated that a virus triggered infection. This, in turn, was believed to predispose the animals to secondary bacterial infection, which largely accounted for the severity of the disease and the ensuing losses. *Pasteurella* species were considered to be the most likely agents. Accordingly, *pasteurella* bacterins and antiserums were produced and widely used. Gradually their efficacy became questioned. Although bacterins containing *Pasteurella* alone, and in combination with other organisms, are still available, their value, in the opinion of most veterinarians, has not been demonstrated. *Pasteurella* antiserums are no longer produced.

Isolation of the PI-3 virus fulfilled a prediction made years before the fact. The most optimistic hope held was that

this hypothetical, long-sought-for virus would prove to be
the sole cause of the disease, or at least the major etiologic
component. It was a great disappointment, therefore, when it
was found to be a relatively weak pathogen which sometimes
produced mild infection, but which more often produced no
clinical evidence of disease whatever. Furthermore, vaccines
consisting of either the viable or inactivated virus failed to
provide any clear evidence of a protective effect.

In attempts to define the role of PI-3 virus in shipping
fever by direct means, the virus was inoculated into cattle by
various routes prior to, after, and simultaneously with other
viruses, *Pasteurella*, mycoplasma, and chlamydia, singly or in
various combinations. These inoculations were accompanied in
many instances by application of various forms of physical and
physiologic stress. Some reports indicated that a syndrome
similar to typical shipping fever was produced, but others
indicated the reverse. In view of these contradictory findings,
there is still no agreement as to the precise cause or causes
of the syndrome, or general acceptance that it has been
reproduced by experimental means. Unfortunately, until this
is accomplished, shipping fever will undoubtedly remain the
enigma which it now is.

Incidence

During 1972, a relatively light year for losses, over
350 000 head of feeder cattle died from shipping fever,
representing a loss of 76 million dollars. Treatment and
veterinary services amounted to an additional 19 million
dollars. If decreased productivity due to sickness and poor
performance as a result of the disease are also included, the
figure is estimated to be almost 300 million dollars (Fleming,
1973).

The high incidence of shipping fever is reflected in the
fact that over 90% of the large feedlots, ie those marketing
over 1 000 cattle per year, reported losses from the disease
during 1972. The apparent influence of transportation on the

incidence is indicated by the occurrence of the disease in almost 60% of western feedlots, which cattle enter after hauls of up to 2 000 miles. This compares to less than 30% in the south eastern part of the country where hauling is minimal as most cattle are fed locally.

Etiologic factors

In a recent survey conducted in Colorado (Jensen et al., 1976) on a population of over 400 000 head of yearling feedlot cattle during a one year period, slightly more than 5% became sick, of which 18.9% died. Sixty-four per cent of the deaths were due to respiratory tract infection, the great majority (75%) being attributed to shipping fever pneumonia. Almost 72% of the fatalities occurred within 45 days after entering the feedlot, probably reflecting the stress of hauling and adapting to feedlot conditions. The effects of unfavourable environmental conditions are indicated by a disease incidence for the fall and winter months double that for the spring and summer.

Pasteurella species, mycoplasma, saprophytic bacteria, and IBR virus were isolated from cultured lungs. *Pasteurella* and mycoplasma predominated. These agents, rarely present in pure culture in the lung, were usually found together with either one or two of the other agents mentioned. Eighteen per cent of the lungs yielded IBR virus, but PI-3 virus was not recovered. Since no serologic studies were conducted, it is not known what other agents might have been present during the early stages of the infection. However, serologic and isolation data from a large state veterinary diagnostic laboratory in another part of the country indicated a much greater prevalence of IBR than PI-3 infection in feedlot cattle affected with respiratory disease. *P. haemolytica* and *P. multocida* were isolated most frequently, but mycoplasma were rarely recovered (Eugster, 1977). These findings, made in two states which lead in the number of feedlots and cattle fed, are probably indicative of the respiratory disease situation in feedlot cattle throughout the country. Failure to isolate adeno- and rhinoviruses in either study emphasises the fact that they are difficult to recover, requiring special techniques which are not ordinarily included in routine viral diagnostic operations.

MISCELLANEOUS RESPIRATORY TRACT DISEASE ENTITIES

In this category are included naturally occurring respiratory tract infections ranging from mild to severe, from which a variety of agents has been isolated. Their role in these infections is uncertain, as they are isolated only rarely, and they produce either asymptomatic or mild clinical disease only on experimental inoculation. However, since several have been found in combination with other disease agents in sick animals, it is possible that they may cause dual infection.

Bovine rhinoviruses

These viruses, first isolated in Germany and England, were recovered later in the USA and subsequently in Japan. Although most serologic surveys reveal that they cause widespread infection in areas where they have been isolated, the rarity with which they are recovered indicates that, in the great majority of cases, infection is subclinical, or the viruses are readily missed by routine culture techniques.

The first rhinoviral isolation in the USA was from an apparently healthy calf in Maryland (Mohanty and Lillie, 1968). Experimental inoculation of this virus produced mild clinical disease in some calves, and occasionally mild pneumonic lesions. A subsequent survey in the state revealed a high prevalence of antibody to the virus but no evidence of clinical infection. In an outbreak of shipping fever, a rhinovirus was isolated and incriminated by serologic means of playing a causal, rather than an associated, role in the infection (Rosenquist, 1971). Subsequently, rhinoviruses were recovered, together with PI-3 and bovine viral diarrhoea (BVD) viruses, from cattle with acute respiratory disease (Rosenquist and Dobson, 1974).

These contradictory findings might be ascribed partially to differences in subjective clinical evaluations, or to the possibility that the isolates studied were of different serotypes, possessing different degrees of pathogenicity. Several serotypes have already been identified, but probably many more exist.

Bovine adenoviruses

Bovine adenoviruses were isolated in the USA during the late 1950's, and subsequently from healthy as well as sick cattle in many parts of the world. Serologic surveys and isolation studies indicate that they are present in widely separated areas of the USA. While adenoviruses are studied widely in Europe, studies in the USA have been conducted mainly in the laboratory of Dr. D.E. Mattson at Oregon State University. His studies of the disease in a large breeding herd of beef cattle over a 4-year period perhaps provide a representative picture of the disease as it occurs in the USA. (Mattson, 1973).

The disease appears about midway through the calving period in calves 7 to 10 days old. The morbidity, higher in calves of first-calf heifers than in those of older cows, eventually reaches 70 to 80% with a mortality rate of about 8%. The onset is manifested by respiratory signs, followed by gastrointestinal involvement. The virus is recovered readily from the conjunctiva and nasal secretions of most sick calves, but not from the intestinal tract. Scattered foci of consolidation indicate that replication of the virus occurs also in the lungs. Most serotypes are recognised in the USA, but serotype 3 is most frequently associated with clinical infection.

While the extent of adenoviral infection in this country is uncertain, these viruses appear to be a major cause of pneumonenteritis in calf-rearing establishments in California. Preventive measures are being developed in Europe, but such developments in the USA are still in the preliminary stages.

Bovine respiratory syncytial viral infection

BRS viruses were isolated originally in Europe, later in Japan, and more recently in the USA (Smith et al., 1974). The American isolate was recovered from feedlot calves in Iowa, where it was found that over 80% of the cattle from various areas of the state were seropositive. A survey in Alabama revealed that 67% of apparently healthy cattle, and almost 100% of the calves tested were seropositive. Under conditions designed to encourage respiratory infection, seroconversion occurred in almost 100% of exposed calves in which clinical respiratory disease ensued. However, a high rate of sero-conversion also occurred in a herd in which clinical respiratory disease was not observed (Rossi and Kiesel, 1974).

Experimental BRS viral infection is sometimes characterised by transient fever, accompanied by coughing and a slight nasal discharge. Small areas of consolidation are sometimes present in the lungs. The extent of the infection in the USA is not known. However, since it occurs in several widely separated areas of the country, indications are that it is probably widespread, although as a subclinical or mild infection.

Mycoplasmal respiratory infections

Mycoplasma organisms were first isolated over 20 years ago from cattle in the USA affected with shipping fever. In a recent survey they were found either alone or in combination with other bacteria and viruses in the lungs of 50% of feeder cattle which died of shipping fever pneumonia (Jensen et al., 1976). In another study, *M. bovigenitalium*, combined with either attentuated PI-3 virus or a chlamydial agent, caused a marked febrile response, respiratory distress, and moderate to severe lung lesions in calves. However, as chlamydia *per se* are able to induce these changes, the above findings do not necessarily incriminate mycoplasma as being etiologically involved in respiratory tract infections. Moreover, in view of the ubiquitous nature of these agents, it is not unusual that they were present in pneumonic lungs of feeder cattle, although not

necessarily as an etiologic entity. At the present time,
opinion is sharply divided regarding the role of mycoplasma in
bovine respiratory infections, other than in pleuropneumonia.
They are considered by some to be of no etiologic significance;
but others believe that, in combination with other bacteria or
viruses, they enhance the severity of respiratory tract disease.

Chlamydial pneumonia

Chlamydia are ubiquitous, and cause a variety of
infections in man and the lower animals on a worldwide basis,
with respiratory tract infection occurring most frequently.
Chlamydial pneumonia of cattle is reported widely from
European countries; but, judging by the scarcity of similar
reports in the American literature, it apparently is an uncommon
infection in the USA.

A chlamydial isolate was recovered during the late 1960's
from the lungs of calves with signs of respiratory infection
(McKercher, 1966). The isolate caused a sharp febrile
response which was more rapid and more pronounced by intratracheal than by intranasal exposure. Clinical signs consisted
of mild depression, inappetence, nasal discharge, and dry
rales. Several repeat exposures at 6-week intervals evoked
much the same type response, although somewhat milder. The
agent was recovered readily from the nasal secretions, but
contact calves did not develop signs of infection. Areas of
consolidation were observed in the lungs of some calves 1 to 3
weeks after the last exposure, and histopathologic lesions were
present in all lungs. Following repeated exposure, complement-
fixing antibody titres did not exceed 1/20, while the clinical
response to reexposure indicated a lack of immunity. These
findings correspond closely to those reported from Canada
(Wilson and Thompson, 1968).

The consistency with which the above mentioned isolate
produced clinical infection by experimental means makes this
agent suspect of playing a primary role in enzootic pneumonia
of calves.

EPIDEMIOLOGY OF BOVINE RESPIRATORY INFECTIONS

Because of their complex etiology, compounded by the
influence of ever changing environmental factors, any attempt
to elucidate the epidemiology of bovine respiratory infections
is destined to end as an exercise in speculation. IBR, being
caused by a single viral agent, is an exception.

IBR usually breaks out in feedlots shortly after the
introduction of replacement stock. This has led to speculation
that the virus is introduced in latently infected animals in
which it becomes activated as a result of stress associated
with transport and adjustment to feedlot conditions. Latent
IBR infection has been demonstrated in cattle after clinical
recovery from the disease. Subsequently the infection was
activated in convalescent cattle by the administration of large
doses of corticosteroid, and by adrenocorticotropic hormone
(ACTH). It was demonstrated also that calves, vaccinated with
inactivated IBR virus and later challenged with virulent
virus, became shedders when injected subsequently with ACTH
(Sheffy and Rodman, 1973). It is conceivable, therefore, that
stress equivalent to, or greater than, that induced experimentally may occur under natural conditions resulting in activation
of latent infection and spread of the disease.

This situation raises the possibility that cows latently
infected either through natural exposure or as a result of
vaccination with live IBR virus prior to conception, might
abort as a consequence of the stress of pregnancy activating
the latent infection. Modified live IBR virus vaccines for
nasal administration are used quite widely in the USA. Despite
claims that they are devoid of arbortifacient properties, there
is some reluctance to use them in pregnant cattle. The
temperature-sensitive IBR mutant vaccine (Zygraich et al.,
1974), now available in the USA, would be a much safer product
in such animals. It would appear also to be an ideal product
for use in cow-calf operations, as the calves are usually

vaccinated while still being nursed by their pregnant mothers.

Abortions have occurred due, presumably, to spread of the conventional vaccine virus from the calf to its susceptible dam by contact.

Apart from the herpesviruses, there is no evidence that respiratory tract viruses of cattle cause latent infection. Latency, however, is one of the unique features of chlamydial infections, particularly in avian species, with man being an interloper host. Latent chlamydial infections occur also in mammalian species, but they are less well understood. Although several ruminant species harbour a chlamydia as an innocuous enteric infection, these strains are not known to be pathogenic. There is evidence, however, that cats, on recovery from feline pneumonitis, become chronic carriers of the agent and suffer relapses. Since chlamydia cause respiratory infections in cattle, it is possible that latent infection occurs on clinical recovery, and might play a role in the epidemiology of chlamydial pneumonia.

DISCUSSION

Many infectious diseases are caused by single disease agents, whereas others are syndromes, eg abortion, enteritis, and encephalitis, each of which is caused by any of several different agents acting independently. However, with the single exception of IBR, respiratory infections also constitute a syndrome, due, apparently, to infection with an etiologic complex consisting of a variety of agents. When inoculated individually into a susceptible host, however, the latter either fails to reproduce the characteristic clinical syndrome, or produces only mild signs of infection. Thus, their role as individual agents of disease remains in doubt.

A possible explanation for this behaviour is that each agent, *per se*, is a relatively weak pathogen; and only when

acting synergistically, and possibly under restrictive
environmental conditions, is the total effect sufficient to
precipitate the natural syndrome. In dealing with shipping
fever particularly, these features pose an added dimension of
complexity to the problem. In view of this possible situation,
failure to reproduce the typical shipping fever syndrome by
experimental means might not appear unreasonable. Healthy
animals, maintained under ideal conditions, are invariably
used in experimental transmission studies. In naturally
occurring shipping fever outbreaks, however, the animals most
susceptible to infection because of stress, presence of the
appropriate complementary microbial flora, absence of immunity,
and factors as yet undetermined, become infected first. From
these foci the causative agents spread by contact acquiring,
as they pass rapidly through great numbers of animals, increased
virulence. Eventually all but the more resistant become
infected. By comparison, experimental infection is a one-step
effort in which a few animals, at the most, are exposed to
agents under conditions which provide them little opportunity
to express their full pathogenic potential.

With respect to their role in disease the status of the
respiratory tract viruses isolated subsequent to IBR and PI-3
viruses, is unclear. It appears unlikely that they are
important pathogens *per se*, but may be contributing factors to
disease under appropriate situations. The fact that they
exist as multiple antigenic and, therefore, possibly immunogenic
types also creates difficulties in determining their true
role in disease, as some serotypes may be pathogenic and others
not. Also, there undoubtedly are still other respiratory tract
agents that have not been isolated thus far because of the
current lack of the necessary technology to do so. Nonetheless,
as long as they remain undetected, they will continue to frustrate
efforts to elucidate further the etiologic aspects of the
bovine respiratory disease complex. In view of this situation,
it is probably no surprise that progress in the elucidation and
control, particularly of shipping fever, has been so limited.

It is becoming increasingly apparent, however, that the approach to the problem in the past was much too narrow and incoordinated. Etiologic studies, whereas of foremost importance, are unlikely to succeed unless supplemented by efforts in areas peripheral to the main problem. The attack must be launched from a much broader base, and entail multidisciplinary efforts on a coordinated team effort. Only when the roles played in respiratory disease by microbial synergism, stress, nutrition, genetic background, and environmental factors have been defined will it be possible to evolve control measures on a firm, logical basis.

Such an effort could assume the proportions of a crash programme. But despite the important issues at stake, it would be impossible to embark on such an ambitious undertaking today because of the lack of adequate support for animal disease research in the USA. However, as the gap between food supply and demand inexorably widens the point will ultimately be reached when a serious effort will have to be made to overcome the deficit. Since increased production of animal proteins is limited by the availability of grazing land and fodder, some of the deficit will have to be made up by other means, such as by reducing losses due to disease. However, more effective means of disease prevention and control than those now available will be needed. Such means can be evolved only through continued research.

REFERENCES

Eugster, A.K. 1977. Personal communication.

Fleming, B. 1973. Beef, 10, No. 2, p. 12.

Jensen, R. (and 11 co-authors) 1976. J. Am. vet. Med. Ass. 169, p. 500.

Mattson, D.E. 1973. Am. J. Vet. Res. 34, p. 623.

McKercher, D.G. 1966. Unpublished data.

Mohanty, S.B. and Lillie, M.G. 1968. Proc. Soc. exp. Biol. Med. 128, p.850.

Rosenquist, B. D. 1971. Am. J. Vet. Res. 32, p. 685.

Rosenquist, B.D. and Dobson, A.W. 1974. Am. J. Vet. Res. 35, p. 363.

Rossi, C.R. and Kiesel, G.K. 1974. Infect. Immuno. 10, p. 293.

Sheffy, B.E. and Rodman, S. 1973. J. Am. Vet. Med. Ass. 163, p. 850.

Smith, M.H., Frey, M.L. and Dierks, R.E. 1974. Vet. Rec. 94, p. 599.

Wilson, M.R. and Thompson, R.G. 1968.. Res. Vet. Sci. 9, p. 467.

Zygraich, N., Huygelen, C. and Vascoboinic, E. 1974. Develop. Biol. Stand. 26, p. 8.

DISCUSSION

O.C. Straub *(West Germany)*

I would like to ask Dr. Lomba if he knows the times at which the colostrum was sampled, and when the samples were taken for examination. Also, at what intervals and in what quantities was the colostrum given to the calf?

F. Lomba *(Belgium)*

The colostrum is collected within ten minutes after calving and is distributed according to the Brussels school - 1 litre in the first hour, 1 litre at the fifth hour and 1 litre at the ninth hour.

O.C. Straub

So you only tested the ten-minute colostrum and not the nine-hour colostrum?

F. Lomba

Yes.

O.C. Straub

In our experience, as far as the virus is concerned, the antibodies cross the barrier up to the twelfth hour, no matter how much we give, but the composition at the twelfth hour is different from what it is at the ninth hour, or ten minutes after birth. If you work on this before the seminar next year which was mentioned by Mr. L'Hermite, I think it is quite important to watch how the composition changes between ten minutes and nine hours.

F. Lomba

When we were checking globulins in colostrum we found, in suckled calves of milking cows, that at the end of the first 24 hours immunoglobulins and antibodies had almost entirely disappeared, even in non-suckled quarters.

O.C. Straub

Yes, I think that is quite important. I would like to say

to Dr. Dannacher that I was not surprised that his dairy farms had more serologically positive animals. Do you not think that it is due more to IPV, since we cannot differentiate between antibodies where there are a few types of IBR and IPV?

G. Dannacher *(France)*

Yes, clinically in these two dairy farms there was very little illness, except perhaps mastitis.

O.C. Straub

IPV can cause mastitis as we know, so I would say that it is due more to IPV than to IBR from an immunological point of view. The same is true for Dr. Thornberry. I think he probably has the same problem, because when I visited Ireland we found out that a few insemination stations also had positive bulls. I think you also have a problem with the IBR/IPV situation in Ireland, and at present you probably have more IPV than IBR. I am curious to find out about your mucosal disease-virus diarrhoea subject. Do you think that you have a respiratory BVD or MD, or do you really have a virus diarrhoea?

H. Thornberry *(Ireland)*

I think we have more virus diarrhoea than respiratory diseases.

O.C. Straub

It is different in our part of the country, as I will explain tomorrow. It was a pity from our point of view that they officially adopted the VD. We think we should not forget about MD, although that is normally used for Marek's disease, but we would like to interpret it as mucosal disease. I was also interested in your note as far as multi-valant intranasal attenuated viruses are concerned. On the Continent we have a difficult time convincing officials that we could use live attenuated viruses. We think their use is justified. We would say, however, that you cannot mix all viruses because some, such as the IBR virus, and the adenoviruses, cause the induction of interferon. Interferon will, of course, prevent the action of the other attenuated viruses and would be followed by an immunity against it. If we use attenuated viruses we must be very careful what sort of mixture we use.

I think Italy is in a very difficult situation because it imports more animals than any other country in Europe, and we all agree that West Germany, France and East Germany contribute to its disease situation. I think that the contribution by Dr. Rognoni has shown the importance of transportation. We have transported animals just to find this out. For example, during one day we have transported six animals for four hours. We repeated this three times during the day, giving a total transportation time of twelve hours. On another day we transported them twice for six hours at a time, and on another day we transported them continuously for twelve hours. Apart from the clinical symptoms, the changes in the blood composition were drastic. We can appreciate that Italy has problems because of the way that animals are imported into the country.

As far as stress is concerned, we can confirm the results given in Professor McKercher's paper. We have given Prednisolone to animals which had a field virus strain of IBR/IPV. Out of 18 animals, 17 shed the virus after 3 - 4 days. Those animals might not have antibodies but they harbour the virus and all we have to do is give them Prednisolone and the virus is dropped.

R.N. Gourlay (UK)

I would like to ask Professor Aalund a question. I was interested to see that he reports the difference in the mortality rate between male and female calves. I wondered if this also applies in respiratory disease? If this is so, are there any population or management reasons which could account for this difference in mortality?

O. Aalund (Denmark)

Yes, this was also true for the respiratory diseases. On this particular farm the reason was that they were treating the female calves in a better way, and the others were just put into a kind of feedlot system on the farm.

P. Pignatelli *(Italy)*

My question is perhaps not very scientific but I think it is in the spirit of this part of our seminar. I would like to know, or to hear any comments, on what kind of scientific controls other people use, for imported animals only, to prevent the arrival of respiratory diseases.

L.H. Thomas *(UK)*

I will answer it very quickly - I would suggest you do not import them!

I am disappointed that we have not heard more data on disease incidence, and the epidemiology, in this session. I suspect that others have found the same difficulty as I in obtaining such data. Since we have heard so much on diagnosis in this session, and especially on virus diagnosis, I would like to make a cautionary, perhaps even a controversial comment on this subject. I would like to repeat the comment which I made in the opening to my talk. I do not believe it is meaningful to attempt diagnosis until we have firmly established which microorganisms are pathogens for the bovine respiratory tract. I might exempt IBR virus from this, because I have no experience of this particular organism, but I believe that all we can learn from such exercises is that certain viruses are common in the cattle population of Europe and the USA. I believe we have known this for some long time.

H.M. Pirie *(UK)*

I would like to follow up Dr. Thomas's general point. Take a disease whose aetiology we know, for instance lungworms, as was mentioned by one or two people, and by Dr. Thomas himself. I wondered how they found the incidence to which they referred. Was it based on post mortem, or clinical examination of the animals? Dr. Frerkin gave a figure for the incidence of lungworms in Germany as a whole, which would probably be an underestimate since it is based on an examination of the lungs of slaughtered animals. Even in Britain, where lungworms are undoubtedly an important problem, the incidence of lungworms in abattoirs is very low, because they shed the worms. So, if you are trying to assess the situation in the field, this can be very difficult.

B. Martin *(UK)*

I have gained the impression from this morning's session that we are dealing with a common respiratory disease problem. The mortality is running at about 10%, and it is appearing between one and three months of age. It occurs mainly during the winter months, even in sunny countries such as Italy.

The use of colostrum in epidemiological studies may well be something which we have been failing to give attention to in the past. One wonders what various viruses such as PI3, reo's, and even the adenoviruses, with the possible exception of some of the strains of adenovirus, are doing. How are they involved in this syndrome of respiratory disease? What about the rhino-viruses - how serious is the problem of rhinovirus infection? We have not answered that. IBR certainly seems to be a common infection, and one which is causing serious disease. We are very interested in this new syndrome described in the Netherlands called 'pinkengriep' which seems to involve two viruses, res-piratory syncytial virus and PI3. We would certainly like to hear more about it later in the seminar.

SESSION 2A

PARASITIC AND ADULT

Chairman:

J.M. Asso

Co-ordinator:

D.R. Snodgrass

THE PNEUMONIAS OF ADULT CATTLE

I.E. Selman

Department of Veterinary Medicine, University of Glasgow
Veterinary School, Bearsden Road, Bearsden, Glasgow, Scotland.

ABSTRACT

For the last eight years, a group of us in the above school have been involved in a clinico-pathological study of respiratory disease in adult cattle. During this time we have carried out clinical and pathological examinations on approximately 300 animals and in most cases we have also visited their farms of origin in order to obtain first-hand background information. In all, we have encountered around 15 different respiratory disorders, most of which we are able to differentiate one from another on clinical and epidemiological considerations alone. For the purposes of this paper, however, discussion will be limited to the more common of these, namely fog fever, farmer's lung, parasitic bronchitis, chronic suppurative pneumonia, diffuse fibrosing alveolitis and pulmonary thrombo-embolism arising from thrombosis of the caudal vena cava. The clinical and, where appropriate, epidemiological features of these conditions will be described: their pathology will be discussed by my colleague, Dr. H.M. Pirie. Aetiological considerations will be limited to one or two of the more interesting and, perhaps, controversial disorders.

INTRODUCTION

The following paper is based upon an on-going clinico-pathological field study of respiratory disease in adult cattle which was started in 1969. The cattle were all referred to us by practising veterinarians, most of whom were working in the west and south-west of Scotland and the north-west of England. The animals were all over 2 years of age and, in addition to carrying out detailed clinical and pathological examinations, visits were made to most of the farms from which the animals originated in order to ascertain their histories and background, to examine other animals and to purchase further interesting cases whenever necessary. Although we have also examined a large number of post-mortem specimens as a service for general practitioners, these have not been included in this paper since we were never able to examine them in life.

The range and type of disorders which we have encountered are summarised in Table 1.

TABLE 1

THE PREVALENCE OF SPECIFIC PULMONARY DISEASES OF ADULT CATTLE EXAMINED IN THE UNIVERSITY OF GLASGOW VETERINARY SCHOOL BETWEEN JULY, 1969 AND JUNE, 1975.

Diagnosis	Number of cases
Individual problems	
Chronic suppurative pneumonia	77
Diffuse fibrosing alveolitis	53
Thrombosis of the caudal vena cava	23
Pulmonary neoplasia	3
Milk allergy	2
Other conditions	9
Group problems	
Fog Fever	62
Parasitic bronchitis (1) patent disease	5
(2) reinfection syndrome	18
Farmer's lung	43
Total:	295

INDIVIDUAL ANIMAL PROBLEMS

1) Chronic suppurative pneumonia

Since we are usually not able to differentiate clinically
between cases of chronic bronchopneumonia, multiple lung
abscesses and bronchiectasis singly or in combination, we find
this a useful term to include all such abnormalities.

The condition is common in cattle of all ages and usually
the history is of weight-loss and coughing for a period of
weeks or months although occasional animals may be presented
with signs of an apparent sudden-onset due to exacerbation of a
chronic suppurative focus within the chest. In a small proportion
of cases it is possible to associate the condition with an
earlier episode of acute pneumonia but often the true cause is
never established.

Typical cases are dull, thin and only intermittently
febrile. Coughing is always present, sometimes accompanied by
the production of mucus, but tachypnoea is by no means a
consistent feature. Thoracic pain may be obvious or detectable
on percussion but dull areas are rarely demonstrable. When
present, rhonchi are almost always limited to the cranio-ventral
chest. Halitosis is usually only a feature of the small
proportion of cases which progress to necrotising bronchopneumonia, this latter situation usually being characterised by
sudden deterioration, marked dullness, fever, pain and death
within a few days.

2) Diffuse fibrosing alveolitis (DFA)

Diffuse fibrosing alveolitis usually affects cattle over
six years of age and has been encountered in both beef and dairy
herds. The history is usually of a chronic and progressive
problem ranging from a few weeks to two years in duration; when
occasional cases of an apparent sudden-onset have been referred
to us, further examination has almost always indicated a longstanding disorder- the animals being thinner than others in the
group and the owners frequently recalling coughing and/or

respiratory signs after mild exercise for weeks or months.

Typical cases are thin but remarkably bright considering the severity of their respiratory signs and appetite is usually good. Depression and inappetance are only seen in severe terminal cases with clinical signs of congestive cardiac failure due to *cor pulmonale*. Coughing is always present and tachypnoea with very marked hyperpnoea are also found, even at rest. On auscultation, rhonchi are usually present over both lung fields and crackles may be heard in the cranioventral chest. Fever and thoracic pain are not a feature of DFA.

The aetiology of DFA in cattle is unknown. In view of the fact many affected animals have precipitating antibodies to *Micropolyspora faeni* it is possible that these may have arisen as a result of chronic farmer's lung (see below). In support of this is the fact that many animals have been admitted from herds with a farmer's lung problem. However, a considerable number of otherwise typical cases are sero-negative which suggests that on occasions, other aetiological factors may be involved.

3) Thrombosis of the caudal vena cava

Approximately 50% of cases have a history of respiratory signs of only a few days duration with rapid deterioration; while in others, a weight-loss and coughing have been noted for weeks or months before referral.

Tachypnoea, shallow breathing and coughing are always present and many cases show signs of severe intra-thoracic pain. Haemoptysis is present in approximately 50% of cases on admission and usually develops within a few days in the rest. Cases deteriorate rapidly once haemoptysis is present and the majority of animals are dead or have been slaughtered within 10 days of being admitted. As a consequence of haemoptysis, there is often mucosal pallor, blood stains are commonly to be found on or around the animal and many also exhibit malaena. Wide-spread rhonchi are frequently detectable on admission and tend to become even more pronounced with deterioration as does thoracic pain. Hepatomegaly is detectable in about 50% of cases on admission and becomes more prevalent, and obvious, with time.

The pulmonary lesions in this condition arise as the result of emboli being carried to the lung from a thrombus which is situated in the vena cava in the region of the liver. This thrombus is usually formed following erosion of a large hepatic abscess through the wall of the vena cava.

GROUP PROBLEMS

1) Fog Fever

Fog fever is an acute respiratory distress syndrome with minimal coughing which occurs in adult beef-type cattle shortly after a change to better, often lush, pasture in the autumn. It is therefore similar, if not identical, to acute bovine pulmonary emphysema (ABPE) as seen in North America.

Almost all outbreaks of fog fever arise within two weeks of moving hungry cattle from bare to lush pastures, such as hay or silage aftermath and consistently affects fat beef cattle, particularly Hereford types. The morbidity rate varies but often approaches 50%; clinical severity is also variable but 30% of severely affected animals die, usually within two days of the onset of clinical signs. In severe cases there is gross dyspnoea, with a loud respiratory grunt, frothing at the mouth and mouth breathing. On ausculation, inspiratory and expiratory sounds are usually soft and crackles are only occasionally detected. Severe cases may improve dramatically after three days and in these animals and in others which have not shown severe signs (and which may not be immediately apparent to the inexperienced observer) it is quite common to note only tachypnoea and hyperpnoea although at this stage harsh respiratory sounds are to be heard on auscultation. Subcutaneous emphysema may also occur in a few convalescing animals. In addition to these signs of respiratory disease within an affected group,

there is also a tendency for the demeanour of the group to
change with the animals becoming more tranquil. Coughing is
never a dominant feature in affected individuals nor in the
group as a whole.

While the aetiology of fog fever is still in some doubt,
there is now abudant evidence to support the view that it arises
as the result of intoxication by a pasture constituent. The
constituent in question is very likely to be the naturally-
occurring amino acid, L-tryptophan, which is converted to the
highly toxic compound 3, methyl indole by the action of ruminal
micro-organisms.

2) Parasitic bronchitis: the patent disease

Parasitic bronchitis is a familiar and common problem of
immature grazing cattle in Britain, even though the disease may
easily be prevented by vaccination with irradiated *Dictyocaulus
viviparus* larvae. There is no clinical or experimental evidence
to support the view that a true age immunity occurs and we have
encountered several outbreaks of classic (patent) parasitic
bronchitis in adult dairy cattle. This situation may arise
when groups of cattle are moved from regions or farms free of
D. viviparus to pastures on which this parasite is a problem. In
both instances, a particular age group may be affected within
the adult herd. The presenting signs of the patent disease are
dramatic drop in milk yield and widespread and frequent
coughing. In individuals, the main signs are depression, anorexia,
frequent coughing and marked tachypnoea; rhonchi and loud
crackles are often audible over much of the caudul lung fields.
Deaths are not at all uncommon. *D. viviparus* larvae are present
in the faeces - up to 500 larvae per gram is not unusual.

3) Parasitic bronchitis: the reinfection syndrome

This condition occurs on farms on which parasitic bronchitis
is endemic but usually only develops when adult milking cows
graze with, or on fields contaminated by, immature cattle with
the patent disease. It has been suggested that the waning

immunity of the adult animals is partially overcome by the
heavy lungworm challenge and the respiratory signs arise as
the result of a small number of larvae gaining access to the
lungs before they are destroyed by the hosts' immune systems.
Commonly, respiratory signs occur 14 to 16 days after cattle
are introduced to contaminated fields and the presenting signs
are again a dramatic drop in milk yield and persistent coughing.
In severely affected individuals, frequent coughing, marked
tachypnoea and dullness may be obvious but affected animals
remain alert and often maintain their appetite. Auscultation
reveals only harsh respiratory sounds. Deaths have not been
encountered in this syndrome. Since egg-laying adults are
absent or few in number, *D. viviparus* larvae are not found in the
faeces.

4) Farmer's lung

Farmer's lung is an allergic respiratory disease which
develops after exposure to the dust of mouldy hay, cereals or
other vegetable matter containing the spores and metabolic
products of *M. faeni* and other thermophilic actinomycetes. The
disease is a problem in man and cattle in the western parts of
Britain, since these are the areas with the highest summer
rainfall. In these regions hay is frequently baled at a high
moisture content (ie well in excess of 30%), overheating is
inevitable and, as a consequence, a thermophilic microflora
becomes dominant.

In Britain farmer's lung disease has been confirmed only
in adult cattle. Clinical signs usually become obvious during
the winter housing period although chronic cases may not be
detected until just after they are turned out in the spring.
The disease is more common in dairy cattle than beef animals.
The possibility that the farmer or farm workers might also be
affected should not be forgotten.

Clinical signs of farmer's lung disease may develop
suddenly, but this form is only rarely seen in more than one
animal in a herd at any time. However, successive acute cases

may occur throughout the winter, hence the decision to regard farmer's lung as a group problem.

The clinical features of the acute form of the disease are sudden onset of dullness, decreased appetite and fall in milk yield (where appropriate). A variable degree of respiratory distress is present and coughing occurs, although this latter sign is often overlooked by the owner. On auscultation, crackles may be heard cranio-ventrally. Fever is not a constant finding under field conditions, perhaps because, in provocation studies, the febrile reaction has been found to occur 4 to 6 hours after antigen exposure and lasts for only a few hours.

Chronic farmer's lung cases may have a history of excessive weight-loss and coughing for several winters with remissions during each grazing season. Other animals may have been recognised as chronic pulmonary cases but eventually may suffer an acute crisis as a result of recent heavy exposure to antigen, unaccustomed to exercise, or to the development of congestive cardiac failure. The clinical features of chronic farmer's lung are weight-loss and, where appropriate, reduced milk yield and there is usually frequent coughing, sometimes with the production of green mucus; affected animals are tachypnoeic and hyperpnoea is often very obvious. There is no alteration in thoracic resonance and no obvious or detectable thoracic pain. Auscultation may reveal harsh crackles in the cranio-ventral thorax and widespread rhonchi. In both forms of the disease, precipitins to *M. faeni* are found in the serum although the disease cannot be diagnosed on their presence alone.

DISCUSSION

It is fortunate that the three major respiratory disorders of adult cattle which we have encountered can usually be differentiated on clinical grounds since information regarding their histories and backgrounds is often of little diagnostic significance. Diagnostic errors have not been common when we have been differentiating between the three most common disorders but mistakes have occurred when we must have been dealing with the much less commonly encountered disorders. Thus, two of the three cases with primary pulmonary tumours in the series were wrongly diagnosed as chronic suppurative pneumonia and the single case of pulmonary tuberculosis we have seen since 1969 was diagnosed as DFA. Some cases of pulmonary thrombo-embolism have been diagnosed as chronic suppurative pneumonia, that is before haemoptysis has been detected, once this has been seen, however, diagnosis is simple.

In contrast, the clear and intimate association between the group disorders which have been described and husbandry patterns and practices must be re-emphasised. As a result, a clinician's approach to differential diagnosis must be based upon a sound understanding of management techniques. Moreover, he must always operate around a balanced appraisal of what is probable as opposed to what is merely possible; clearly such a balance may well be subject to national or regional variation. When diagnostic errors have occurred in the group disorders they have, again, not involved a confusion of the conditions which have been described above. On a very few occasions we have been presented with syndromes which fit into the above classification but which, after detailed investigation, prove not to have been due to the conditions described. For example, on two occasions, a clinical diagnosis of reinfection husk has been made but pathological investigations have revealed lesions not consistent with that condition. It is possible that these were examples of an undescribed disorder. However, as clinical and epidemiological findings were so strongly in favour of a diagnosis of reinfection husk it seems more likely that the individuals examined pathologically did not have what we currently consider to be typical lesions of the reinfection syndrome. Similarly, we have investigated one incident which proved to be due to an extrinsic allergic alveolitis but where none of the animals were sero-positive to *M. faeni*; extensive serological testing completely failed to identify the allergen responsible. Very recently, we have investigated an outbreak of

coughing in a housed dairy herd in which many cases developed
transient haemoptysis. All animals quickly and spontaneously
recovered and a retrospective diagnosis of infectious bovine
rhinotracheitis was made on examination of paired sera.

Possibly the most significant obstruction to the advance-
ment of knowledge in the field of respiratory disease in adult
cattle has been the confusion which has arisen from the
indiscriminate and haphazard use of such terms as *pasteurellosis*,
fog fever and atypical interstitial pneumonia. In our opinion,
little or nothing can be gained from discussions in which the
term 'fog fever' is applied to a number of manifestly different
syndromes; similarly, it seems pointless to group the pathology
of these, and other syndromes, under a heading such as 'atypical
interstitial pneumonia' - despite its obvious pathological
convenience - when so often their pathological features are
vastly different. So often it is obvious that confusion has
also arisen as the result of a lack of dialogue between
clinicians, pathologists and others.

We feel that integrated studies such as we have carried
out have resulted in a much clearer picture of the types and
patterns of certain adult bovine pulmonary diseases. Despite
the fact that much has still to be learned and in some instances
the aetiology of certain disorders have still to be defined, at
least it is now possible to systematically examine individual
cattle and outbreaks with some confidence that a sound diagnosis
can be made, based upon clinical and epidemiological findings.

REFERENCES

Breeze, R.G., Pirie, H.M., Dawson, C.O., Selman, I.E. and Wiseman, A.
     1975. Folio vet. Lat. 5, p. 95.

Pirie, H.M., Breeze, R.G., Selman, I.E. and Wiseman, A. 1976. Proceedings
     9th International Conference of World Associated Buiatrics, Paris,
     p. 475.

Selman, I.E., Wiseman, A., Pirie, H.M. and Breeze, R.G. 19 . Vet. Rec.
     93, p. 180.

Selman, I.E., Wiseman, A., Pirie, H.M. and Breeze, R.G. Vet. Rec. 95, p.139.

Selman, I.E., Wiseman, A., Petrie, L., Pirie, H.M. and Breeze, R.G. 1974.
     Vet. Rec. 94, p. 459.

Selman, I.E., Wiseman, A., Breeze, R.G. and Pirie, H.M. 1976. Vet. Rec.
     99, p. 181.

Wiseman, A., Selman, I.E., Pirie, H.M. and Breeze, R.G. 1976. Proceedings
     9th International Conference of World Associated Buiatrics, Paris,
     p. 467.

THE PULMONARY LESIONS CHARACTERISTIC OF PARASITIC BRONCHITIS AND THE COMMONER PNEUMONIAS OF ADULT CATTLE IN BRITAIN

H.M. Pirie

Department of Veterinary Pathology, University of Glasgow
Veterinary School, Bearsden Road, Bearsden, Glasgow, Scotland.

ABSTRACT

Parasitic bronchitis and pneumonia is mainly a disease of animals put onto infected pastures for the first time in their lives, therefore, in most instances young cattle under one year of age are affected. Adult cattle may develop significant pulmonary lesions, however, leading to clinical disease because either they have not been exposed before, which is unusual, or their immunity has waned. The lesions characteristic of Dictyocaulus viviparus infection in the completely susceptible animal and those that occur during reinfection are described.

In Britain the most important respiratory disease of adult cattle grazing is fog fever. The pulmonary lesions seen in this condition are any combination of pulmonary congestion and oedema, hyaline membranes, hyperplasia of alveolar epithelial type II pneumonocytes and interstitial emphysema. Since pulmonary congestion and oedema or interstitial emphysema can occur on their own or with other pneumonias, it is important to consider the whole spectrum of lung pathology in any individual case before making a diagnosis. In addition the diagnosis of fog fever also depends on a consideration of the clinical history particularly in relation to the time of year and change of pasture. Other conditions producing severe pulmonary damage leading to acute respiratory distress are considered and it is pointed out that in most of these the pulmonary pathology makes differentiation from fog fever easy eg diffuse fibrosing alveolitis.

The lesions of bovine farmer's lung and diffuse fibrosing alveolitis in cattle with and without precipitins to Micropolyspora faeni are also described.

The conditions referred to already are important because several animals may be affected in a herd at any one time and they are common.

Other pulmonary lesions which may be clinically significant in adult cattle are chronic suppurative pneumonia, necrotising pneumonia, bronchiectasis, pulmonary thrombo-embolism, pulmonary tumours and pleurisy. The relationship of these conditions within the spectrum of broncho-pulmonary disease in adult cattle is briefly discussed.

INTRODUCTION

Bronchopulmonary disease is common among adult cattle in Britain, judging from the fact that almost 300 cases were referred to one group of investigators during a recent six year period (Wiseman et al., 1976). This figure is an under-estimate of the prevalence of these conditions since only animals that were available for postmortem examination were included. The lesions found in them confirmed that several distinct clinical and pathological entities can be recognised in adult cattle. Some of these such as fog fever and bovine farmer's lung may involve groups of animals whereas others such as chronic suppurative pneumonia tend to be discovered as single cases. It is important to keep these single cases in perspective however and they should not be discounted as unimportant since overall they made up 25% of the total adult cattle with respiratory disease in this series (Wiseman et al. 1976).

Although the pathology of 'husk' - parasitic bronchitis and pneumonia - will be summarised in this paper it should be emphasised that the largest proportion of cases of 'husk' in Britain is seen in bovine animals put onto infected pastures when they are under one year of age. This does not mean that infection by *Dictyocaulus viviparus* does not occur in adult animals with the production of clinical signs. Eight per cent of the 300 cases referred to earlier were diagnosed as parasitic bronchitis.

As well as providing an understanding of the immune and inflammatory reactions occurring in bovine lungs, a knowledge of the lesions that develop in these groups of animals ie young animals grazing, adult animals grazing and adult animals indoors, has practical applications. In many situations it enables a definitive diagnosis to be made and this can be followed by appropriate advice on prophylaxis or therapy.

Most of the conditions to be dealt with are comprehensively illustrated in the paper by Breeze et al. (1975_1) and other aspects of these problems have been discussed recently (Pirie, 1977).

Parasitic Bronchitis and Pneumonia (Husk)

The pathology of parasitic bronchitis and its correlation with the clinical disease were described in detail by Jarrett et al. ($1975_{1, 2}$ and 1960). The uncomplicated disease is considered to pass through four phases:

1) the penetration phase

2) the prepatent phase

3) the patent phase and

4) the postpatent phase.

Animals do not have clinical signs or pulmonary lesions during the penetration phase, which lasts from one to seven days after infection and is the period during which the infective larvae are migrating to the lungs. Infected cattle may die during any of the other three phases whenever the basic pulmonary lesions become extensive or complications develop. These complications are either massive pulmonary oedema, severe interstitial emphysema or secondary bacterial infection. The degree of lung damage is directly related to the larval challenge in ordinary infections and in most cases of husk can be attributed to the parasite itself.

The prepatent phase is from day eight to day 25 after infection and during this time larvae cannot be detected in the faeces of an infected animal. Heavy infestations may produce death towards the end of this phase due to interstitial emphysema. At postmortem the most striking finding is interstitial emphysema almost masking the other changes and parasites may be difficult to see in the bronchi because they are either small larvae or immature adults. The basic lesions associated with this phase of the disease are alveolitis produced by eosinophils, macrophages

and giant cells; a bronchiolitis with eosinophils in the
bronchiolar walls and plugging their lumina; and an early
bronchitis with eosinophils the main cell present. Larvae
may be seen associated with these reactions in the alveoli,
the bronchioles and the bronchi by microscopy. Bronchiolar
obstruction by cells and parasites leads to collapse of related
alveoli and this is thought to be an important part of the
disease process at this stage. When the bronchiolar obstruction
is not complete it may lead to increased airway resistance and
if this is widespread, as in severe infections, it will
facilitiate the development of widespread interstitial emphysema.

The patent phase of husk is from day 26 to day 55. During
this time mature worms are present in the bronchi and caudal
trachea and larvae can be detected in the infected animal's
faeces. Animals die during this stage from the extensive
pneumonic lesions that develop and also from the complications
of severe interstitial emphysema with or without extensive
pulmonary oedema. Hyaline membrane formation may occur if
there is pulmonary oedema and focal areas of alveolar epithelial
hyperplasia may be found microscopically. The basic lesions are
a bronchitis and a pneumonia, principally affecting the diaphragmatic lobes of the lungs, associated with mature parasites lying
in a frothy white exudate within the lumina of bronchi. Microscopically a variety of lesions is seen in the bronchi including
hyperplasia of the epithelium, infiltration of the lamina
propria by eosinophils and plasma cells and mature parasites in
the lumen surrounded by variable amounts of mucus, eosinophils
and other inflammatory cells. In the pneumonic areas the typical
reaction is one in which aspirated first stage larvae and eggs
in the alveoli and bronchioles are surrounded by multinucleated
giant cells and macrophages;dense focal accumulations of the
eosinophils and polymorphs also occur. Additional bronchiolar
lesions found during this phase are hyperplasia of the epithelium
and polypoid projections into the bronchiolar epithelium, and
bronchiolar polyps may persist for a considerable time and are a
useful indication of pulmonary damage by *D. viviparus*.

The postpatent phase of the disease extends from day 56
onwards, it may last until day 90 although the original
description stated day 70. No larvae are detected in the
faeces of animals during this period since the parasite burden
has either been expelled completely from the lungs or reduced
to a very low number. In most animals the clinical signs are
diminishing and pulmonary lesions are resolving or healing by
localised fibrosis often around bronchi and bronchioles.
However in a proportion of cases, usually stated to be twenty-
five per cent, there is an exacerbation of clinical signs
following the development of diffuse alveolar epithelial
hyperplasia, a lesion that can be described as a proliferative
alveolitis. The reason for this is not known. Pulmonary
oedema and interstitial emphysema may also supervene in these
cases and then the animal will die from acute respiratory
failure. It is important to realise that although the
pulmonary pathology of these animals superficially resembles
that of fog fever (Selman et al., 1973; Pirie et al., 1974)
in these cases not only are there residual lesions from the
patent phase of husk but the animals are younger than those
typically affected by fog fever and there is a history of
respiratory disease prior to the onset of the terminal clinical
syndrome.

In particular situations, another significant lesion seen
in animals exposed to *D. viviparus* is pulmonary lymphocytic
nodules, 2.0 - 4.0 mm in diameter and grey or grey with greenish
yellow centres. These nodules are essentially masses of lymphocytes that have accumulated around a dead larval or adult lung
worm. The nodule with the greenish yellow centre is an earlier
phase and has this appearance because the centre is the degenerat-
ing parasite surrounded by eosinophils. These nodules are an
indication that either the animal has been vaccinated in recent
months with X-irradiated lungworm larvae (Jarrett and Sharp,
1963; Pirie et al., 1971[1]) or there has been reinfection of an
immune animal (Jarrett et al., 1960; Michel et al., 1976; Pirie
et al., 1971[1]; Breeze et al., 1975[1]) or that the animal has been
treated with an anthelmintic (Jarrett et al., 1962). The lungs

of animals that have been reinfected usually have dense
infiltrates of eosinophils in the connective tissue of the
pleura, the interlobular septa, the walls of the bronchi and
the lumena of the bronchi. The collections in the bronchi
sometimes appear as greenish-yellow plugs of mucus and
inflammatory cells.

In adult cattle husk is either seen as the reinfection
phenomenon with pulmonary lymphocytic nodules or less commonly
as a primary infection. The pulmonary lesions in the latter
instance are the same as those in the uncomplicated forms of
the disease in young animals. The clinical signs in reinfection
often appear to be out of proportion to the amount of lung
damage as assessed in animals that have been slaughtered for
investigative purposes.

Acute Respiratory Distress Syndrome

Adult cattle with respiratory difficulty that is sudden in
onset can be classified broadly into two groups. One group is
homogeneous in terms of its lung pathology and has a combination
of lesions that have been referred to as the bovine acute
respiratory distress syndrome (ARDS) (Breeze et al., 1976_1),
whereas the second group is heterogeneous pathologically being
composed of animals with pulmonary lesions varying from reinfection
husk to pulmonary thrombo-embolism (Breeze et al., 1975_2). The
lesions characteristic of ARDS are any combination of:

1) pulmonary congestion and oedema

2) hyaline membranes

3) alveolar epithelial hyperplasia and

4) interstitial emphysema.

It is important to have a combination of these lesions because
pulmonary congestion and oedema, alveolar epithelial hyperplasia
and interstitial emphysema have been found as separate entities
in adult bovine lungs and probably then represent a different

process from ARDS. The acute respiratory distress syndrome has been found in cattle in a variety of situations but the most important in adult cattle in Britian is fog fever (Selman et al., 1973, 1974[1]). These lesions have been regarded as obligatory for the diagnosis of fog fever but they are not pathognomonic (Pirie et al., 1974).

There are interesting and probably significant differences between the pulmonary lesions of cases of fog fever that have died from the lung damage and those that have been slaughtered after being severely ill for several days (Pirie et al., 1974). Animals that died had haemorrhages in the laryngeal, tracheal and bronchial mucosae, severe pulmonary congestion and oedema, hyaline membranes, severe interstitial emphysema and moderate epithelial hyperplasia of the type 2 pneumonocytes (Breeze et al., 1975[3]) and less severe pulmonary congestion and oedema, less advanced interstitial emphysema and usually no haemorrhages in the mucosae of the conducting airways and larynx. As far as is known these lesions can resolve completely.

Bovine Farmer's lung

Housed adult cattle in Britain develop a type of extrinsic allergic alveolitis known in man as farmer's lung (Pirie et al., 1971[2]; Wiseman et al., 1973; Wiseman et al., 1976). Similar problems have been described in Switzerland (Nicolet et al., 1969; Pauli et al., 1971), and France (Espinasse 1972). This mouldy hay pneumoconiosis is usually due to the inhalation of dust containing *Micropolyspora faeni* and precipitating antibodies to this organism can be found in cattle sera (Nicolet et al., 1972; Pirie et al., 1972; Dawson et al., 1977).

The lungs of bovine farmer's lung cases are not readily available for examination since animals do not usually die from this disease unless they have what is thought to be an advanced chronic form of the condition, diffuse fibrosing alveolitis (Wiseman et al., 1976). When confirming farmer's lung in an animal with precipitating antibodies to *M. faeni* by pathological examination of the lungs it is important to ensure that the

pulmonary lesions conform to those required for the diagnosis
of the disease in man since precipitating antibodies could be
present in animals with other pulmonary conditions. The
lesions characteristic of the disease are:

a) interstitial infiltrates in the alveolar walls of
lymphocytes, plasma cells and macrophages

b) bronchiolitis obliterans and

c) epithelioid granulomas in which organisms cannot be
seen.

After recent exposure to the dust of mouldy hay neutrophils may
be seen in the alveolar walls and in severe chronic cases there
is fibrosis of the alveolar interstitium which is focal at first
but then progresses until the lungs are diffusely involved
(Wiseman et al., 1976; Pirie et al., 1976).

A variation of the lung damage produced by mouldy hay is
seen in some cattle which have, in addition to the lesions
described, epithelioid granulomas containing fungal elements
identical to *Asperigillus* spp. (Wiseman et al., 1973). A similar
type of lesion has been seen in Norway (Oksanen 1972).

Diffuse Fibrosing Alveolitis

Diffuse fibrosing alveolitis (DFA) is a term defined on a
pathological basis that has been used to categorise a bovine
pulmonary syndrome that can be recognised clinically and
pathologically (Pirie and Selman 1972). The term is useful
because these cases are quite distinct pathologically from
other chronic pneumonias of cattle (Breeze et al., 1975[1]; Pirie
et al., 1976). Clinical cases are found indoors and outdoors.
Characteristically the lungs are diffusely involved by an
immunological and an inflammatory process that results in
cellular thickening and fibrosis of the alveolar walls; large
mononuclear cells are often present in the alveolar airspaces
and there may be hyperplasia of type 2 pneumocytes or metaplasia
of the alveolar epithelium so that it contains ciliated and

mucous secreting cells. The dominant changes are in the
alveoli but a variable degree of bronchitis can be found as
indicated by strands and globules of excess thick mucus within
bronchi. Cor pulmonale due to pulmonary hypertension develops
in about 12% of cases and these animals eventually go into
congestive cardiac failure.

Two broad categories of DFA can be recognised, one consists
of dairy cows which have precipitating antibodies to *M. faeni*
and the other of beef cattle which do not have precipitating
antibodies to *M. faeni*. The former are probably advanced
farmer's lung cases and resemble 'Urner Pneumonie' described
in Switzerland by Fankauser and Luginbuhl (1960), the aetiology
of the latter group is not known.

Taken together, bovine farmer's lung and both groups of
diffuse fibrosing alveolitis constitute an important section
of adult bovine bronchopulmonary disease since they account for
about 33% of all cases (Wiseman et al., 1976).

Bacterial Pneumonias
    Lung damage attributed to invasion by pathogenic bacteria
is seen in adult cattle indoors and outdoors. Usually only one
animal within a group is affected and consequently, with the
exception of pulmonary tuberculosis, these cases do not receive
a great deal of attention. Nevertheless as was pointed out
earlier, the total number of animals which are involved puts
these conditions in a significant position within the spectrum
of pulmonary disease in adult cattle.

When animals are seen with these conditions the lesions are
usually well developed and easily recognised. Over half the
lungs may be consolidated, the consolidation extending from the
anterior lobes caudally. Apart from a few exceptions the basic
reaction is that of an exudative pneumonia, the alveoli and
bronchioles being packed with a population of inflammatory cells
in which neutrophils and macrophages usually predominate although
the cellular characteristics of the population change with

the stage of the disease. There is also a variable degree of congestion and oedema of alveoli and bronchioles. Areas of suppuration progressing to abscess formation or areas of coagulative necrosis are often found and occasionally may develop. Many of these reactions are chronic and are accompanied by fibrosis of the interlobular septa and the pulmonary parenchyma. The latter is not focused on alevolar septa as in DFA.

Severe necrotising pneumonias sometimes occur in animals with mucosal disease and these may be due to the aspiration of infected material from oral or pharyngeal ulcers that have become secondarily infected with bacteria. A severe acute exudative interstitial pneumonia of the type considered to be caused by *Pasteurella* spp. is sometimes found in adult cattle and this can be fatal. The pulmonary lesions in these animals are characterised by fibrinous exudation within the alveoli and interlobular septa, and the cut surface of the lung has a marbled appearance; thrombosis of blood vessels is often a notable feature. Although tuberculosis is not common in Britain it should be remembered that it may manifest itself as a pulmonary disease and occasional cases still occur (Wiseman et al., 1976). Finally, anthrax is another important disease that can affect the lungs and recently it was reported to be the cause of a respiratory illness in four dairy cows two of which died (Bell and Laing, 1977).

Bronchiectasis

Bronchiectasis can be responsible for clinically detectable chronic pulmonary disease. The bronchi of the cranial and middle lobes of the lung are usually affected although the bronchi of the cranial segments of the diaphragmatic lobes may also be damaged. When the disease is fully developed, which is not uncommon, the alveolar tissue in affected segments is completely destroyed by the dilating bronchi and the lung lobes are converted to a series of branching dilated tubes filled with thick mucopus and surrounded by fibrous tissue. The pathogenesis of bronchiectasis in cattle is not known and it is usually assumed

to be due to incompletely resolved bronchopulmonary infections
earlier in life. The cranial distribution suggests that
respiratory infections occurring indoors might be important.

Pulmonary Tumours

Primary pulmonary tumours may produce clinical disease in
cattle. Therefore in addition to their significance in
comparative oncology they have to be differentiated from other
respiratory problems. They can, for example, produce enough
pulmonary damage to cause acute respiratory distress. One
survey (Anderson and Sandison, 1968) of all the cattle slaughtered
at 100 abbatoirs during one year in Britain found lung tumours
occurring at a rate of 19 per million cattle slaughtered. All but
one of these tumours were in animals over 2 years of age. The
tumours included well-differentiated adenocarcinomas, squamous
and oat cell carcinomas and several anaplastic types. Virtually
all of the tumours had metastasised to the bronchomediastinal
lymph nodes and some had also spread to the liver and kidneys.
There was no regional geographical incidence of the tumours.
Secondary lung tumours were twice as common as primary tumours
and just less than half of these were lymphosarcoma.

Pleurisy

Pleurisy may result from infection with *Mycobacterium tuberculosis* but most cases are now due to traumatic penetration of
the thorax by a foreign body passing cranially from the reticulum.
When this happens a fibrinopurulent pleurisy which is often
unilateral can be produced. The pleural spaces may be filled
with fluid pus amounting to as much as 6 to 8 litres, in some
animals and this compresses and collapses the lung.

Pulmonary Thrombo-embolism

There are two lesions mainly responsible for pulmonary
thrombo-embolism in cattle, one is bacterial endocarditis and
the other is thrombosis of the posterior vena cava. The
pathology of the former cases is centred on the cardiac lesions
and the pulmonary emboli do not appear to play a major part in
the functional disturbance (Fisher and Pirie, 1965) whereas the

pulmonary changes are a very significant component of the disease in the latter cases (Selman et al., 1974_2; Breeze et al., 1976_2). The thrombus in the vena cava is usually infected therefore two categories of pulmonary lesion develop:

a) embolic suppurative pneumonia and

b) pulmonary vascular damage leading to massive intra-pulmonary haemorrhage and fatal haemoptysis.

The vascular lesions are in the arterial side of the circulation and consist of arteritis, endarteritis and aneurysm formation. The walls of damaged arteries rupture and blood escapes into the bronchial tree where it is readily detected at postmortem as are the large globular concentric masses of intrapulmonary haemorrhage.

It is not known why there is such a dramatic difference between the sequelae of pulmonary embolism from bacterial endocarditis and those from a thrombus in the posterior vena cava. It has been suggested that significant pulmonary hyper-tension may be more liable to develop in the latter situation when the heart is normal. Animals with this condition accounted for 8% of the cases seen by Wiseman et al. (1976).

CONCLUSIONS

Parasitic bronchitis and pneumonia is the most important respiratory disease of young cattle grazing in Britain. The pathogenesis of the disease is complex but several distinct forms are identifiable. Respiratory disease is important in adult cattle and it is essential for clinical and laboratory investigatory dealing with these problems to differentiate the diseases that are now recognised if correct and adequate advice is to be given.

REFERENCES

Anderson, L.J. and Sandison, A.T. 1968. Br. J. Cancer, 22, p. 47.

Bell, W.J. and Laing, P.W. 1977. Vet. Rec. 100, p. 573.

Breeze, R.G., Pirie, H.M., Dawson, C.O., Selman, I.E. and Wiseman, A. 1975[1]. Folia Vet. Lat. 5, p. 95.

Breeze, R.G., Pirie, H.M., Selman, I.E. and Wiseman, A. 1975[2]. Vet. Rec. 97, p. 226.

Breeze, R.G., Pirie, H.M., Selman, I.E. and Wiseman, A. 1975[3]. J. comp. Path. 85, p. 147.

Breeze, R.G., Pirie, H.M., Selman, I.E. and Wiseman, A. 1976[1]. Vet. Rec. 98, p. 138.

Breeze, R.G., Pirie, H.M., Selman, I.E. and Wiseman, A. 1976[2]. J. Path. 119, p. 229.

Dawson, C.O. Wiseman, A., Pirie, H.M. and Breeze, R.G. 1977. J. comp. Path. 87, p. 287.

Espinasse, J.M. 1972. Proceedings 7th International Congress on Diseases of Cattle: London.

Fisher, E.W., and Pirie, H.M. 1965. Ann. N.Y. Acad. Sci. 127, p. 606.

Fankhauser, R. and Luginbuhl, H. 1960. Schweizer Arch. Tierheilk. 102, p. 47.

Jarrett, W.F.H., McIntyre, W.I.M. and Urquhart, G.M. 1957[1]. J. Path. Bact. 73, p. 183.

Jarrett, W.F.H., Jennings, F.W., McIntyre, W.I.M., Mulligan, W., Sharp, N.C.C. and Urquhart, G.M. 1960. Vet. Rec. 72, p. 1066.

Jarrett, W.F.H., Jennings, F.W., McIntyre, W.I.M., Mulligan, W. and Urquhart, G.M. 1975. Vet. Rec. 69, p. 1329.

Jarrett, W.F.H., McIntyre, W.I.M. and Sharp, N.C.C. 1962. Am. J. Vet. Res. 23, p. 1183.

Jarrett, W.F.H. and Sharp, N.C.C. 1963. J. Parasit. 49, p. 177.

Michel, J.F. and Mackenzie, A. 1965. Res. Vet. Sci. 6, p. 344.

Nicolet, J., de Haller, R. and Scholar, H.J. 1969. Pathologia Microbiol. 34, p. 252.

Nicolet, J., de Haller, R. and Herzog, J. 1972. Infect. Immun. 6, p. 38.

Oksanen, A. 1972. Nord. Vet Med. 24, p. 281.

Pauli, B., Luginbuhl, H. and Gerber, H. 1971. Proc. 4th Int. Symp, Davis. p. 241. Hans Huber, Bern, Stuttgart, Vienna.

Pirie, H.M. 1977. Vet. Rec. 101, p. 255.

116

Pirie, H.M., Breeze, R.G., Selman, I.E. and Wiseman, A. 1974. Vet. Rec. 95, p. 479.

Pirie, H.M., Breeze, R.G., Selman, I.E. and Wiseman, A. 1976. Proceedings 9th International Congress on Diseases of Cattle: Paris, p. 475.

Pirie, H.M., Dawson, C.O., Breeze, R.G., Wiseman, A. and Hamilton, J. 1971_2. Vet. Rec. 88, p. 346.

Pirie, H.M., Dawson, C.O., Breeze, R.G., Selman, I.E. and Wiseman, A. 1972. Clin. Allergy, 2. p. 181.

Pirie, H.M., Doyle, J.J., McIntyre, W.I.M. and Armour, J. 1971_1. In Pathology of Parasite Diseases, Purdue University Press, Indiana, p. 91.

Pirie, H.M. and Selman, I.E. 1972. Proc. Roy. Soc. Med, 65, p. 987.

Selman, I.E., Wiseman, A., Petrie, A.L., Pirie, J.M. and Breeze, R.G. 1974_2. Vet. Rec. 94, p. 459.

Selman, I.E., Wiseman, A., Pirie, H.M. and Breeze, R.G. 1973. Vet. Rec. 93, p. 180.

Selman, I.E., Wiseman, A., Pirie, H.M. and Breeze, R.G. 1974_1. Vet. Rec. 95, p. 139.

Wiseman, A. Selman, I.E., Dawson, C.O:, Breeze, R.G. and Pirie, H.M. 1973. Vet. Rec. 93, p. 410.

Wiseman, A., Selman, I.E., Pirie, H.M. and Breeze, R.G. 1976. Proceedings 9th International Congress on Diseases of Cattle: Paris, p. 467.

DICTYOCAULOSIS IN GERMANY

H.J. Bürger and V. Bunke

Institut für Parasitologie, Tierärztliche Hochschule Hannover,
Bunteweg 17, 3000 Hannover 71, Germany.

ABSTRACT

Infections with Dictyocaulus viviparus are among the most hazardous diseases of calves during the second half of the grazing season. Spring-born calves brought to pasture in July or later are especially prone to become sick.

The transmission of the infection from one generation of calves to the following one has been looked at by means of faecal examinations of yearling calves, by performing larval counts on herbage samples and by grazing tracer calves.

PREVALENCE AND LOSSES

Infections with *Dictyocaulus viviparus* are among the most hazardous diseases of calves during the second half of the grazing season. The parasite is distributed throughout Germany, infections being more prevalent in the lowlands of the north. Detailed overall information on the prevalence of the parasite, the incidence of disease, and losses due to it, are not available.

Total annual losses have been estimated in Belgium to be approximately 600 m Belgian francs (Pouplard, 1967). In the Democratic Republic of Germany 22 000 of approximately 2 m young cattle died from dictyocaulosis or had to be slaughtered (Hiepe, 1964). Sixty per cent to 70% of farms were reported to have lungworm infections in young cattle in the district of Schwerin; 10% of the animals had to be killed on some farms, and up to 50% on individual farms (Gräfner et al., 1965). We recorded 2 deaths and 6 emergency slaughters among 36 first-season male calves on one farm in August 1977.

Reduced weight gains are usually assumed to be present in *Dictyocaulus* infections. However, there is no information on food conversion rates in affected cattle. This does not only concern the prepatent and patent phase of the disease, but also its postpatent phase. This time may be of special importance as the epithelium of the alveoli may consist of thickened gland-like cells in a considerable proportion of animals for a long time (Urquhart et al., 1973). Whether oxygen exchange and food utilisation are different in these chronically affected animals is not known.

EPIDEMIOLOGY

Four factors concerning the transmission and onset of disease are of prime importance:

1. Good immunity is induced by *Dictyocaulus* in cattle. This

becomes evident by resistance to challenge infections and
by accelerated elimination of worms from the lung of
immune animals (Michel and MacKenzie, 1965). Consequently
in endemic areas disease is usually restricted to calves
in their first grazing season. It does, however, also
occur in cattle in their second grazing season and even in
cows. Diseases in older cattle occurred on several occasions
in the Hannover area. The high incidence of dictyocaulosis
in older cattle in summer 1977 may be explained by the
fact that infections were not very widespread during the
summer of 1976 and 1975 (both exceptionally warm and dry)
thus preventing immunisation of the calves.

2. Viability of all larval stages on pasture is relatively
short (Rose, 1956; Jørgensen, 1977; own observations).
Infectivity seems to be even more limited (Tomanek and
Prochazka, 1968; Cornwell and Jones, 1970). This means
that high infection risks inducing disease are usually
restricted to short periods while low continuous infections
inducing immunity may occur for a much longer time.

3. The requirements for the development of infective
third-stage larvae and their translation (that is the
process whereby larvae in faeces become infective larvae
on herbage) (Spedding and Michel, 1967) are now well
understood. Optimal conditions providing sufficient
numbers of larvae to cause disease seem to be very limited;
temperature, moisture and aeration of faecal pats are
expected to be among the most important factors (Rose,
1956).

4. Transmission may be brought about in several ways; the
relative importance of these is controversial.

(a) Inhibition of development of larvae at the early
fifth stage in the lungs was demonstrated a long time ago
and was interpreted as a diapause-like phenomenon (Taylor
and Michel, 1953). However, its epidemiological significance
as a factor of creating silent carriers has been emphasised
recently (Gupta and Gibbs, 1970; Supperer and Pfeiffer, 1971

Pfeiffer, 1976). Inhibition was demonstrated to occur in
the field in autumn (Gupta and Gibbs, 1975). It could be
induced experimentally after storing infective larvae at
low temperatures (4 to 7°C) for a couple of weeks (Gupta
and Gibbs, 1975; Pfeiffer, 1976; Inderbitzin and Eckert,
1976; Inderbitzin, 1976) thus simulating weather conditions prevailing in autumn. It is important to note that
these inhibited larvae seem to accomplish their development
in spring and start to produce larvae at that time.
Excretion of D. *viviparus* larvae in spring by animals which
had been infected during their first grazing season and had
stopped shedding larvae in the winter (Frick, 1964; Supperer
and Pfeiffer, 1971; Eisenegger and Eckert, 1975; Gupta and
Gibbs, 1975) can be interpreted along these lines. This
may also be suggested by our own data which were obtained
by occasionally Baermannising faecal samples during the
course of experiments on parasitic gastroenteritis in
calves. Output of D. *viviparus* larvae was demonstrated in
cattle at the end of their first grazing season and for
some time after housing (Table 1). It then stopped for
some months, but was demonstrable again in a few animals
in March or April. An alternative interpretation of
these findings may consider newly acquired infections
but this possibility seems unlikely although it cannot
be ruled out with certainty.

Other authors demonstrated the output of larvae throughout
the winter (Wetzel, 1948). Whether lungworms get through
the winter as inhibited or non-inhibited stages, it is
important that a considerable percentage of cattle carry
Dictyocaulus in winter. Surveys of lungs from endemic
areas in northern Germany or Scotland revealed 28 or 30%
infections in animals after their first grazing season
or 6 to 4%, respectively, in older cattle (Enigk and
Düwel, 1962; Urquhart et al., 1973). Thus contamination
of pastures may readily originate from carrier animals
at the beginning of a new season.

TABLE 1

OUTPUT OF *Dictyocaulus viviparus* LARVAE BY CALVES AT THE END AND AFTER THEIR FIRST GRAZING SEASON

Year	Group	Number of Calves	Number of Positive Calves in								
			Aug.	Sept.	Oct.	Nov.	Dec.	Jan.	Febr.	Mar.	Apr.
1966	Bb	34	24	30	1	3	0	0	0	1	1
1967	Bf	10	9	1	0	0				1	
1967	Br	10	6	2	1	2				1	
1968	Bf	9	0	0	0	1	0	0	0		
1968	Br , Brb	18	0	0	0	3	1	1	0		
1970	Bf	10	7	2							0
1970	Br , Bfr	21	14	8							0
1970	K	20	1								0
1973	Bbf	22	12	10	1						1
1973	Br	12	9	3							0

Further support for the importance of carrier cattle
comes from an evaluation of the management of experimental
first-season calves and their infection with *D. viviparus*
(Table 2). Ten of 12 groups of cattle became infected or
even affected during their first grazing season if they
were temporarily kept on pastures which had been stocked
by second-season heifers or steers in the preceding
weeks or months. In only two groups grazed according to
this management system were lungworms infections not
noticed (Table 2a). On the other hand, infections became
evident in only 2 of 12 groups of first-season calves
restricted to pastures which had not been stocked by
older cattle during the current season. While these
data suggest that second-season cattle play an important
role in transmitting *D. viviparus* infections to the next
generation of calves, a few cases cannot be explained
by this method of transmission.

(b)   Overwintering of larvae on pastures has been
demonstrated in some parts of northern Germany, in the
Oldenburg and Hannover area (Enigk and Düwel, 1961) as well
as in the Schwerin district (Gräfner et al., 1965).
Investigations using a new technique for the detection
of larvae in herbage samples (Jørgensen, 1975) also
revealed *D. viviparus* larvae on pastures in the Hannover
area in spring 1977. However, two tracer calves put on
one of these pastures were free from lungworms at
necropsy. Similar experiments with tracer calves revealed
no spring contamination with infective larvae in
Switzerland (Eisenegger and Eckert, 1975), in England
(Soliman, 1952; Michel and Parfitt, 1955), in Belgium
(Vercruysse, 1952), in Florida (Porter, 1941) or in
Alabama (Porter, 1942). However, survival through the
winter and infectivity of overwintering larvae in spring
has unequivocally been proven in the west of Scotland
(Jarrett et al., 1955) and in Quebec (Gupta and Gibbs,
1970). Calves grazing pastures not yet stocked in the
current season in the north-west of Germany excreted

TABLE 2A

PASTURE MANAGEMENT OF FIRST-SEASON CALVES AND *Dictyocaulus viviparus* INFECTIONS: CALVES GRAZING PASTURES PREVIOUSLY USED BY OLDER CATTLE

Year	Group	Number of Calves	Sex	Larvae in Faeces	Calves Coughing	Calves Sick and Treated
1965	Bx	35	O	n.d.	?	-
1965	Kb	18	♀	n.d.	?	-
1966	Bb	35	O	+	+	+
1967	Bf	10	O	+	-	-
1967	Br	10	O	+	-	-
1970	Bf	10	O	+	+	+
1970	Br,Bfr	22	O	+	+	+
1970	K	27	♀	+	-	-
1971	Bbf	11	O	n.d.	+	-
1971	Br	10	O	n.d.	+	-
1973	Bbf	22	O	+	+	-
1973	Br	12	O	+	+	+

n.d. = not done, + = positive, - = negative, ? = unknown.

124

TABLE 2B

PASTURE MANAGEMENT OF FIRST-SEASON CALVES AND *Dictyocaulus viviparus* INFECTIONS: CALVES GRAZING PASTURES PREVIOUSLY USED BY OLDER CATTLE

Year	Group	Number of Calves	Sex	Larvae in Faeces	Calves Coughing	Calves Sick and Treated
1968	Bf	9	O	-	-	-
1968	Br,Brb	19	O	+	-	-
1969	Bf	10	O	-	-	-
1969	Br,Brb	20	O	-	-	-
1972	Brf	13	O	-	-	-
1972	Br	13	O	-	-	-
1973	K	16	♀	+	-	-
1974	K	17	♀	-	-	-
1975	Ke	7-10	♀	n.d.	-	-
1975	Ki	8-21	♀	n.d.	-	-
1976	Ke	4-10	♀	n.d.	-	-
1976	Ki	11-20	♀	n.d.	-	-

n.d. = not done, + = positive, - = negative.

Dictyocaulus larvae in July indicating survival of larvae
(Enigk and Düwel, 1961).

In summarising these results, there remains the
impression that overwintering of infective larvae may
occur under certain conditions in some privileged areas
of Europe giving rise to infections in the next
generation of calves.

(c) Transmission by game animals (roe deer, fellow deer,
red deer) is another means of infecting cattle (Enigk
and Hildebrandt, 1969; Gräfner et al., 1969). While
Gräfner et al. (1969) emphasise the importance of roe deer
as a source of infection for cattle, Pfeiffer (1971)
considers this possibility as a minor risk. It is not
known whether inhibition of development occurs in game.
This would be of considerable epidemiological importance.
However, *D. viviparus* was more prevalent in roe deer and red
deer on Czechoslovakian hills in May than at any other
time of the year (Erhardova-Kotrla and Kotrly, 1973).

(d) Transmission during the housing period has been
demonstrated (Enigk and Düwel, 1962; Gupta and Gibbs, 1970;
Pfeiffer, 1971); these infections may even induce fatal
disease in young cattle under favourable conditions
(Gupta and Gibbs, 1970; Simionescu and Talos, 1974).
Whether indoor transmission may occur under modern
conditions of fattening calves and older cattle is not
known.

INTERFERENCE WITH OTHER PATHOGENS

The possible role of *Dictyocaulus* larvae as a vehicle for
any virus is obscure. It is conceivable that *Dictyocaulus* may
hide, protect and conserve any of these agents.

Furthermore, it is unresolved whether *Dictyocaulus* in the

lungs may create any predilection sites for the intrusion of
other pathogens. It may be added that larvae of other
helminths which pass the lungs in the course of their
development *(Strongyloides, Bunostonum, Toxocara, Fasciola)* may also
be suitable candidates for providing infection sites and/or
aggravating other diseases.

REFERENCES

Cornwell, R.L. and Jones, R.M. 1970. Res. Vet. Sci. 11, p. 484.

Düwel, D. 1971. Tierärztl. Umschau 26, p. 152.

Eisenegger, H. and Eckert, J. 1975. Schweiz. Arch. Tierheilk. 117, p. 255.

Enigk, K. and Düwel, D. 1961. Tierärztl. Umschau 16, p. 415.

Enigk, K. and Düwel 1962. Dtsch. Tierätztl. Wschr. 69, p. 72.

Enigk, K. and Hildebrandt, J. 1969. Zbl. Vet. Med. B. 16, p. 67.

Erhardova-Kotrla, B. and Kotrly, A. 1973. Fol. Parasit. (Praha) 20, p. 41.

Frick, W. 1964. Angew. Parasit. 5, p. 111.

Gräfner, G., Krause, H., Blum, H. and Danailov, J. 1965. Mhft. vet. Med. 20, p. 204.

Gräfner, G., Eichhorn, G. and Benda, A. 1969. Mhft. vet. Med. 24, p. 412.

Gupta, R.P. and Gibbs, H.C. 1970. Can. Vet. J. 11, p. 149.

Gupta, R.P. and Gibbs, H.C. 1975. Can. Vet. J. 16, p. 102.

Hiepe, T. 1964. Wiss. Zschr. Humboldt-Univ. Berlin, math. naturw. R. 13, p. 605.

Inderbitzin, F. and Eckert, J. 1976. Z. Parasitkde, 50, p. 218.

Inderbitzin, F. 1976. Vet. Med. Dissert. Zurich.

Jarrett, W.F.H., McIntyre, W.I.M., Urquhart, G.M. and Bell, E.J. 1955. Vet. Rec. 67, p. 820.

Jørgensen, R.J. 1975. Vet. Parasit. 1, p. 61.

Jørgensen, R.J. 1977. Personal communication.

Michel, J.F. and MacKenzie, A. 1965. Res. Vet. Sci. 6, p. 344.

Michel, J.F. and Parfitt, J.W. 1955. Vet. Rec. 67, p. 229.

Pfeiffer, H. 1971. Wien. Tierätztl. Mschr. 58, p. 14.

Pfeiffer, H. 1976. Wien. Tierärztl. Mschr. 63, p. 54.

Porter, D.A. 1941. J. Parasit. 27, Suppl. 22.

Porter, D.A. 1942. Proc. Helminth. Soc. Wash. 9, p. 60.

Pouplard, L. 1967. Econ. Med. Anim. 8, p. 337.

Rose, J.H. 1956. J. comp. Path. 66, p. 228.

Simionescu, F. and Talos, V. 1974. Angew. Parasit. 15, p. 101.

Soliman, K.N. 1952. Br. vet. J. 108, p. 167.

Spedding, C.R.W. and Michel, J.F. 1957. Parasitology 47, p. 153.

Supperer, R. and Pfeiffer, H. 1971. Berl. Münch. Tierärztl. Wschr. 84, p.386.

Taylor, E.L. and Michel, J.F. 1953. J. Helminth. 27, p. 199.

Tomanek, J. and Prochazka, Z. 1968. Docum. vet., Brno, 7, p. 247.

128

Urquhart, G.M., Jarrett, W.F.H., McIntyre, W.I.M., Poynter, D. and Peacock, R. 1973. In Helminth diseases of cattle, sheep and horses in Europe. Robert MacLehose and Co. Ltd., University Press, Glasgow, p. 23.

Vercruysse, R. 1952. Vlaams Diergeneesk. Tijdschr. 21, p. 183.

Wetzel, R. 1948. Mhft. vet. Med. 3, p. 141.

ALLERGIC PATHOPHYSIOLOGY OF BOVINE LUNG

P. Eyre

Pharmacology Laboratory, Department of Biomedical Sciences,
Ontario Veterinary College, University of Guelph, Ontario ,
Canada.

ABSTRACT

*In mammals in general (including cattle), lung from sensitised
subjects liberates histamine and slow-reacting substance of anaphylaxis
(SRS-A) as principal primary mediators upon challenge with specific
antigen. Additionally, other mediators such as leucotactic factors,
kinins and prostaglandins are produced. The principal sources of these
inflammatory chemicals are mast cells and leucocytes. In ruminants, in
addition to the abovementioned substances, 5-hydroxytryptamine (serotonin,
5HT) and dopamine are evolved.*

*The pulmonary inflammatory response so induced is subject to
intricate systems of checks and balances (feedback-modulation) caused by:*

*1) autonomic neurohormones such as acetylcholine, adrenaline and
noradrenaline, by corticosteroids, each liberated locally or
systemically as a result of trauma, and by*

2) local and systemic actions of the chemical mediators themselves.

*Modulation of the allergic inflammatory response of cattle is
radically different from that in other mammals. In the latter β-sympatho-
mimetics inhibit mediator release whereas α-sympathomimetics and cholinergic
agonists cause enhancement. In cattle all sympathomimetic drugs (α and β)
inhibit, whereas dopamine enhances mediator release from lung. Paradoxically
all sympathomimetics except dopamine enhance histamine release from bovine
leucocytes. Dopamine and carbachol are without effect. Histamine itself
inhibits histamine release, as does serotonin.*

*It may be that catecholamines, while directly inhibiting lung
histamine release, simultaneously increase leucocyte histamine release.
Thus the leucocyte, being a uniquely mobile cell, may operate a negative*

histamine 'feedback' ie reducing further mediator release from tissues. It is possible that during allergic inflammation histamine acts (typically) as a mediator of inflammation, the severity of which might be rendered self-limiting as with increasing concentration, histamine became inhibitory in action. Therefore, the use of antihistaminic drugs might prove to be not merely ineffectual but potentially detrimental.

Further research is required to elucidate more clearly the mechanisms described.

INTRODUCTION

Several important respiratory diseases of cattle may be associated with a state of hypersensitivity (Breeze et al., 1975). Sufficient knowledge now exists to permit a general description of the chemical mediators of bovine immediate-type hypersensitivity, together with aspects of the pathophysiological modulation of their synthesis and release (Aitken and Sanford, 1972; Sanford and Evans, 1975; Eyre et al., 1973; Burka and Eyre, 1974; Holroyde and Eyre, 1976[1,2]). It is appropriate to consider how the new information might assist the better understanding of certain respiratory disease syndromes of adult cattle.

The intrinsic biochemical reactions of bovine lung to trauma differ greatly from those of other species described so far. Thus it is of interest to compare the pathophysiology of respiratory hypersensitivity in cattle with that in a more 'typical' mammal. The guinea pig model and the human subject will be used for comparison purposes.

Chemical mediators of immediate-type hypersensitivity (Figure 1).

Lung from sensitised subjects (bovine, guinea pig, and human) liberates histamine and slow-reacting substance of anaphylaxis (SRS-A) as principal primary mediators, on challenge with appropriate allergen (Eyre et al., 1973; Burke and Eyre, 1976; Austen and Orange, 1975). Other primary mediators such as platelet-activating factor (PAF), eosinophil chemotactic factor (ECF) and neutrophil chemotactic factor (NCF) are released from tissues of many mammals including man (Austen and Orange, 1975). These agents may also arise from bovine tissues, but so far they have been positively identified. Basophil leucocytes release the same primary mediators on allergenic challenge (Ishizaka et al., 1972). Bovine basophil-rich leucocyte suspensions are known to liberate histamine on challenge (Holroyde and Eyre, 1975). Other chemical mediators have not been measured.

In cattle and sheep, in addition to histamine and SRS-A,

132

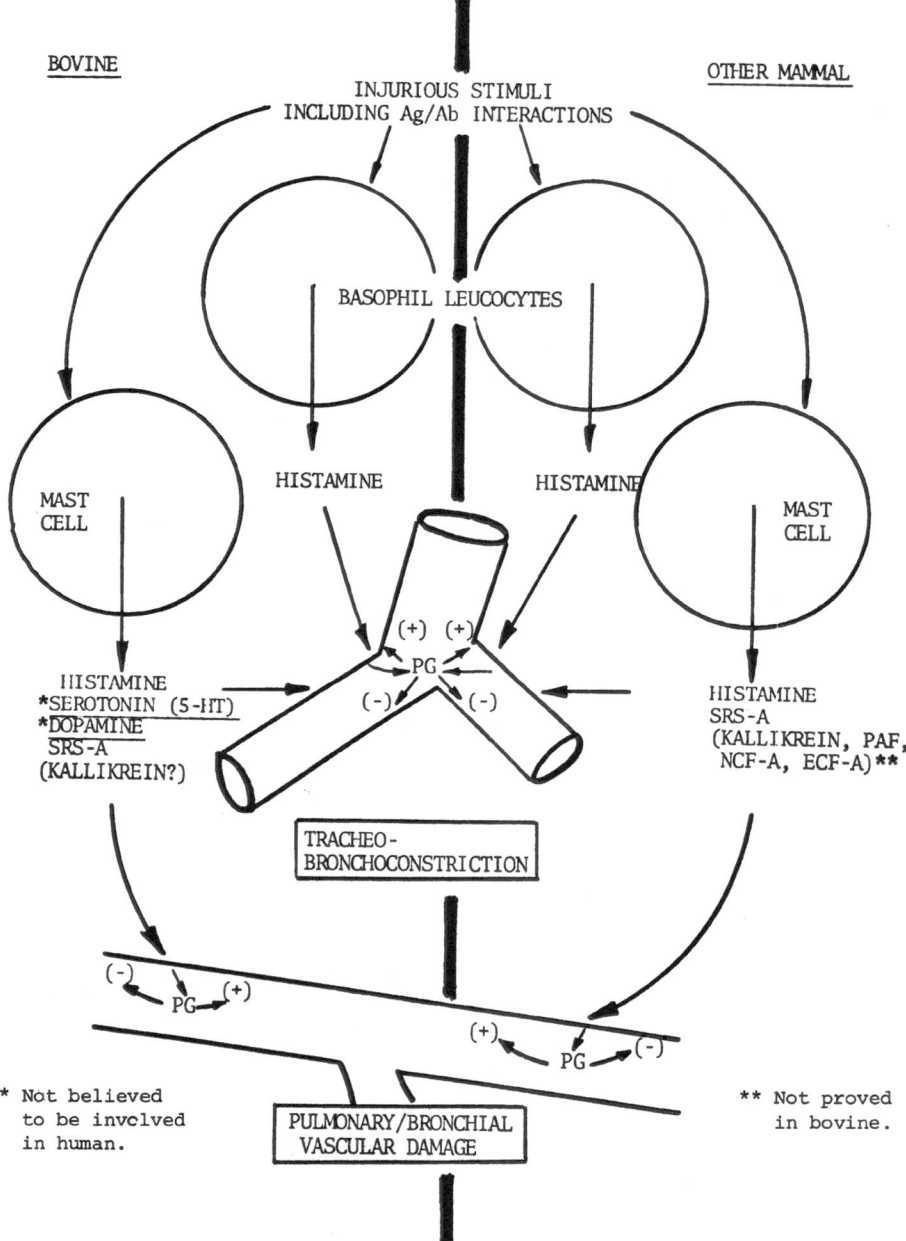

Fig. 1.   Comparisons of chemical mediators of inflammation.

two further amines: 5-hydroxytryptamine (5-HT, serotonin) and
dopamine are evolved antigenically from sensitised lung
(Eyre, 1971; 1972). Serotonin is believed to be a participant
in hypersensitivity reactions of the rat and mouse but not of
guinea pig or man. Dopamine is apparently unique to hypersensitivity of the ruminant species (Eyre, 1971).

Prostaglandins(PG) (formed from fatty acid substrate in
cell membranes which have been 'damaged' by other chemical
mediators) and kinins which are derived enzymatically (kallikrein) from plasma proteins, are considered to be secondary
mediators. They have been identified in all species so far
investigated.

Extensive studies with pharmacological antagonists
suggest that the vasoactive lipids (eg SRS-A and PG) are of
greater overall significance than the biogenic amines in the
chemical mediation of immediate hypersensitivity in cattle
(Aitken and Sanford, 1972; Eyre et al., 1973). Indeed,
histamine, serotonin and dopamine may serve more as modulators
of the allergic response rather than true primary mediators.

Interrelationships and 'feedback' mechanisms of mediators and
autonomic neurohormones. Figure 2.
The inflammatory reaction is subject to intricate
systems of checks and balances caused by:

1) local and systemic effects of the chemical mediators
themselves and

2) by autonomic neurohormones such as acetylcholine,
adrenaline and noradrenaline and by corticosteroids
liberated as a consequence of the initial trauma.

In most mammals (including man and guinea pig), adrenergic
(sympathetic) control of release of mediators of anaphylaxis has
a consistent pattern. Beta agonists such as adrenaline and
isoprenaline inhibit the release of histamine and SRS-A from

134

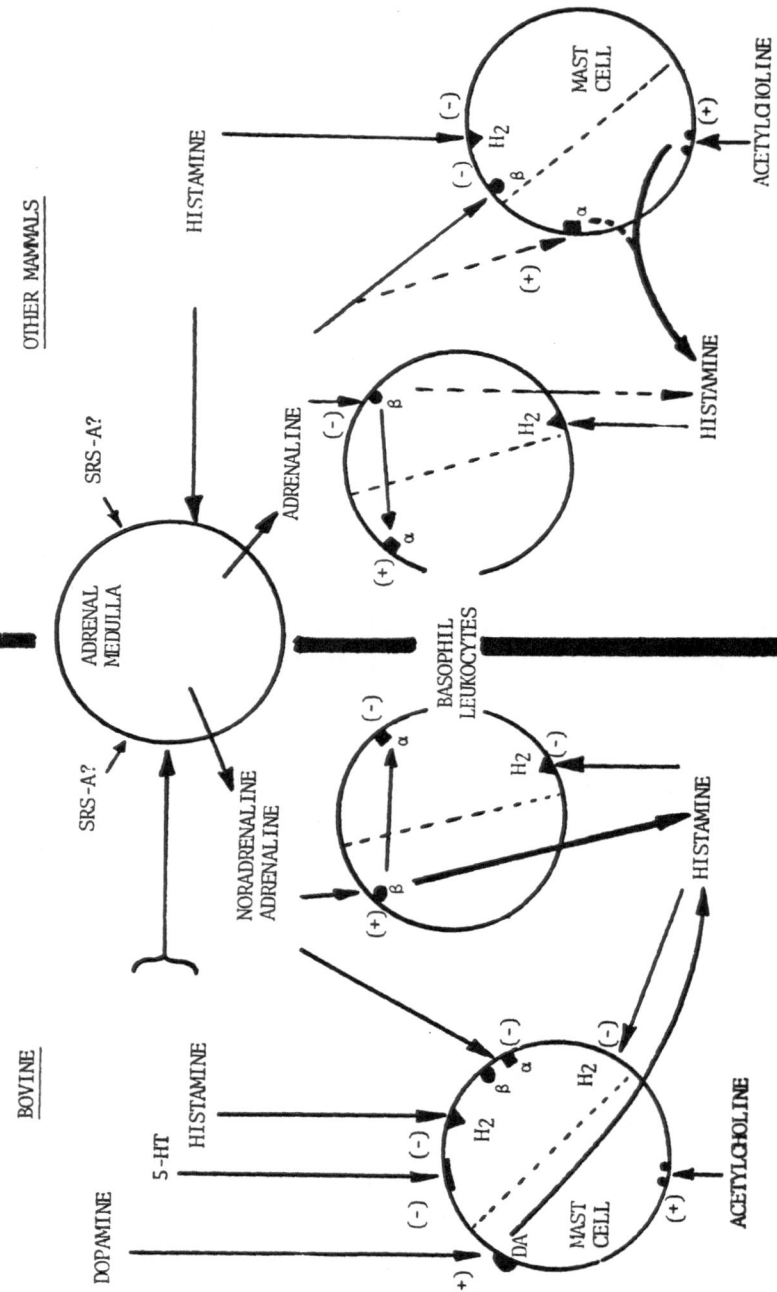

Fig.2. Comparisons of pathophysiological 'feedback' modulation by chemical mediators and autonomic neurohormones.

leucocytes and pulmonary mast cells (Lichtenstein and Margolis, 1968). The mechanism may operate by means of stimulating adenylate cyclase and increasing levels of cyclic adenosine 3',5' monophosphate (cyclic AMP). Alpha agonists such as noradrenaline and phenylephrine, and cholinergic stimulants (eg acetylcholine and carbachol) enhance the release of histamine and SRS-A from pulmonary mast cells, but not from leucocytes (Orange et al., 1971; Kaliner et al., 1972). Alpha agonists inhibit cyclic AMP function, whereas cholinomimetics stimulate guanylate cyclase and increase cellular levels of cyclic guanosine 3',5' monophosphate (cyclic GMP).

In bovine lung by contrast, stimulation of either α or β adrenoceptors leads to inhibition of mediator release (Burka and Eyre, 1976; Burka et al., 1976). Cholinergic stimulation causes enhancement as in other species. Dopamine which may stimulate α,β or specific dopaminergic (DA) receptors strongly enhances the release of chemical mediators and operates through the specific DA-receptor in cattle (Burka et al., 1976). In contrast dopamine preferentially stimulates β-adrenoceptors in human lung and therefore inhibits histamine release (Assen and Schild, 1971).

Both adrenaline and noradrenaline (10^{-8} to 10^{-4} M) stimulate β-receptors and enhance histamine release from basophil-rich suspensions of bovine leucocytes. This mechanism is biphasic since higher concentrations (10^{-4} to 10^{-3} M) of these agonists inhibit mediator release through α-adrenoceptor stimulation. Mediator release from bovine leucocytes is unaffected by either dopamine or carbachol (Holroyde and Eyre, 1976_1).

Release of mediators is modulated by the mediators themselves. It has been known for some time that histamine inhibits the further release of histamine from lung and leucocytes. The mechanism appears to operate through an elevation of intracellular cyclic AMP concentrations caused by stimulation of

adenylate cyclase via the histamine H_2-receptor. The response
is antagonised by metiamide - a new histamine blocking drug
(Bourne et al., 1971; Lichtenstein and Gillespie, 1973). Our
preliminary findings in the bovine indicate that the negative
feedback actions of histamine are biphasic; low concentrations
(10^{-9} to 10^{-7} M) causing potentiation of histamine release and
higher concentrations (> 10^{-7} M) causing inhibition (unpublished
observations).

Serotonin (5-HT) inhibits histamine release from bovine
leucocytes at all concentrations (10^{-9} to 10^{-3} M). This may
be important in view of the proven release of 5-HT from
sensitised bovine lung, although it is not known whether 5-HT
is also released from bovine leucocytes (Holroyd and Eyre,
1976[2]). The influence of 5-HT feedback in hypersensitivity
in other animals and in human allergy is not known, atlhough
one would not be surprised if it were absent in most species
in view of the proposed lack of importance of 5-HT in hypersensitivity of mammals apart from rats anc mice.

REFERENCES

Aitken, M.M. and Sanford, J. 1972. J. comp. Path. 82, p. 247.

Aitken, M.J., Sanford, J. and Evans, D.P. 1975. Res. Vet. Sci. 18, p. 41.

Assem, E.S.K. and Schild, H.O. 1971. Int. Archs. Allergy appl. Immun. 40, p. 576.

Austen, K.F. and Orange, R.P. 1975. Am. Rev. resp. Dis. 112, p. 423.

Bourne, H.R., Melmon, L.K. and Lichtenstein, L.M. 1971. Science, 173 p.743.

Breeze, R.G., Pirie, H.M., Dawson, C.O., Selman, I.E. and Wiseman, A. 1975. Folia vet. Lat. 5, p. 95.

Burka, J.F. and Eyre, P. 1974. Can. J. Physiol. Pharmac. 52, p. 1201.

Burka, J.F. and Eyre, P. 1976. Int. Archs. Allergy appl. Immun. 50, p. 664.

Burka, J.F., Eyre, P., and Holroyde, M.C. 1976. Br. J. Pharmac. 58, p. 445.

Eyre, P. 1971. Br. J. Pharmac. 42, p. 423.

Eyre, P. 1972. Archs. Int. Pharmac. Therapie. 199, p. 245.

Eyre, P., Lewis, A.J. and Wells, P.W. 1973. Br. J. Pharmac. 47, p. 504.

Holroyde, M.C. and Eyre, P. 1975. Am. J. Vet. Res. 36, p. 1801.

Holroyde, M.C. and Eyre, P. 1976_1. Immunology, 31, p. 167.

Holroyde, M.C. and Eyre, P. 1976_2. Europ. J. Pharmac. 37, p. 397.

Ishizaka, T., deBernardo, R., Tomioka, H., Lichtenstein, L.M. and Ishizaka, K. 1972. J. Immun. 108, p. 1000.

Kaliner, M.A., Orange, R.P. and Austen, K.F. 1972. J. Exp. Med. 136, p. 556.

Lichtenstein, L.M. and Gillespie, E. 1973. Nature (London), 244, p. 287.

Lichtenstein, L.M. and Margolis, S. 1968. Science, 161, p. 902.

Orange, R.P., Austen, W.G. and Austen, K.F. 1971. J. Exp. Med. 134, p. 1361.

O.C. Straub *(West Germany)*

You mentioned drooling as a symptom of fog fever, Dr.
Selman. I am frequently asked why a sick animal drools. If
the animal has rabies it drools because it is paralysed. If it
has IBR it will drool because it may have pain in the trachea,
or because the salivary glands are nervously affected. Why do
they drool in fog fever - are they afraid to swallow?

I.W. Selman *(UK)*

I do not know what the answer is. I think it is simply because they are so distressed and they are not able to swallow.
They stand with their heads hanging down, and I think they are
just unable to swallow saliva. It is not pulmonary fluid which
is coming out - it is saliva. It is only the very severe cases
which develop this symptom.

K. Petzoldt *(West Germany)*

Is the oral intake of mouldy hay necessary to induce Farmers
Lung disease?

I.W. Selman

No, it is a disease which arises as a result of inhalation
of the allergen, not the ingestion of it. It is the inhalation
which takes place during feeding time. It is definitely the
spores of *Micropolyspora faeni* which bring about the disease. It
has been calculated that humans working in a dusty environment
can inhale and retain six million spores per minute. Obviously
cattle inhale more. This is a major problem. The hay is so
mouldy that when the farmers are feeding the hay the whole
atmosphere goes blue.

J. Asso *(France)*

Is it possible to get this kind of disease from silage?
Silage is very often in a mouldy condition.

I.E. Selman

As far as we know there is no Farmers Lung-like disease in cattle which results from the inhalation of allergens from silage. Farmers can, if they have the capital, bring themselves out of a Farmers Lung situation which is involving both them and the cows, by changing to silage feeding. Unfortunately, in the upland areas farmers frequently do not have the money to do this.

H.J. Breukink *(Netherlands)*

Dr. Selman, I missed one particular disease in your lecture and that was the acute form of pulmonary emphysema due to re-infestation of lung-worms, which looks a bit like fog fever. Do you see that type of acute allergic pulmonary emphysema due to re-infestation of lungworms?

I.E. Selman

I think you are quoting the Weisman view.

H.J. Breukink

Of course, because we have seen quite a lot of that.

I.E. Selman

We have challenged recovered proven fog fever cases with large numbers of proven viable larvae, as he did, and we did not produce anything in terms of clinical response, and when we post mortemed the animals some 14 to 16 days later, we found occasional nodules, the sort of things which will be described later by Dr. Pirie as part of the reinfection syndrome. We regularly see this nodular form of the disease, the reinfection husk. We have not seen what Weisman has described. In many cases I think it is tempting to assume that he was giving pretty heavy challenges and was in fact producing prepatent husk - the prepatent form of the disease. I do not think that he checked very carefully to ensure that he was not producing this form of the disease - he was not absolutely certain of the immune status of his calves, and I am not now quite sure what his challenges were, but I think what he described sounded much more like prepatent husk - which again will be described by Dr. Pirie. But I know the work you are referring to (Weisman, 1970)

L.H. Thomas *(UK)*

I wonder if I could tempt Dr. Pirie to speculate on the
aetiology of diffuse fibrosing alveolitis. I know that he has
mentioned that it may be a progression of Farmers Lung, but what
else might there be to the story?

H.M. Pirie *(UK)*

I do not know. In the other beef animals they do not have
precipitins and it is not really known why they get this disease.
Some workers have considered that there may be immune complexes
deposited in the alveolar interstitium, but as far as I am aware
this has not been confirmed. It is thought that there may be an
early stage of pulmonary oedema in a mild form which mainly
affects the alveolar interstitium, and this could allow complexes
into it which could move on to this diffuse fibrosis. We have
not been able to confirm this in cattle. There are other similar
types of pulmonary pathology in man and most of them are preceded by a non-fatal pulmonary oedema.

J. Asso *(France)*

Is it true to say that spores of *Micropolysporum faeni* do not
come inside the lung when you have these epithelioid granulomas
centred around the organism?

H.M. Pirie

It is thought that there may be antigens of the organism
in the granulomas, although you do not see the organism itself.
The organism does not grow in the lung because it requires a
higher temperature. There is one theory that it may germinate
slightly, and some of the enzymes actually initiate the damage.

J. Asso

Dr. Bürger, what is the immunological status of the animals
which are carriers? Do you think that you will be able to find
antibodies?

H.J. Bürger

We have not looked at these animals to see if they have antibodies or not, but I think they will have.

J. Asso

And that means that maybe in the Spring there is some decrease in these antibodies. Is this possible?

H.J. Bürger

It might be, but I do not know of any report on this.

J. Asso

Is it possible to find complement fixing antibodies?

H.J. Bürger

Yes, it is possible to find antibodies, but it has not
been looked at in animals in this situation.

J. Asso

One other thing which I do not completely understand is about
overwintering - when you cool the larvae, do you maintain them
outside the animal, or do you inoculate them in the animal?

H.J. Bürger

They cool them in the refrigerator outside the animal,
and then they infect the animal, and then they get inhibition
of the larvae.

J. Asso

That means that the larvae which are in the lung all winter
have been kept during the autumn.

H.J. Bürger

In the field, this inhibition will occur by picking up larvae
in October/November, which have been outside during this cold
weather. I do not think it is known yet the exact temperature
at which these larvae have to live, but it has been shown that
at $4^{\circ}C$ to $7^{\circ}C$ these larvae will become inhibition-prone.

I.E. Selman

Where do you think these inhibited larvae sit when they
are in the animal, throughout the winter?

H.J. Bürger

There is a report from Austria that they found them in the small bronchioli as fifth stage larvae. We are looking at this at the moment, just trying to get lungs throughout the winter, and to get the larvae out.

I.E. Selman

Were they not producing any clinical reaction in these terminal bronchioles?

H.J. Bürger

As far as I know, nobody has looked at this.

P.W. Wells *(UK)*

Dr. Eyre, when you say that some of the antihistaminics may not be beneficial, do you mean that the antihistaminics which block the H-1 receptor will be the ones which are not beneficial?

P. Eyre *(Canada)*

This is a question of the differences between the H-1 and the H-2 receptors. These are not the H-2 receptors that immunologists talk about. Receptors, to a pharmacologist, are chemical structures in and on cells which are capable of responding when attached to a particular drug. They are simply chemical monitors which have a specificity for a drug molecule. There are two kinds of histamine receptor in the body. One is the one which everyone knows about - the bronchoconstrictor, the vasodilator, and so on - that sort of reaction. In the last four or five years a second type of histamine receptor has been discovered. These types of receptors are the so-called H-2 receptors. These are the ones which are operating on the mast cell. But we do have some evidence that in cattle there are H-1 receptors on the mast cells as well, so that there are two quite different types of histamine receptors. I deliberately did not discuss these, because in general you might not be familiar with all the background to the work which has been done on histamine in the last few years. But the antihistamines which a veterinary clinician would be using in the field may or may not inhibit

these particular mechanisms. We do not actually know. We have
obtained some evidence recently that H-1 receptors, which are
used clinically, may have an effect on the further release of
histamine and other chemical mediators as well. Dr. Wells is
asking whether this mechanism is ordinarily blocked by the
antihistamines which the veterinarian might use in practice.
The answer is that I am not completely sure at this stage, because we have not completed the work. There is good evidence
that some of them do alter the release of histamine from mast
cells, and it should be looked at rather carefully. With this
kind of knowledge, antihistamines should be re-evaluated.

J. Asso
    Do you have the same chain of events in the Arthus phenomenon?

P. Eyre
    I do not think that the Arthus phenomenon, which is essen-
tially an allergic vasculitis, is necessarily biochemically
identical to what I have been talking about. I have concentrated
on the immediate type, according to Gell and Coombs classification, type 1 allergy, as opposed to the so-called type 3, or
Arthus phenomenon. But the Arthus reaction certainly has elements
in it which are essentially similar to the ones I have been
describing - the release particularly of prostaglandins and
kinins by immune complexes. Complement did not come into this
at all. Complement is important, and is known to be a direct
cause of leaky blood vessels, and may even cause broncho-con-
striction. It releases histamine, and has been shown to do so.
I had rather included complement as part of my trauma, which is
an over-simplification, I admit.

K. Petzoldt *(West Germany)*
    May I ask you about another type of receptor on the muscle
surface. Do you have any information about the IgE receptor
and its inter-relationship with H-2 or H-1 receptors?

P. Eyre
    I am sure you are all familiar with the work which has been

done - most of it in Germany, and some in my laboratory some
years ago - on bovine reaginic antibodies. There certainly are
receptors on bovine mast cells, and on bovine basophils which
attract reagins. Subsequent exposure to the allergen to which
the animal was originally sensitised will produce the reactions
which we have been talking about. I do not think there is a
direct interconnection between the IgE receptor and the H-2
receptor. The receptor which is associated with IgE or with
the reagen is a specific receptor for immunoglobulin. That gives
rise to a series of biochemical events which release histamine
and cause prostaglandin biosynthesis and so on. The histamine
receptor is a quite separate entity, physically and chemically.
I do not wish to imply that this histamine is acting on immunological receptor mechanisms - it is not. Histamine is actually
working through membrane bound adenylate cyclase. By stimulating
adenylate cyclase, which is a ubiquitous enzyme in most cell
membranes, it increases the intracellular levels of cyclic AMP,
and it is the cyclic AMP which then shuts off the biochemical
reaction which is giving rise to the release of histamine and
prostaglandin. That is how it operates. I know that the IgE
also influences cyclic nucleotide levels in cells, but by
different mechanisms, and so do prostaglandins. There is an
indirect, not a direct connection.

H.M. Pirie

As a pathologist I have been getting rather excited about
what you have been saying. I agree with most of it - I think
we have to think about inflammation in the lung in this manner.
On the other hand, before we dash home and sell our microscopes,
I think we should remember that, if we throw away the cells, we
are left with what has been described as inflammatory soup and
a tangled web of mediators, which can be pretty indigestible.
Inflammation is as much an interplay between cells. You have to
identify the cells.

P. Eyre

I did not say that you should not. In fact I said very
specifically and very carefully that, in order to do this job,

you have to be able to recognise this thing accurately clinically.
You have to be able to recognise it accurately from a pathological point of view, and you have to do the right microbiology to
identify the offending organism. I agree with that. But why
are these cells which you see, as a pathologist, responding in
that way that they do? They are probably responding along concentration gradients of chemotactic factors. This is the kind
of point which I am trying to make. What I am really saying
is that, underlying what you see and what the clinician sees,
there is a whole world of biochemical changes which are essentially ignored. I will stick to that and will not be diverted
from that point of view, but it does not detract from what you
or anyone else is doing. We are merely working on different
levels.

REFERENCE

Weisman, J. 1970. Infection with *D. viviparus* in cattle and the relation to
  fog fever. PhD Thesis, Univ. of Utrecht.

SESSION 2B

ENVIRONMENT

Chairman:

J.M. Asso

Co-ordinator:

D.R. Snodgrass

INFLUENCE OF ENVIRONMENT ON RESPIRATORY DISEASE

A. Wiseman

University of Glasgow Veterinary School, Department of
Veterinary Medicine, Bearsden, Glasgow, Scotland.

ABSTRACT

The development of respiratory disease in cattle is dependent upon
the response of the individual animal to various environmental factors
acting either independently or in concert. Only the effect of environmental factors which are known to be associated with respiratory disease
in cattle will be considered here.

It is not surprising that the environment is closely associated
with the onset of respiratory disease since the respiratory system is
continuously under challenge from the inhalation of potentially pathogenic
material. Infectious agents are transferred from animal to animal via
the aerosol route and infectious respiratory diseases are common and
represent an important source of economic loss particularly in intensive
calf rearing enterprises. Bacteria, mycoplasmas and viruses have all
been implicated in the aetiology of infectious respiratory disease in
cattle at one time or another, but the repeated failure of infection with
micro-organisms alone to produce clinical respiratory disease has led to
the adoption of the hypothesis that environmental factors such as a sudden
drop in temperature or transportation, are necessary to allow these agents
to express their full pathogenicity probably by decreasing the resistance
of the animal to infection.

Respiratory disease can also result from certain dietary regimes;
farmer's lung may develop following the feeding of mouldy hay over a
period of months. A sudden change from bare to lush pasture can precipitate
the onset of fog fever and only grazing animals are likely to develop
parasitic bronchitis.

The interaction of environmental factors (climate, topography, feeding
and management practices) in the development of respiratory disease in cattle
will be presented with specific reference to farmer's lung disease.

INTRODUCTION

The environment has been defined as the aggregate of surrounding things, conditions and influences that can affect an organism. The influence that environmental factors may have on the development of respiratory disease will be presented from three aspects:

1) physical factors which can act directly or indirectly,

2) social factors and

3) economic factors.

Influence of physical factors
(a) Acting directly
As a result of a clinico-pathological field investigation of acute respiratory disease carried out at the Glasgow Veterinary School, it has been established conclusively that fog fever is a disease of adult beef-type cattle that usually occurs within 14 days of a change to lush pasture in the autumn (Selman et al., 1974).

When susceptible calves are allowed to graze permanent pasture during their first summer, then they will inevitably develop parasitic bronchitis as a result of their becoming infected with the lungworm *Dictyocaulus viviparus*. If dairy cows are given access to pastures on which calves with parasitic bronchitis have previously grazed, then they too can develop clinical parasitic bronchitis (Selman et al., 1975). These two conditions exemplify the importance of obtaining an accurate grazing history while investigating outbreaks of respiratory disease in grazing cattle.

In cattle housed for the winter, the feeding of mouldy hay can result in the development of a respiratory disease clinically, epidemiologically, pathologically and serologically identical to farmer's lung in man (Pirie et al., 1971; Wiseman et al., 1973). Farmer's lung in cattle has only been confirmed in certain areas of western Britain and it is particularly prevalent in the Lake District of England, an area renowned for its scenic beauty and regular summer rainfall. Since this condition exemplifies the theme of this seminar, the environmental factors that influence the development of farmer's lung in cattle will be discussed in more detail.

About 80% of the grass that is conserved in Britain is made into hay (Boden, 1970). In the wet western upland areas, it has been estimated that hay will dry properly under natural conditions only one year in every four (Raymond et al., 1972). The rest of the time the hay is likely to be baled and/or stored with a moisture content greater than 30%. It will subsequently heat, become mouldy and develop a thermophilic microflora dominated by actinomycetes, in particular *Micropolyspora faeni* (Festenstein et al., 1965). The inhalation of mouldy hay dust over a prolonged period can result in the development of hypersensitivity to *M. faeni* and clinical farmer's lung (Pepys, 1969).

The feeding of mouldy hay to cattle is undoubtedly associated with the development of clinical farmer's lung because more cases were admitted following the very poor hay-making summer of 1974 than during any other winter. As part of the acute respiratory disease survey mentioned above, the prevalence of precipitins to *M. faeni* was ascertained in 19 herds and, at the end of the winter housing period, a significantly higher prevalence of precipitins was found in herds in which clinical farmer's lung had been confirmed than in the others (Table 1). The frequency of coughing in the herds was also closely associated with the prevalence of precipitins to *M. faeni* (Table 2). When the herds were grouped according to the farmer's assessment of the mouldiness of the hay, there was a very highly significant difference between the prevalence of precipitins in the group given moderately mouldy hay compared with that fed slightly mouldy hay (Table 3). Therefore, the overall prevalence of precipitins to *M. faeni* in a herd of cattle

TABLE 1

THE RELATIONSHIP BETWEEN THE PREVALENCE OF PRECIPITATING ANTIBODIES TO
Micropolyspora faeni IN 19 HERDS OF ADULT CATTLE AT THE END OF THE WINTER
HOUSING PERIOD AND THE PRESENCE OF CONFIRMED FARMER'S LUNG.

Farmer's lung confirmed				Farmer's lung not confirmed				
No. herds	No. sampled	No. positive	%	No. herds	No. sampled	No. positive	%	Significant difference
10	536	291	54	9	442	143	32	+, P<0.001

TABLE 2

THE ASSOCIATION BETWEEN THE PREVALENCE OF PRECIPITATING ANTIBODIES TO
Micropolyspora faeni IN 19 HERDS OF ADULT CATTLE AT THE END OF THE WINTER
HOUSING PERIOD AND THEIR FREQUENCY OF COUGHING.

Frequency of coughing	No. herds	No. cattle sampled	No. cattle positive	%	Significant difference
+	4	282	55	20	+, P<0.001
++	10	430	196	46	
+++	5	266	183	69	+, P<0.01

TABLE 3

THE ASSOCIATION BETWEEN THE PREVALENCE OF PRECIPITATING ANTIBODIES TO
Micropolyspora faeni IN 19 HERDS OF ADULT CATTLE AT THE END OF THE WINTER
HOUSING PERIOD AND THE MOULDINESS OF THE HAY THEY WERE FED.

Slightly mouldy hay				Moderately mouldy hay				
No. herds	No. sampled	No. positive	%	No. herds	No. sampled	No. positive	%	Significant difference
6	383	129	34	13	595	305	51	+, P<0.001

at the end of the winter housing period is a reliable indication of the severity of their recent exposure to mouldy hay but is only a guide to the probability of there being clinical farmer's lung disease in the herd.

During the winter there was a significant rise ($P < 0.05$) in the prevalence of precipitins and a significant fall ($P < 0.001$) during the summer grazing period. This latter change in the precipitin status was particularly marked in the cattle less than six years old (Dawson et al., 1977). This together with the presence of a good correlation between age and prevalence of precipitins ($r = 0.9835$) indicates that the effect of repeated exposure to mouldy hay dust is cumulative.

In the same area, dairy cattle are housed for a longer period during the winter than are beef cattle and a higher proportion are tied in byres. A combination of these two factors is the obvious explanation for there being a higher incidence of farmer's lung in dairy than in beef cattle. However, in the county of Westmorland, the disease is particularly common in beef cows since many are still housed in small, traditional, very poorly ventilated field-houses.

Although a statistically significant correlation was not found between the total monthly rainfall during June or July or August and the making of mouldy hay, there was a fairly close association between the number of raindays in July and the making of slightly or moderately mouldy hay. This lack of a good correlation is not surprising since rainfall during the summer varied greatly from area to area although during a very wet summer a large proportion of the hay will undoubtedly be mouldy. However, it is not possible to assess critically the decision making ability of the individual farmer and this is of crucial importance to the making of good hay. Farmer's lung in cattle provides a very good example of how environmental factors acting in concert can affect the development of a respiratory disease.

Respiratory signs are also seen in milk allergy which is
the result of a type 1 hypersensitivity reaction to alpha-
casein (Campbell, 1971). Clinical signs develop after milk
has been allowed to accumulate in the udder and Channel Islands
breeds seem to be particularly susceptible.

(b) Acting indirectly

These are often classed as 'stress factors' and are said
to act by decreasing the animal's ability to resist infection.
The combined action of environmental stressors and infectious
agents has given rise to the idea that infectious respiratory
disease, particularly in calves, has a multiple factor
aetiology. This concept has achieved credibility largely as a
result of work involving shipping fever in North America
(Sinha and Abinanti, 1962) or transit fever as it is called in
this country (Hepburn, 1925). In this condition, chilling and
transportation together with weaning and mixing all contribute
significantly to the severity of the disease that develops
following viral and bacterial infections.

A sudden drop in environmental temperature is often
followed by episodes of acute respiratory disease within 24 to
72 h. While this is most obvious in calves being reared in
modern intensive units, sudden onset cold and wet conditions
have been shown to precipitate infectious respiratory disease
in single suckled calves that had never been housed (Wiseman
et al., 1976). It has been suggested that cold causes latent
respiratory infections to flare-up and that the animals
huddling together to counteract the cold facilitates the spread
of infectious agents. Castration and dehorning which have also
been associated with the development of respiratory disease
incidents in calves, may also act in this way whereas the acute
respiratory distress which follows vaccination with brucella,
lungworm or mixed commercial bacterial vaccines is probably
the result of a pulmonary anaphylactoid reaction.

There is some evidence that the absorption of large
amounts of colostral immunoglobulin is associated with a delayed

onset of tachypnoea in the early stages of cuffing pneumonia
and also with a lower incidence of severe respiratory disease
(Thomas and Swann, 1973). Protection against respiratory
pathogens could be afforded by specific and/or non-specific
factors in the colostrum or perhaps calves which had not
experienced the ravages of severe colibacillosis might be
better able to withstand the challenge from inhaled respiratory
pathogens.

Influence of social factors

As referred to above, the weaning and the crowding
together of large numbers of single suckled calves accustomed
to an extensive outdoor life, plays an important part in predisposing these calves to shipping fever. In modern calf-
rearing enterprises, large numbers of two to four week old
animals are purchased and then reared together under one roof.
The host of infectious agents which these calves have brought
in can easily spread by the aerosol route because of their
close proximity. It is this bringing together of large numbers
of similarly aged calves from different farms and then allowing
them to share the same air space that is at the heart of the
pneumonia problem on intensively calf-rearing farms.

On these units, crowding is still judged by the floor
space or cubic space allocated per calf. Yet, Breeze et al.
(1945) found that in naval barracks crowding, as judged by
the number of men per room, was more important in determining
the incidence of respiratory disease than the floor space or
cubic space per person. Therefore, control of calf pneumonia
is more likely to be achieved by decreasing the numbers that
are housed together while at the same time increasing the
ventilation rate to reduce the number of infectious agents per
unit volume of inhaled air.

Influence of economic factors

The general economic climate affects the incidence of
respiratory disease by, for example, determining the number of
calves that are reared. An adverse economic climate will also

lead to a cessation in the use of preventative measures such
as vaccination and routine treatment with anthelmintics.

The incidence of farmer's lung disease will be influenced
by the availability and price of fodder; when this is high
very mouldy hay has to be fed to milking cows rather than
being given to young stock or to 'dry' cows out of doors.

The market price of cows culled from a beef or dairy
herd will have an important bearing on the length of their
productive life. When the price is low, cows will be kept
longer and more cases of conditions such as chronic farmer's
lung will be recognised. This may lead to false conclusions
being drawn when comparisons are made in the disease incidence
in different years.

CONCLUSIONS

Experimental studies of respiratory disease in cattle have
concentrated mainly on the microbiological aspects of the
problem to the almost complete exclusion of the effects of
environmental factors. As a result, the state of knowledge
regarding the influence of environment on the incidence of
respiratory disease, particularly of an infectious origin, is
similar to the position in man. This was aptly summarised by
Andrews (1964) when he stated that "we do not yet understand
how seasonal and other factors affect the incidence of colds
and influenza".

In the future, experiments must be designed to examine
the interaction between combinations of infectious agents and
environmental factors. If not, then an understanding of the
pathogenesis of syndromes such as the pneumonias of housed
calves will be virtually unattainable.

REFERENCES

Andrews, C.H. 1964. Science, 146, p. 1274.

Boden, S.M. 1970. Dairy Farmer, Ipswich, April, p. 47.

Breese, B.B., Stanbury, J., Upham, H., Calhoun, A.J., Van Buren, R.L. and
     Kennedy, A.S. 1945. War Med. 7, p. 143.

Campbell, S.J. 1971. J. Allergy clin. Immunol. 48, p. 230.

Dawson, C.O., Wiseman, A., Pirie, H.M. and Breeze, R.G. 1977. J. comp. Path.
     87, p. 287.

Festenstein, G.N., Lacey, J., Skinner, F.A., Jenkins, P.A. and Pepys, J.
     1965. J. gen. Microbiol. 41 p. 389.

Hepburn, W. 1925. Vet. Rec. 37, p. 201.

Pepys, J. 1969. In hypersensitivity diseases of the lungs due to fungi and
     organic dusts. S. Karger, Basel.

Pirie, H.M., Dawson, C.O., Breeze, R.G., Wiseman, A. and Hamilton, J. 1971.
     Vet. Rec. 88, p. 346.

Raymond, F., Shepperson, G. and Waltham, R. 1972. Farming Press, Ipswich.

Selman, I.E., Wiseman, A., Pirie, H.M. and Breeze, R.G. 1974. Vet. Rec.
     95, p. 139.

Selman, I.E., Wiseman, A., Pirie, H.M. and Breeze, R.G. 1975. Vet. Annual,
     15, p. 16.

Sinha, S.K. and Abinanti, F.R. 1962. Adv. Vet. Sci. 7, p. 225.

Thomas, L.H. and Swann, R.G. 1973. Vet. Rec. 92, p. 459.

Wiseman, A., Selman, I.E., Dawson, C.O., Breeze, R.G. and Pirie, H.M. 1973.
     Vet. Rec. 93, p. 410.

Wiseman, A., Selman, I.E., Pirie, H.M. and Harvey, I.M. 1976. Vet. Rec.
     98, p. 192.

INFLUENCE OF ENVIRONMENT ON RESPIRATORY DISEASE

D.G. McKercher

School of Veterinary Medicine, University of California, Davis,
California, USA.

ABSTRACT

In the USA the influence of environment on respiratory tract
infections is most dramatic in the case of feeder cattle. Such animals
are invariably at the mercy of the elements, usually under natural or
artificially created conditions which predispose to, and promote the
spread of, respiratory infections. The major health problem in these
animals is a disease complex known as 'shipping fever'. Despite long-
term efforts to bring this condition under control, it continues to
extract a high economic toll from the feeder cattle industry. The environment can also influence disease in a more subtle manner. By redirecting
the invasion route normally taken by a virus, particularly by members of
the herpesvirus group in attacking the host, the pathogenic potential of
the virus is increased, with the emergence of additional clinical
expressions of disease.

In the constant struggle between the environment and living things, life can survive only by adapting to the changing conditions. Those forms which do so successfully survive, whereas those which fail in the process, perish. The fossilised remains of the myriad forms of life which existed on the earth in past ages bear mute witness to the fate of those, both large and small, which could not cope with their hostile surroundings. Contemporary animal life represents species which evolved from primitive ancestors that survived by virtue of natural selection, superior mental capabilities, and possibly fortuitous external circumstances.

Present day animal populations still must cope, to some extent, with natural environmental situations inimical to their survival. This applies particularly to wildlife, which must contend not only with natural disasters such as drought, flood, fire, and disease which directly affect food supply, shelter, living space, and health, but to an even greater extent with their natural enemies, not the least of which is man himself. This is all too apparent in today's lengthening lists of endangered species. In contrast, man has sheltered his domestic animals from the stresses of the natural environment, mainly to increase the volume and quality of the products provided by them. In so doing, however, he has created artificial environments which, although improving the well-being of the animals, create new problems, especially with respect to disease, which are incompatible with his economic objectives.

ENVIRONMENTAL INFLUENCE ON DISEASE

Indirect

Almost 100 years ago Pasteur demonstrated that the natural resistance of birds to the anthrax organism could be overcome by partially immersing inoculated subjects in cold water. Thus, the first demonstration that stress is an important predisposing factor to disease was provided. Many years later, due largely to the pioneering studies of Selye, the role of stress in disease was well established and, to a certain extent, elucidated.

Although the most marked and spectacular environmental effects are exerted through the medium of stress, management practices may also create environmental conditions which indirectly influence the trends of infectious diseases. Such trends may result in broadening the pathogenic scope of disease agents, culminating in the emergence of new clinical syndromes which may be of greater severity and economic importance than those with which the agents were associated initially. Thus far this phenomenon is known to occur only among the herpesviruses.

In Africa, *Bovine herpesvirus-2*, the so-called 'Allerton' virus (Alexander et al., 1957), causes a condition resembling mild lumpy skin disease. The latter is characterised by the development of small, firm nodules in the skin over much of the body. The virus is believed to be vector transmitted in its African habitat; however, in the United Kingdom this virus causes bovine mammillitis, presumably by invading through test abrasions to which the cattle are predisposed as a result of the cold, damp fall weather while they are still on pasture (Martin et al., 1969). When the virus is inoculated intra-venously, thus simulating vector exposure, the characteristic nodules appear in the skin. It is reasonable to believe that in an environment supporting the appropriate vector, the lumpy skin form of the infection, rather than mammillitis, would occur.

An even more striking example is provided by *Bovine herpesvirus-1*, commonly known as the infectious bovine rhinotracheitis (IBR) virus. The condition which this virus caused initially was a genital infection described in the German veterinary literature, which dates back more than 150 years. Because of its venereal nature, the disease became known as coital vesicular exanthema, and colloquially as 'Blaschenausschlag'. One may wonder whether originally the virus was incapable of producing respiratory infection, or whether it was through lack of opportunity that it failed to do so.

In view of the husbandry practices in those days in central Europe, the latter possibility appears to be the more likely. The herds usually consisted of 1 or 2 cows, just sufficient to fulfill the needs of a family. To obtain maximum utilisation of the limited pasture on the small, plot-like farms, the cattle were tethered while grazing. Thus, they were effectively isolated from each other, and the likelihood of airborne infection occurring was minimal. As the community bull was the sole contact common to all the cows, the genital infection was promoted and perpetuated. When nasal exposure to the virus occurred, as it undoubtedly did from time to time, the immunity resulting from the genital infection would protect against infection of the respiratory tract. Assuming, however, that respiratory infections did occur, the virus, after infecting a particular cow, would reach an impasse through lack of additional animals to infect. It therefore had no opportunity to become established as a respiratory tract pathogen. Thus, the venereal infection was perpetuated because of circumstances favourable to genital infection but unfavourable for infection of the upper respiratory tract.

Since cattle were imported from Europe by the USA through the late 1920's, it is not surprising that the virus was introduced into this country. Neither is it surprising that it initially caused a genital infection, since essentially the same husbandry prevailed in this country, namely closed herds in which natural service was used, as in central Europe. Once in the country, it was inevitable that the virus would be carried to the feedlots of the mid and western states. This is believed, in retrospect, to have occurred during the late 1940's. This occurrence would appear to be of little consequence, as feeder cattle are reproductively inactive. Although essentially impervious to attack via the genital route, such animals were highly susceptible to respiratory tract invasion. Moreover, enormous numbers were available under conditions which promoted rapid and widespread viral exposure, features which, in turn, favour the selection both of viral mutants and genetically

susceptible individuals. Eventually a new clinical entity,
frequently accompanied by conjunctivitis and characterised by
several sequelae, emerged. This syndrome became known as IBR.

Direct

Cattle today are subjected to harsh environmental
conditions created as a consequence of certain production
practices. This situation applies to feedlot operations to a
greater extent than to any other type of animal-production
enterprise. It is estimated by some that up to one-half
million cattle die annually, mainly from respiratory infection,
and especially shipping fever, during and after movement from
the production sites through the feedlots. In view of the
nature of feedlot operations, such high losses are understand-
able.

Practically all beef breed calves in the USA are produced
in so-called 'cow-calf' operations. The calves are generally
born on the range, and remain with their mothers for the first
6 to 8 months of life. They are then weaned and placed on
pasture for 5 to 7 months. After grazing, many are shipped
directly to the large feedlots for finishing. However, probably
the majority reaches this destination after variable periods
in saleyards, holding yards, and backgrounding operations. Many
of these establishments are veritable hotbeds of infection.

Much of the stress to which beef-type animals are exposed
stems from the distant hauling in open trucks and railroad cars,
often under adverse weather conditions. In most instances,
cattle reach the feedlots deyhdrated, fatigued, and in a highly
excitable state. Cattle coming from saleyards and similar
operations are often sick on arrival, or in the preclinical
stages of infection. Those arriving directly from pasture may
require several days or more to become familiar with the automatic
watering and feeding devices, and to the unfamiliar rations.
Within 7 to 10 days the new arrivals are routinely vaccinated,
castrated and dehorned as necessary, branded, dewormed, and
treated for grubs, injected with vitamins, and implanted with

antibodies. These manipulations, often carried out with unnecessary brutality, place further stress on animals already
severely traumatised, both physically and emotionally. While
in the feedlot, climatic factors in the form of heat and dust,
rapid extremes of temperature, and wind, mud, rain, and snow
take their toll. This is largely in terms of respiratory
infection, which frequently terminates fatally in pneumonia.

Dairy cattle are ordinarily subjected to much less severe
stress than are beef breeds because of the relatively favourable
conditions under which they are maintained and handled. However,
under conditions comparable to those endured by beef animals,
respiratory diseases are a common occurrence. This was
demonstrated quite clearly by the fact that the original
outbreaks of IBR in California occurred, not in feedlot cattle
but, rather, in the large dairy herds in the Los Angeles area
(McKercher et al., 1954). In contrast to the usual dairy-type
operations, these herds were maintained in relatively small
corrals, replacements were obtained from distant sources, and
high-energy rations were fed - a situation quite analogous to
that of feedlot operations.

A similar situation arose also when dairy cattle,
collected from various parts of the USA for export, were held
in closely confined quarters in the dock area while the full
quota of the shipment was being assembled. IBR broke out while
the animals were on shipboard en route to Peru, resulting in
considerable mortality and some abortions (McKercher, 1965). It
appears, therefore, that irrespective of the breed of cattle or
the type of operation involved, the associated stress is the
dominant factor in predisposing the animals to infection,
particularly that of the respiratory tract.

PREVENTIVE MEASURES

In an attempt to minimise losses due to shipping fever,
IBR, and other feedlot diseases, the approach eventually evolved
was that of 'preconditioning'. The primary objective of pre-

conditioning is to prepare cattle, while still in the relatively
stress-free atmosphere of the ranches of origin, in such a way
as to counter the effects of stress to which they are exposed
as they move subsequently through the various channels from
the production sites through the feedlots. The main emphasis
is on disease prevention. The programme involves weaning and
vaccination of the calves at least 30 days before sale; dehorning and castrating sufficiently in advance of sale to
ensure healing; and familiarisation of the animals with feedlot-
type rations and feeding methods. Compliance with the Federal
regulations governing the handling of cattle during interstate
shipment by rail or truck is also a requirement (Horlein, 1973).

The programme was adopted about 10 years ago, and was
reasonably well accepted at first. However, failure of processors
to offer premium prices for preconditioned cattle, and scepticism
on the part of some cattle producers and veterinarians as to
whether the programme provided any real benefits, undermined it
to some extent. As a result, probably not more than 10% of
the cattle entering commercial channels today have been preconditioned. (Crenshaw, 1977).

DISCUSSION

It appears that the environment plays both a passive and
an active role with respect to disease. The ability of a certain
environment to maintain a particular arthropod vector, or to
promote a certain type of husbandry practice, may deprive a
disease agent of the route by which it ordinarily invades the
host, forcing it to adopt an alternative route. The result may
be the emergence of a new clinical syndrome, and increased
pathogenic scope on the part of the agent. The consequences
are higher incidence and enhanced severity of disease,
particularly of the respiratory tract.

Despite the fact that stress arising from environmental
conditions, either natural or artificial, plays an extremely
important role in disease, the mechanism by which it exerts its

effects on the body is incompletely understood. It is known,
however, that the homeostasis of the body is disturbed in the
stressed individual, with the resultant release of glucocorticoids from the adrenal cortex. These activate metabolic
regulatory mechanisms which function to restore and maintain
the homeostatic state. On the negative side, the glucocorticoids interfere with the activities of the bursal and thymic
cells, and thus inhibit immune responses. They also activate
latent infection. It is further believed that in response to
chilling, the thermoregulation of the body fails, reducing the
integrity of the nasal mucosa. Mucin secretion and ciliary
activity then become depressed, thus providing an opportunity
for the establishment of infection by way of the respiratory
tract (Phillip, 1972).

Theoretically, preconditioning is a valid approach to the
control of respiratory diseases of cattle, as it endeavours to
counter, by direct and indirect means, the effects of stress,
and by protecting the animals, through vaccination, against the
diseases feeder cattle are most likely to encounter in the
commercial channels. However, while not unsuccessful, the
programme has not lived up to expectations. This is probably
because too much was expected of it, and also because of lack
of cooperation among the various interested groups involved.
Nonetheless, the experience clearly demonstrated that feedlot
diseases, of which the majority is respiratory in nature,
constitute a more complex problem than was originally realised.
We obviously lack full knowledge of the spectrum of etiologic
entities involved, and the nature of their interrelationships
in disease causation; we fail to understand the interplay of
nutrition and stress as predisposing factors in disease; and we
are ignorant of the possible part played by genetic makeup in
disease resistance. It is apparent, therefore, that much
greater cooperative effort among diverse areas of specialisation
is required if an attack on the problem is to be launched on a
sufficiently broad scientific basis. However, no one can foresee when, or if, such an approach will ever be realised. At

the moment, the logical alternative is to utilise the more
successful aspects of the preconditioning programme while
attempts are being made to evolve more efficacious means of
controlling these costly diseases.

In this quest, encouragement might be found in reports
from the field of human medicine regarding antiviral compounds.
Recently The New York Academy of Sciences devoted an entire
conference to this topic. At the time of the first conference,
12 years ago, the attitude of virologists was that 'antiviral
drugs are unlikely and vaccines were the only realistic
solution to viral disease'. Contrast this statement with the
one emanating from the most recent conference of the Academy on
the same topic, 'So many have accepted the antiviral drug
concept that conferences spring up everywhere, and competition
is vigorous' (Herrmann, 1977). Thus, there are realistic hopes
that in the foreseeable future antiviral compounds will come
into their own, revolutionising the handling of viral diseases
as antibiotics did those caused by bacteria.

Another approach to control, not only of viral disease but
of diseases in general, is the development of disease-resistant
strains of cattle by means of genetic engineering. Such studies
in the animal field should produce results relatively rapidly,
as gene pools from populations possessing desirable genetic
material can be readily built up, and the techniques of ovum
and embryo transplantation are becoming increasingly sophisticated.

Such developments, however, require time, and herein lies
the critical issue, vastly more urgent problems might render
relatively insignificant those problems of a more limited nature.
Two major situations currently exist which carry with them the
potential for worldwide catastrophe. As the world's population
explodes at an ever-increasing rate, the demands for food, but
not the supply, keep pace. This crisis, coming at a time when
not only are the reserves of unreplenishable resources indispensable
to life being depleted at an alarming rate, but when we might

well be on the brink of major climatic changes, is giving
rise to widespread anxiety. There are unmistakable indications
that, on a worldwide basis, the weather is changing. Widespread drought in North America, Africa, and Europe over the
past several years is causing deep concern on the part of
climatologists. Some are of the opinion that these changes
portend an era of weather patterns which could deprive
agricultural regions of once reliable rainfall. Such a major
climatic shift could persist for years, or more hopefully,
could be a short-term phenomenon although occurring more
frequently than in past decades. In either case, agricultural
productivity would drop drastically.

The probability of having to produce double the amount of
food now produced annually in order to feed the anticipated
world population of eight billion people by the end of this
century or early in the next, is a formidable prospect. Moreover, with most of the arable land of the world already under
cultivation, and with a diminished and uncertain supply of fresh
water on a worldwide scale, it becomes a challenge of awesome
proportions. Under these circumstances such an inefficient
feed converter as the cow could well be an early casualty. For
a time, the lush grasslands of the tropics might stave off the
inevitable, but this possibility is also fraught with problems.
Indigenous tropical forage lacks the nutrients required for
normal growth of livestock, (Wayman et al., 1973) and the
excessive heat and humidity of the tropics depress reproduction
(Jöchle, 1972). Moreover, the disease load for European breeds
of cattle in such areas would be prohibitive.

The prospects of being able to cope successfully with the
problems created by over-population and diminished food supply
are not encouraging. Shortages will increase, certain basic
items will disappear completely, and life will assume a simplicity
and primitiveness unknown for generations. In parts of the
world at least, present-day food-producing animals such as the
cow, the pig, and the sheep may well be replaced, as one economist
predicted, by more prolific breeders, better feed converters,

and more versatile producers such as the goat, the rabbit, and
the chicken.

REFERENCES

Alexander, R.A., Plowright, W. and Haig, D.A. 1957. Bull. epizoot. Dis. Afr.
   5, p. 489.

Crenshaw, G.L. 1977. Personal communication.

Horlein, A.B. 1973. J. Am. Vet. Med. Ass. 163, p. 825.

Herrmann, E.C. 1977. Ann. N.Y. Acad. Sci. 284, p. 1.

Jöchle, W. 1972. Int. J. Biomet. 16, p. 131.

Martin, W.B., James, Z.H., Lauder, I.M., Murray, M., and Pirie, H.M. 1969.
   Am. J. Vet. Res. 30, p. 2151.

McKercher, D.G. 1965. Unreported data.

McKercher, D.G., Moulton, J.E., Madin, S.H. and Kendrick, J.W. 1957. Am.
   J. Vet. Res. 18, p. 246.

Phillip, J.I.H. 1972. Vet. Rec. 90, p. 552.

Wayman, O., Campbell, C.M., Reimer, D., Donoho, H.R. and Nakamura, R. 1973.
   Int. J. Biomet. 17, p. 135.

SOME FACTORS INFLUENCING RESPIRATORY DISEASE IN GROWING BULLS AND THE EFFECT OF TREATMENT ON LIVEWEIGHT

A.H. Andrews

Veterinary Department, Meat and Livestock Commission, Queensway House, Bletchley, Milton Keynes, England.

ABSTRACT

The records are presented of 1 240 animals which underwent central bull performance testing at two test centres (A and B) between January 1972 and December 1976. This showed that the introduction of a management system under which bulls were kept in small groups for the first month after entry resulted in less respiratory conditions than when animals were held in larger groups. At both centres the disease was greatest in October to December; with successive decreases in July to September, January to March, and the lowest level in April to June. About 50% of the cases occurred within four weeks of entry to both centres with over 25% within two weeks of entry. Cattle weaned 15 days or longer before entry at either centre were probably (p = < 0.05) less likely to have respiratory disease during the first month of test than those weaned 14 days or less. Three batches of data were examined to investigate the effect of treatment on final weight. In each batch, weight differences between performance test groups proved to be significant. However, although the mean weight of treated bulls was less than that of untreated ones, the differences were not significant. It is suggested that the overall final test weights of treated and untreated bulls do not reflect the disease situation in individual animals. Further work is therefore necessary to quantify the severity of the disease and its effect on performance.

INTRODUCTION

About one quarter of the beef produced in Great Britain
comes from the progeny of beef suckler cows. These are the
source of about 1 200 000 suckler calves raised annually for
beef. Many of these calves, born in the autumn and spring, are
kept on the farm of birth until transferred to other farmers
for fattening through the traditional autumn calf sales. This
movement however predisposes to respiratory upsets commonly
termed 'shipping' or 'transit fever' when the animals reach
the second farm. The dairy herd calves, which account for 41%
of home produced beef as well as dairy breed replacements, are
also susceptible to respiratory diseases - commonly termed
enzootic pneumonia. This calfhood type of respiratory disease
is more common than transit fever but the latter condition is,
nevertheless, a major disease problem for the beef producer.

Under the Meat and Livestock Commission's Central Bull
Performance Testing programme between 450 and 500 young weaned
bulls enter the five testing centres at intervals throughout
the year from many different farms. It is therefore not
surprising that respiratory conditions similar to those on
farms which buy suckler calves are encountered in these testing
centres, where considerable attention is paid to their
prevention and control to avoid interruptions of the testing
programme.

A previous report (Andrews 1976) discussed factors
associated with respiratory disease at these testing centres
and the results of investigations which confirm some of these
findings are presented. Preliminary studies of the influence
of respiratory disease on liveweight are also reported.

MATERIALS AND METHODS

Some 1 240 bulls passed through the two bull performance
testing centres (A and B) between January 1972 and December
1976. During this period three management systems as summarised

in Table 1 were used at these two centres. System 1 was used
between January 1972 and April 1973 at both centres. Under
System 2, introduced at both centres in June 1973, the through-
put of bulls was increased by reducing the age at entry and
the test period was lengthened so that the animals left the
centre at the same age as under System 1. Centre A continued
on System 2 until December 1976 as no alternative system was
feasible there. In accordance with the normal practice at MLC
performance testing centres the bulls were subjected to weekly
weighings, a health control routine was maintained, and treatments for disease were carefully recorded. System 3 was
introduced in January 1974 at Centre B only and was still in
operation in December 1976.

TABLE 1

MANAGEMENT SYSTEMS AT CENTRES A AND B DURING 1972 - 1976

	Period:	
System 1 (Centres A & B)	Jan 72 to Apr 73	Groups of bulls introduced every 2 - 4 months at 7 months of age, housed singly throughout the test until departure at 13 months of age
System 2 (Centres A & B) (Centre A only)	Jun 73 to Dec 73 Jan 74 to Dec 76	Groups of bulls introduced monthly at 6 months of age, group housed for 3 months and then singly for the final 4 months of test
System 3 (Centre B only)	Jan 74 to Dec 76	Groups of bulls introduced monthly at 6 months of age, housed in twos and threes for the first month and then group housed for 3 months. During the final 3 months of test the bulls were housed singly.

Bulls were considered to have respiratory disease if
they exhibited dyspnoea or hyperpnoea, inappetance and pyrexia.
In many cases there was a mucoid or muco-purulent nasal
discharge, and intermittent coughing was also often present.

The sick animals were generally first noted by the stockman, but diagnosis was confirmed by the centre veterinary surgeon who was responsible for instituting a course of treatment, each of which was considered as a single case or outbreak of disease. When an individual bull had more than one course of treatment at an interval of 7 days or longer, the second course was classed as a new case of disease. Routine sampling for isolation of micro-organisms or for serology was not carried out. Owners of bulls entering performance test were requested to supply information about the previous management and health of the bull and these data were examined further in those test groups in which respiratory disease occurred.

At both centres individual weekly weight records were examined for the groups of bulls performance tested between January 1972 and December 1974. The volume of data and the limitations of the computer programme required the information from Centre B to be divided into two batches and from Centre A only the data for the period when most respiratory disease occurred, was used.

RESULTS

The number of treatments for respiratory disease between January 1972 and December 1976 are shown in Table 2. The introduction of System 2 produced an over four-fold rise in respiratory outbreaks at both centres in the period June to December 1973 when compared with that under System 1. Utilising System 3 at Centre B halved the number of outbreaks during 1974 while those at Centre A were similar to previously. It is apparent that in the first three years of the study the level of disease was lower at Centre A then Centre B, whereas the position reversed in 1975 and 1976 while System 3 was in operation at the latter.

A. Factors related to the incidence of respiratory disease

A study of the overall records of respiratory disease in

TABLE 2

THE LEVEL OF TREATMENT FOR RESPIRATORY DISEASE AT THE TWO PERFORMANCE
TESTING CENTRES (CENTRES A AND B) FROM JAN 1972 TO DEC 1976.

Period	Centre A			Centre B		
	System	bulls at start of test	% treatments for respiratory disease	System	bulls at start of test	% treatments for respiratory disease
Jan 1972/ Apr 1973	1	176	8.0	1	120	16.7
Jun 1973/ Dec 1973	2	97	44.3	2	70	85.7
Jan 1974/ Dec 1974	2	154	45.5	3	114	46.5
Jan 1975/ Dec 1975	2	139	43.9	3	108	23.2
Jan 1976/ Dec 1976	2	148	37.2	3	114	21.9

relation to certain factors has revealed the following:

1) Management - the previous study (Andrews 1976)
indicated that System 3 whereby bulls were held in groups
of three or less for the first month after entry
considerably reduced respiratory disease levels. The
new system had then only been in operation for a year but
the subsequent two years' results (Table 2) at Centre B
confirm that finding. The general level of treatments
in 1975 and 1976 was about half that in 1974 and approached
that under System 1 when bulls were all individually housed.

2) Interval between centre entry and disease onset - The
number of respiratory disease treatments in each week
following entry between 1972 and 1976 are shown in Figure
1. The data for the first 26 weeks are based on all the
1 240 cattle which entered, whereas the last four weeks
relate only to the monthly intake groups (944 cattle).
Some 48.6% of respiratory treatments at Centre A and 58.5%

at Centre B occurred within the first four weeks of entry
and 35% of all cases at Centre A and 28.4% at Centre B
were within two weeks of entry. The monthly group intake
data showed that the majority of outbreaks (37.1% of
total at Centre A, 34.4% at Centre B) after the first
month of entry occurred during the group housing period.

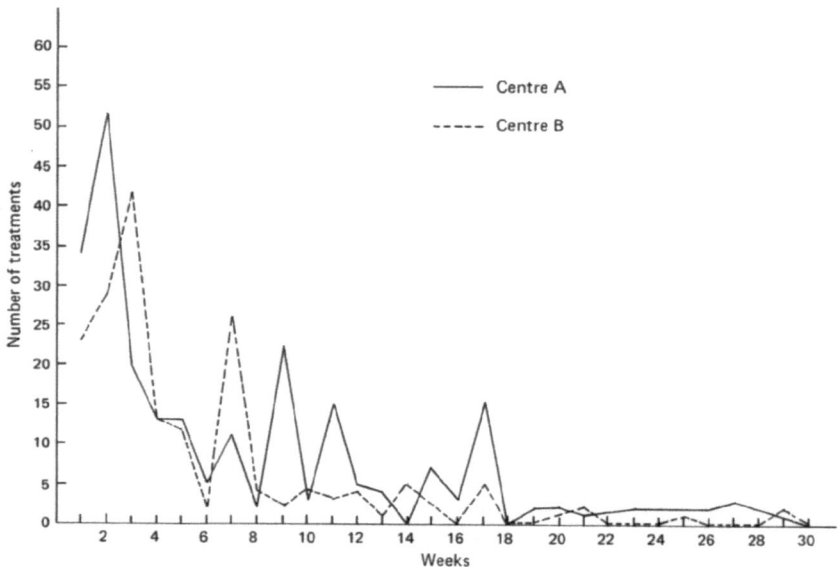

Fig. 1   The numbers of treatments for respiratory disease in each week
following entry to the performance testing centre

3) <u>Season</u> - The number of respiratory disease outbreaks
as a percentage of animals at risk between 1972 - 1976
are shown in Figure 2. At both centres more disease
(8.6% at Centre A, 8.8% at Centre B) occurred in the
second half of the year (July to December) than the
first half (1.4% at Centre A, 1.7% at Centre B). Examination of the quarterly records at both centres showed
the same order of severity with the following rising level
of incidence: April to June (0.4% at Centre A, 1.3% at
Centre B); January to March (2.2% at Centre A, 2.1% at
Centre B); July to September (3.2% at Centre A, 6.8% at

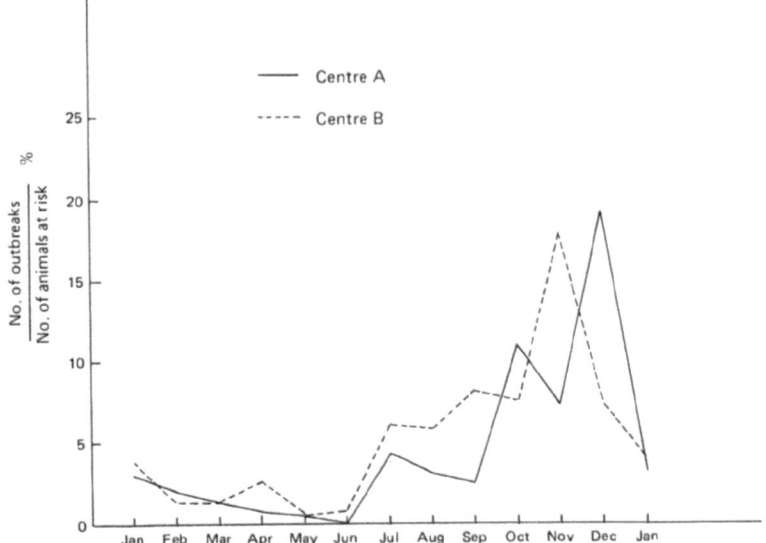

Fig. 2 The number of respiratory disease outbreaks as a percentage of the number of animals at risk for each month of the year

Centre B); October to December (12.8% at Centre A, 10.8% at Centre B). The same sequence was obtained when using only the data from the monthly intake groups for the three year period between January 1974 and December 1976 namely, April to June (0.6% at Centre A, 1.6% at Centre B); January to March (2.6% at Centre A, 2.8% at Centre B); July to September (4.8% at Centre A, 5.1% at Centre B); October to December (14.8% at Centre A, 8.7% at Centre B). Most disease outbreaks occurred in the month of December at Centre A and in November at Centre B. The month with least disease was exactly 6 months previously at both centres, ie June at Centre A and May at Centre B.

4) <u>Pre-test management</u> - Whether the animal suckled its dam or a nurse cow and whether or not it received creep

feed did not seem to influence the level of respiratory disease. However, at both centres, there was a relationship between time of weaning prior to entry and the incidence of respiratory disease during the first month of test (see Figure 3). Utilising x^2 test, these bulls at both centres which were weaned less than 14 days were more likely ($p =< 0.05$) to develop respiratory disease during the first month of performance test than those weaned 15 days or more.

B. Study of the effect of respiratory disease treatment on end of test weight

The possible relationship between respiratory disease treatment and weight of bulls at end of test was investigated in three batches of data - one from Centre A and two from Centre B as explained earlier. The programme was designed to investigate the effect of treatment on the end of test weight while also taking into account the test group of the animal and its weight at the start of test. The results did not show any consistent interactions between treatment and end of test weight. In some cases there was no effect, whereas in others it appeared to increase weight gain and again in others a weight decrease occurred. The three sets of least squares means data are presented in Table 3, and are taken from models which assumed that the effects were additive with no interactions. Utilising a more complicated model, in which interactions were included, indicated that for the second batch of Centre B data the effect of treatment varied between different test groups. Weight differences between performance test groups proved to be significant for each batch of data. In the three batches the mean end of test weight of treated was less than that for untreated bulls but the difference only approached significance at Centre A with a level of about 7% probability.

DISCUSSION

This further study confirms the previous observations that where groups of young bulls enter a centre each month and have

TABLE 3

THE MEAN WEIGHT IN KG OF CATTLE (TRANSFERRED TO LEAST SQUARE MEANS) FOR
EACH PERFORMANCE TEST GROUP AND UNTREATED AND TREATED ANIMALS

	Centre A		Centre B (i)		Centre B (ii)	
	No. of animals	Mean weight kg	No. of animals	Mean weight kg	No. of animals	Mean weight kg
Test groups	20	461	19	522	7	516
	17	475	19	507	8	529
	19	478	15	512	10	526
	7	482	19	527	6	496
	9	486	19	525	10	494
	12	512	9	559	9	480
	20	488	10	556	10	491
	9	479	6	525	10	489
	17	488	9	537	9	482
	18	466	10	553	9	515
	9	494				
	17	493				
Untreated	119	488	91	536	58	505
Treated	55	479	44	535	30	499
Overall Mean	174	483	135	536	88	502

eventually to be housed in large groups, the incidence of
respiratory disease is reduced if the animals are kept in small
groups of two or three for the first month of test. The
reduction in disease level at Centre B from 46.5% in 1974 to
23.2% in 1975 and 21.9% in 1976 could also be attributed to
the centre manager being convinced of the value of System 3
and therefore implementing the necessary management restrictions
more rigorously.

At Centre A more disease control problems have arisen
because of the variable size of intake groups (either 10 or 20)
and the different building design which allowed too much
common air space.

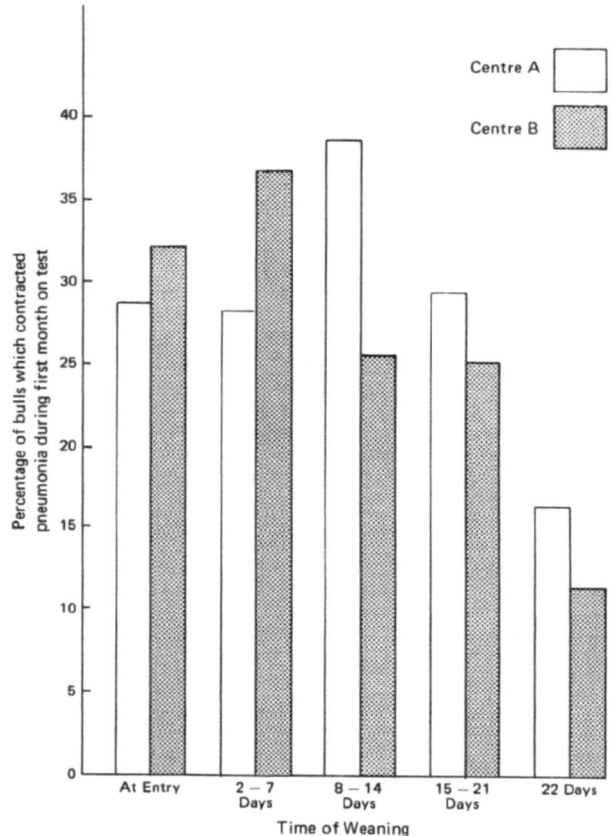

Fig. 3   The effect of time of weaning before entry on the incidence of pneumonia during the first month on performance test

The success of System 3 would appear to be due to the holding of the intake of animals in small groups for the first month as half the disease outbreaks occurred within the first four weeks of entry.   Spread of infection within the intake group was reduced and furthermore, spread to other groups of animals which had been at the station for longer periods was also prevented.

The levels of respiratory disease varied according to the

season of the year. If, as is postulated, the type of disease encountered on MLC Central Bull Performance Test Centres is similar to that of suckled calves, the traditional autumn sale of such animals obviously exacerbates the problem. However weaning of such calves 13 days or more prior to sale might partially reduce respiratory disease levels.

The study of the effect of treatment on the end of test weight showed that treated animals had a lower mean final weight than those untreated, but the difference was not significant. This result must however be qualified in that it was possible that several bulls had clinical disease and were not treated and others had sub-clinical disease and so were included in the untreated category. It was also possible that some animals treated for respiratory disease did not in fact have the condition. As the animals were not slaughtered the use of treated and untreated groups appeared to be the best method of dividing the data as no other objective measurement was available for classifying the disease in animals. If the animals had been taken to slaughter four groups could have been used, namely, treated with respiratory lesions, treated without respiratory lesions, untreated with respiratory lesions and untreated without respiratory lesions. The other problem was to quantify the severity of the disease; some bulls showed more severe signs of disease than others and some cases, not necessarily the same, took longer to recover while still requiring the same amount of treatment. Postmortem examination, not possible in this work, could have indicated the degree of lung damage. Further work is in progress to try to evaluate the severity of disease and its effect on weight gain.

ACKNOWLEDGEMENTS

It is a pleasure to acknowledge the assistance of Mr. D. Jones in performing the analysis of the effects of treatment on liveweight and the most helpful advice of Dr. D.R. Melrose.

REFERENCE

Andrews, A.H. 1976. Vet. Rec. <u>98</u>, p. 146.

STUDIES OF CALF RESPIRATORY DISEASE IN A LARGE COMMERCIAL VEAL UNIT

W.M. Miller, J.W. Harkness, M.S. Richards and D.G. Pritchard
Ministry of Agriculture, Fisheries and Food,
Central Veterinary Laboratory, New Haw, Weybridge, Surrey,
England.

ABSTRACT

An analysis of records of treatment for respiratory disease in a veal unit containing 12 'sheds' of 28 market-bought calves in the south west of England revealed a peak of incidence at 5 weeks after arrival, by 10 weeks it had disappeared. 980 calves entered the unit in the year of the study and only 30 died or were removed as unsuitable.

Three indices of disease were examined, first treatment, new courses of treatment and total number of treatments. Over the study period both secular (increasing) and transient effects were observed. These indicated that extrinsic factors (eg weather or the introduction of a particular pathogen) were also important. Weather parameters from a local meteorological station were examined for possible predisposing patterns. In addition the effect of pen position on disease spread within each of the 12 sheds was examined.

INTRODUCTION

Respiratory disease is a major problem for calf rearers in Great Britain, especially in intensive husbandry systems. Serious financial losses occur as a result of deaths, culling, depressed growth rate and the necessity for veterinary treatments. In the past, research into calf respiratory disease has been focused on the isolation and identification of micro-organisms which have an aetiological role, and the elucidation of the pathological and immunological processes involved. One of the primary objectives of such work has been the development of effective vaccines. Bacteria, viruses and other infectious agents have been implicated (Phillip and Darbyshire, 1971; Gourlay et al., 1970). These agents may act alone or in concert, and their effects can be modified by climatic (Martin et al., 1975) and husbandry (Parker, 1968) factors, by the presence of gaseous pollutants (Mayan and Merilan, 1976) and by the physiological (Roy et al., 1971) and immune status (Thomas and Swann, 1973) of the calf. Particular microclimates facilitate the spread of infection and the survival of micro-organisms (Wray, 1975).

Under field conditions calves are exposed to a variety of infectious agents, which can be isolated from the respiratory tract of both sick and healthy animals, but attempts to reproduce the clinical syndrome under laboratory conditions, even with massive doses of infectious organisms, have generally failed. The nature of the relationships between the micro-organisms involved, the environmental factors and the host animal remains obscure, and there is much current interest in epidemiological studies which seek to analyse these interactions.

This paper reports an analysis of treatment records from a large veal unit, the object being to describe the epidemiology of respiratory diseases in this system, and to develop hypotheses relating to liability to disease and the spread of infection.

MATERIALS AND METHODS

The study was carried out in a veal unit in the west of England which contains some 300 calves under one roof. The animals are penned individually in 12 sheds (Figure 1) each of which contains two facing rows of 14 pens. Each shed is ventilated by a single 38cm diameter fan (thermostatically switched, but with manual speed control) which is fitted in the door 45cm above the ground. The fan draws air from the control passageway and the outlet is a stack at the far end of the shed.

The calves, which are mainly Friesians are supplied from local markets at 7 - 10 days old and 35 - 45 kg (80 - 100 lb) body weight. Batches of 28 calves arrive at intervals of approximately one week. The sheds are stocked in sequence, and the 28 calves remain in the same shed as a single 'crop' until ready for slaughter 15 - 16 weeks later at 180 kg (400 lb) liveweight. All calves are bucket-fed twice daily with warm milk substitute (Volac*). Unsuitable calves are rejected during the first few days and a high standard of management, together with observation at least twice daily, contributes to the low mortality rate. Respiratory disease is virtually the only health problem and is treated promptly with a course of parenterally administered antibiotic. An accurate record is kept of all treatments (transcription of the form of record is shown in Figure 2), and this was the main source of data used in the analysis. Over the study period, the daily record for each crop of 28 calves was processed by a computer programme and four indices of disease were examined:

1. First treatment (ie incidence).

2. New courses of treatment (ie any treatment preceded by at least one day of non-treatment).

3. Total number of treatments.

4. Removal (due to death or unsuitability).

* Volac Ltd., Crayden Old Farm, Wendy, Royston, Herts, England.

184

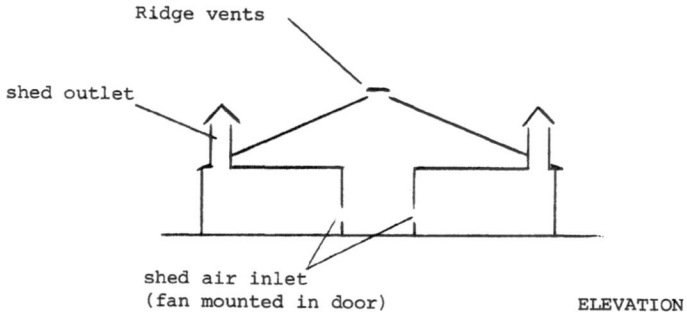

Ridge vents

shed outlet

shed air inlet
(fan mounted in door)

ELEVATION

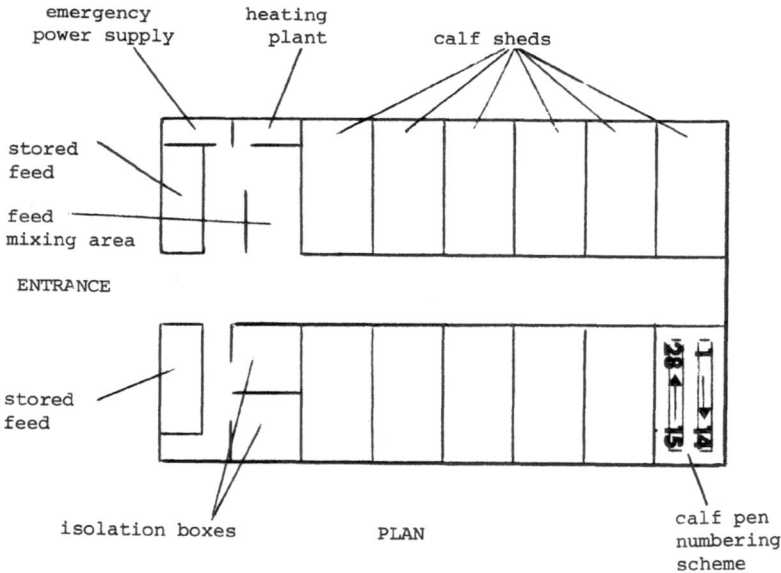

emergency
power supply

heating
plant

calf sheds

stored
feed

feed
mixing area

ENTRANCE

stored
feed

28 ◄ 15

1 ► 14

isolation boxes

PLAN

calf pen
numbering
scheme

Fig. 1. Layout of veal unit.

CALF RESPIRATORY DISEASE TREATMENT RECORD

SHEET No. 1 OF 63

	PEN NUMBER																												TREATMENT DATE Year		Month		Day		START DATE Year		Month		Day		SHED	
Column Number	1	2	3	4	5	6	7	8	9	10	11	12	13	14	15	16	17	18	19	20	21	22	23	24	25	26	27	28	29	30	31	32	33	34	35	36	37	38	39	40	41	42
Row 1																			S										7	5	0	8	0	6	7	5	0	8	0	1	0	5
2																			S										7	5	0	8	0	7								
3		S											S						Ø		S								7	5	0	8	1	5								
4		S											S								S								7	5	0	8	1	6								
5		S											S								S								7	5	0	8	1	7								
6																			S								S		7	5	0	8	2	2								
7													S						S				C				S		7	5	0	8	2	3								
8										S			S						S				C				S		7	5	0	8	2	4								
9										S			S										C				C		7	5	0	8	2	5								
10										S														C					7	5	0	8	2	6								
11																								C					7	5	0	8	2	7								
12																								C			T		7	5	0	8	2	8								
13																											T		7	5	0	8	2	9								
14												S					T												7	5	0	8	3	0								
15												S					T						S						7	5	0	8	3	1								
16												S					T		C				S						7	5	0	9	0	1								
17															S		C		C				C						7	5	0	9	0	2								
18															S		C		C				C						7	5	0	9	0	3								
19		C											C																7	5	0	9	0	9								
20		C											C																7	5	0	9	1	0								
21									S																				7	5	0	9	1	3								
22									S																				7	5	0	9	1	4								
23		S								S	S																		7	5	0	9	2	6								
24		S								S	S																		7	5	0	9	2	7								

REPEAT PUNCH COLS 35-42 BELOW

CODES

Ch (Chloramphenicol)	C
Pb (Penbrittin)	P
St (Streptopen)	S
T (Terramycin)	T
Tr (Trivetrin)	V
Ty (Tylosine)	Y
Died	D
Taken Out	Ø
Replaced	R

Please return forms to: M. Richards, Epidemiology Unit, Central Veterinary Laboratory, New Haw, Weybridge, Surrey. Byfleet 41111 ext. 264

Fig. 2. Treatment record form.

Meteorological data extracted from the returns of two local meteorological stations were also made available to the computer.

STATISTICAL ANALYSIS

To ascertain whether one half of the shed might be more liable to disease than the other, the differences, (D) in the amount of disease between the two halves is calculated for each index of disease for each crop. If there is no difference between halves, the expected value of the sum of D for all crops ($\leq$ D) would be zero. D was calculated for 'left' versus 'right' halves (pens 1 - 14 versus 15 - 28), 'door' versus 'end' (1 - 7 and 22 - 28 versus 8 - 21), and 'middle' versus 'ends' (4 - 10 and 18 - 24 versus 11 - 17 and 25 - 28) (Figure 1). The sum of the squares of the D values for all crops ($\leq$ D^2) was also calculated. The first statistic ($\leq$ D) provides an indication of a consistent excess of disease in one half of the sheds, whilst the second ($\leq$ D^2) detects any tendency for the disease to concentrate in one half, even though the choice of half is not consistent from crop-to-crop and shed-to-shed. For each crop, the corrected sum of squares (CSS) of the amount of disease in each pen was calculated, and the total of these values over all crops was compared with the CSS of the totals in each pen position. An excess of the observed value over the expected indicates that a calf's position in the shed has a consistent effect on liability to disease.

RESULTS

A total of 980 calves in 34 crops passed through the unit during the study period. Thirty calves died or were removed as unsuitable (ie unlikely to thrive under veal unit conditions) during the year of the investigation, and a total of 4 280 doses of antibiotic were administered, as treatment for respiratory disease. 677 animals (69%) had at least one course of treatment.

The relationship between the age of the calves in days after arrival on the farm, and three of the indices of disease (first treatment, new courses of treatment, and total treatments) is shown in Figure 3. The variation in timing and extent of disease in the 34 crops of calves appears in Figure 4. Figure 5 demonstrates the relationship in successive crops between the three disease indices. Figure 6 is a 'cusum' diagram, comparing the cumulative total of new courses of treatment with the number expected on the basis of the age-structure of the calf population present at the time.

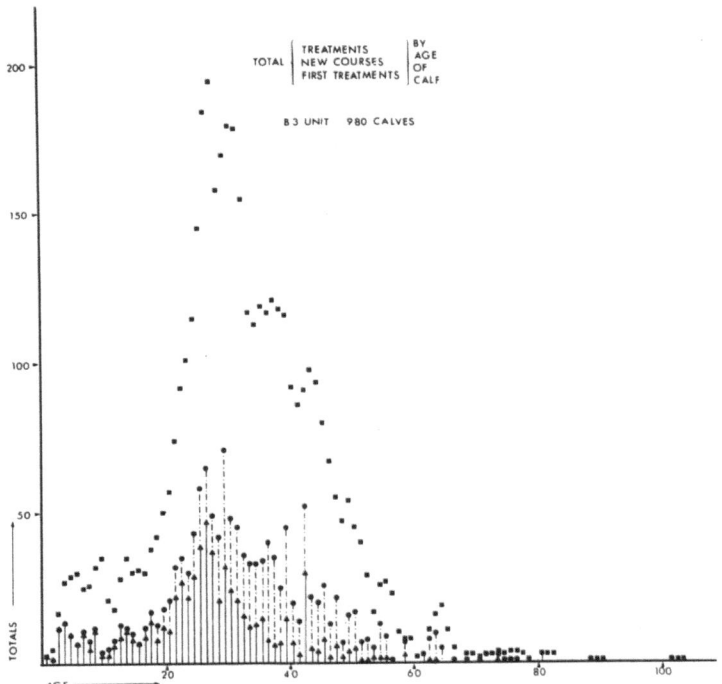

Fig. 3. Relationship between time of arrival on farm and disease indices.

The results of the analysis of the effect of pen position on liability to disease are shown in Table 1. The only significant values are $\pounds D$ for 'left' minus 'right' halves, and $\pounds D^2$

TABLE 1

	Total no.	Total corrected sums of squares		Differences between halves							
				End-door				Left-right			
		observed	expected	£D observed	P	£D² observed	£D² expected+	P	£D observed	P	£D² observed	£D² expected+	P
First treatments	677	156.11	179.61	13	.33	247	186.3	.09	27	.04	207	186.3	.33
New courses	1340	843.43	1368.07	8	.83	3522	1418.7	<.01	80	.03	1902	1418.7	.09
Treatments	4280	15273.43	15296.71	24	.85	44884	15863.3	<.01	414	<.01	21100	15863.3	.11
Removals	30	31.86	26.93	-10	.03	42	31.0	.12	-4	.44	30	31.0	.46

34 crops - 980 calves

P values and expected values are calculated from the randomisation distributions of the 28 values in each crop. (Pitman 1938). For £D the test is two-sided and the expected value is zero; for £D² it is one-sided.

for 'door' minus 'end' halves. The door/end division is that
which divides the house into the two most separated halves,
and thus in effect indicates clustering of disease within a
crop of calves. Both effects were shown most strongly in the
treatment index, but were also evident in the less sensitive
indices.

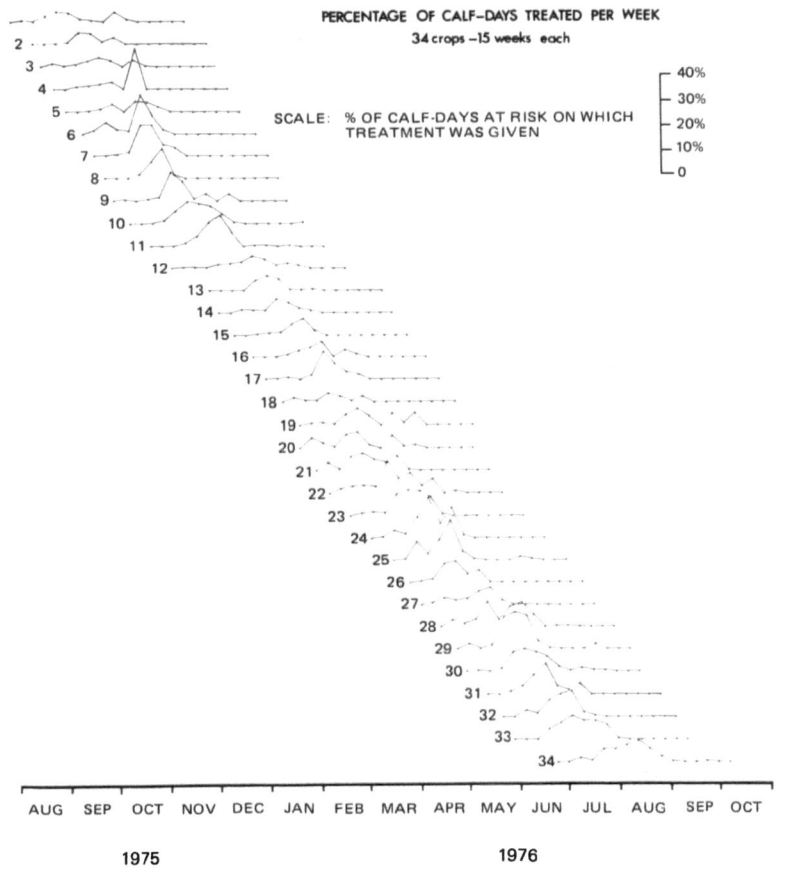

Fig. 4 Variation in timing and extent of disease in 34 crops of calves

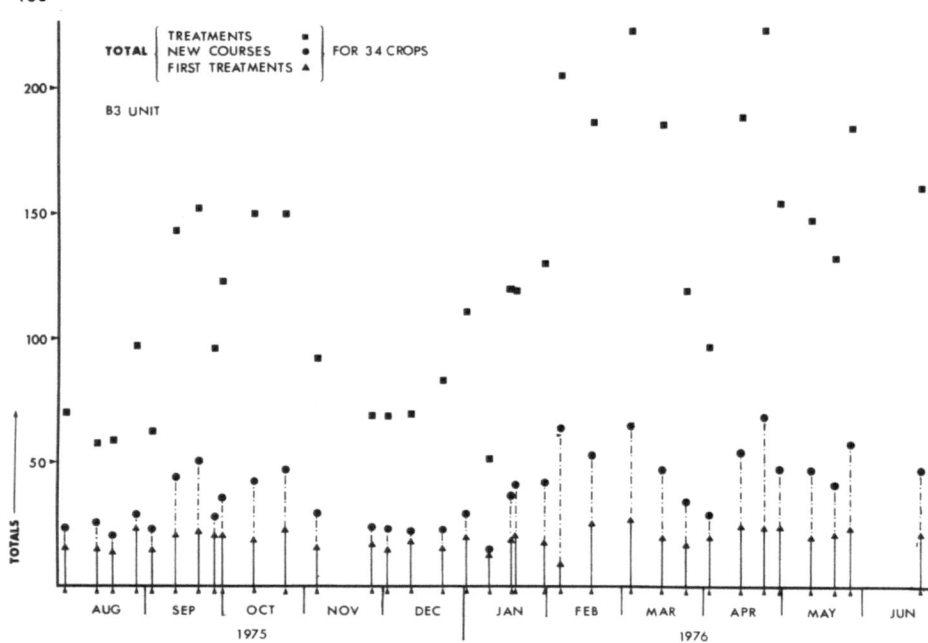

Fig. 5. Relationship in successive crops between the disease indices.

DISCUSSION

Throughout the analyses of the data, the four indices of disease, first treatments, new cases, total treatments and removals, were used. First treatments had the advantage of being less liable to subjectivity than the others, but the population at risk diminished rapidly. Total treatments reflected the severity of clinical disease in individual animals but was liable to have been less accurate, as a result of increased anxiety in the stockman during a serious outbreak of disease. New courses of treatment was a compromise between these two. Removals were too infrequent to serve as a useful index.

The most prominent feature of respiratory disease among these calves was the peak of treatments at about 28 days and the low levels prior to the twentieth and after the fiftieth days

in the unit. Most of the new courses of treatment after the
peak were attributable to recrudescence of disease.

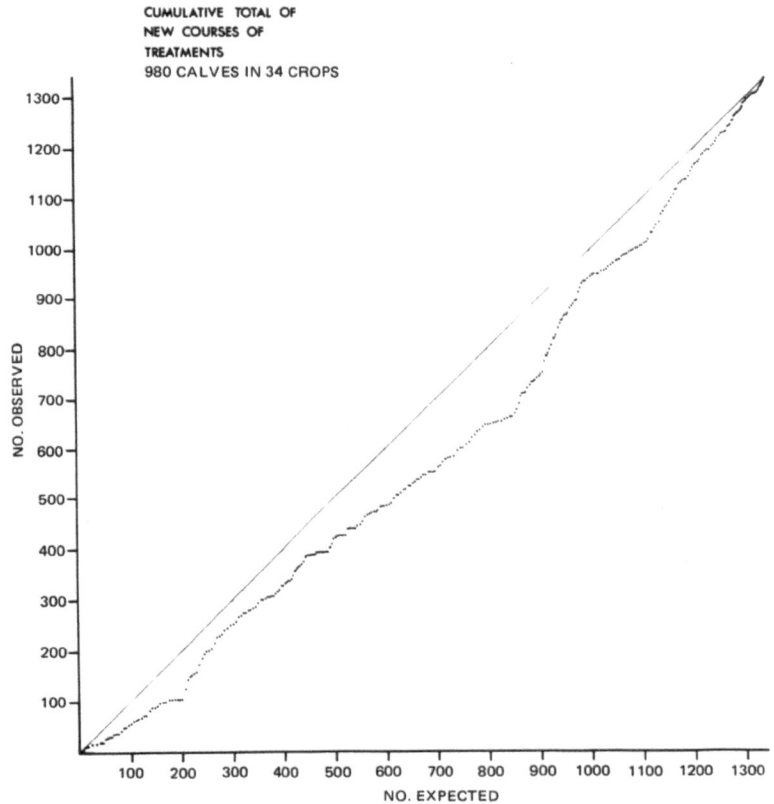

Fig. 6 Comparison of cumulative total of new courses of treatment
with the number expected

Figure 4 shows evidence of an extrinsic factor acting on
all sheds simultaneously in October 1975, April 1976 and early
June 1976. This has the effect of synchronising disease events
in a number of different houses, but in spite of this the age-
dependent effect appears dominant. The synchronising effect
is better shown in Figure 6. It results in the discontinuities
evident in the graph and in basic changes in the trend. This

presentation is particulalry useful where day to day variation
is a problem in time-series data. Unfortunately, the time-
base is non-linear so that comparisons with weather data are
difficult.

The disease records undoubtedly have a subjective basis,
that of the perceived need to treat an animal, but the uniformity
of management, accurate recording and veterinary supervision,
together with data itself, give confidence that the measures
of disease have validity. The rates of treatment are high and
this may have a bearing on the low mortality rate, especially
with early treatment. Obviously, constant veterinary supervision is out of the question, but the information can usefully
form the basis of descriptive epidemiology from which hypotheses
can be generated. These have useful attributes of being likely
to have practical and economic significance.

The data demonstrates a fundamental age-dependent
susceptibility, due perhaps to diminishing maternal immunity,
though no simple relationship exists with the zinc sulphate
turbidity test results, or changes in physiology. This effect
is so dramatic as to dominate all other effects detected during
the analysis and to suggest a single disease syndrome. An
interesting feature of the Veal Unit is that it is constantly
being re-stocked with susceptible animals and one sees a
constant succession of minor epidemics. Susceptible subjects
are always available to maintain the pool of pathogens and new
pathogens are continually being introduced.

Transient synchronising effects probably due to weather
or the arrival of a particularly virulent pathogen are also
seen, but they could be confounded by an increased desire to
treat during serious outbreaks. The plausibility of the weather
hypothesis is to be examined using data from nearby meteorological
stations. In spite of the 'controlled' environment the
desire to maintain a fairly high ambient temperature (16^{0}C)
effectively reduces fresh air exchange and increases relative
humidity and pollution during cold spells. It is difficult to

know whether such environmental changes either increase the
microbiological challenge, or physiological stress on the calves.

The excess of treatments on the left hand side is difficult
to explain; it may reflect a quirk of the ventilation system,
which is identical in each shed, or a predisposition for treatment on that side by the stockman. The latter seems unlikely.
The fact that disease was concentrated in one end of the house
or the other indicates that short-range or contact spread is
likely to be the dominant mode of transmission among these
calves. The data does not show the widespread distribution of
new cases which would be associated with diffuse aerosol spread.
The high relative humidities observed in these sheds may be
a relevant factor but whatever the explanation the findings are
in stark contrast to the widely held view that the aerosol route
is most important in respiratory disease. If it is generally
true that short-range spread is the dominant route, the finding
could have considerable implications for some disease control
strategies.

Respiratory disease has been shown to have a seasonal
pattern (Backstrom and Bremer, 1976) even in 'controlled
environment' buildings. Work is currently in progress to
investigate the relationshp between local meteorological
station data and the 'synchronising effect '. Further investigation of the calf-to-calf spread is planned using a simulation
approach. Provided that a reasonably robust model can be
developed and validated against data from the succeeding year,
it should be possible to draw conclusions on means of spread
and optimal control measures.

194

REFERENCES

Backstrom, L. and Bremer, H. 1976. Svensth Vet. Tiching 28, p. 312.

Gourlay, R.N., MacKenzie, A. and Cooper, J.E. 1970. J. comp. Path. 80, p. 575.

Martin, S.E., Schwabe, C.W. and Frauti, C.E. 1975. Can. J. Comp. Med. 39, p. 377.

Mayan, M.N. and Merilan, C.P. 1976. N.Z. vet. J. 24, p. 221.

Parker, W.H. 1968. Vet. Rec. 83, p. 364.

Phillip, J.I.H. and Darbyshire, J.H. 1971. Adv. vet. Sci. comp. Med. 15, p. 159.

Roy, J.H.B., Stobo, I.J.F., Gaston, J., Ganderton, P., Shotton, S.M. and Oster, D.C. 1971. Br. J. Nutrition, 26, p. 363.

Thomas, L.H. and Swann, R.G. 1973. Vet. Rec. 92, p. 454.

Wary, C. 1975. Vet. Bull. 45, p. 543.

DISCUSSION

J. Asso (France)

Do you not think, Dr. Wiseman, that when we send our very
young children to school we are exposing them to the kind of
problem you mentioned? In one way it is beneficial because it
is better to have whooping cough and measles and so on when you
are young, rather than later.

A. Wiseman (UK)

Providing you survive! I think the condition in young
calves is absolutely identical to the condition you see in school
children. It is the only time one thinks of putting a similarly
aged group of individuals together, and presumably most of them
are completely susceptible to all the various infectious agents
which are going about.

J. Asso

Dr. McKercher, do you think that milk consumption will ever
be reduced? Maybe the future of the cow as a meat producer is
limited, but as a milk producer we need it.

D.G. McKercher (USA)

The goat is also a milk producer and a much better grazer.
In fact, there is a lot of interest in the United States today
in the diseases of goats. I do not know whether this just
happened, or whether people are looking ahead as well, and
planning for a not-so-favourable future.

I thought I might get some argument from the Europeans about
the evolution of IBR. I do not know your views on it, but it
seemed a logical evolution.

O.C. Straub (West Germany)

I got to know about IBR when I was working on it in the
States with Dr. McKercher. When they told us that IPV and IBR
were the same we could hardly believe it. This started the
interest. When I went to Tübingen in 1961 we isolated the IPV,

yet we did not have the IBR. We wondered whether the rapid animal passages had led to IBR, or whether IPV really causes IBR. So we tested a number of strains of IPV, and those strains which we tested as pure IPV strains do not cause disease of the respiratory tract, even if they have the chance, after passage in the tract. Then, as some of you know, we tried electrophoresis to separate them. The idea was that the pH of the genital tract was different from that of the respiratory tract in cattle. We measured the pH, and then I said that there must be some difference in those strains. We started to pick strains and measure them, and we found that there was a difference in the migrating electrophoresis between the typical IPV strain which would not cause IBR, and the IBR strain. You might ask if any new-found IBR strain causes IPV. I can say that it does. All the IBR strains we have so far isolated or checked in Europe have had the capability to produce IPV, but IPV strains do not produce IBR. In other words, the genetic composition of the IBR virus is different from the composition of the IPV. It is a newer one and it has more properties, and has also retained the old properties, and has also retained the old properties such as causing IPV.

Then, as you know, we found it in Australia and California, in encephalitis, and later on in California it was found in abortion. We know that it has caused abortion in other countries as well. Again, we thought there must be a difference and so we did plaque studies. We found some differences. The typical IPV strain caused the smallest plaques within the shortest period of time, whilst the encephalitis strain and the abortion strain produced the largest plaques. We had also taken IBR strains from the United States, and from Italy and a number of other countries but we could not significantly differentiate them by diameters. This is how we found the differences between the various strains, if this is of any value to you.

B. Martin *(UK)*

May I ask Professor Straub for some clarification. Are you saying that, although the IPV strain of virus did not cause disease in the upper respiratory tract, it did not multiply?

O.C. Straub

No, it could multiply but it did not cause disease.

B. Martin

How many passages of the virus did you make in the respiratory tract, and did you try it in animals of different ages?

O.C. Straub

We did a few passages. We took the isolate from the nose and put it into the next animal. We also did it, for example, when we caused mastitis with an IPV virus. Of course you do not need an IBR virus to cause mastitis. We used that virus to see whether the contact cow could pick it up in the nose, and it did. The contact cow would pick up this virus from the mastitis in the nose, but it would not develop signs of IBR. If you do the same with the IBR virus you would get the disease immediately. We had the last severe outbreak of IBR two days ago, and it is really striking. Out of 30 animals, 26 became sick at the same time, on a Saturday morning. Nothing like this happens with IPV. You can hardly recognise it.

B. Martin

I think that in outbreaks of IPV in calves or in contacts one can detect the virus in the upper respiratory tract of the calves, although they do not necessarily show signs of upper respiratory tract infection.

O.C. Straub

My present point of view is that those terrible strains which we have found in the last few years in Europe originated in the New World, and we have gradually acquired them in the Old World. I do not think those passages have occurred in the Old World. The first outbreak was in 1955, so it took approximately six years until the virus was found. I think the strains which were detected in the US would certainly have been detected if we had had them earlier in Europe. The largest outbreak in our country occurred two years ago and we could trace it back from Schleswig-Holstein to Saxony, Holland and Belgium. I think

Belgium was the first country to have it in 1972. It took from 1972 until 1975 to reach us, when we had our first two outbreaks. I think France had outbreaks in 1974. I think we can trace the true IBR back to the New World.

D.G. McKercher

I think they might have come from the New World, but I also think that the virus originally came from Europe. It possibly had to pass through thousands of cattle. I think this is what happened in IBR. This is where it did establish its pathogenicity for the upper respiratory tract. But, if you will recall, the first IPV isolate was made at Cornell. We did cross-immunity tests and these two came up in the cattle. The genital isolate did produce respiratory infection and disease, and vice versa. When I worked in Tübingen I compared the American strains with the genital isolates from Europe and the IPV isolates produced respiratory disease, but not as severe, of course, as the IBR isolates.

O.C. Straub

I have talked to people in South Africa and they have had the same experience. They have compared about 15 IPV strains and they would not cause respiratory disease. We have isolated strains in Germany which do cause respiratory disease, but they are newer strains. The old strains, such as those from the Alpine region, have been in the genital tract for a very long time, and they are very harmless. You hardly ever see them.

D.G. McKercher

Do you not think that the European strains which originally caused IPV now cause IBR because you now have essentially the same situation that we have with feedlots?

O.C. Straub

This situation has arisen only recently. We think that the very virulent strains have not been produced in Europe. I think that they have been introduced.

D.G. McKercher
That is true. I think they were produced in the American feedlots, but from genital strains from Europe. I still think that they were produced in Europe simply by the trend towards highly intensive situations. However, I agree, it will never be settled.

O.C. Straub
No, it will never be settled.

V. Bitsch *(Denmark)*
I am inclined to support the view of Professor McKercher. We have the IBR infection in Denmark and the infection seems to have been introduced originally about 1960 with beef cattle imported from abroad. The infection was spread by artificial insemination centres as a genital infection. Today the infection is under control in artificial insemination centres, but it has spread from the centres into herds in certain districts and areas. Today we have IBR infection in these districts; and we have, with a genital strain of virus, been able to reproduce IBR, not in its classical American form, but nevertheless the virus could produce mild clinical symptoms. I cannot see why the differences which Professor Straub has observed cannot be explained simply by a variation in pathogenicity among strains of IBR virus.

O.C. Straub
Because, as Professor McKercher mentioned, you need the large herds, and we still do not have them in our country. We do not have the feedlot conditions in Germany, so we think that we introduced those strains.

F. Lomba *(Belgium)*
I think this question is worth mentioning. Since 1950 we have been able to demonstrate IPV virus. In 1972 we introduced 48 Holstein cows which were divided into four groups. IBR began there and it spread from there within two or three years. The spread was very easy to follow on the map.

R.N. Gourlay *(UK)*

Dr. Andrews, is it possible to use deaths as a measure of the severity of respiratory disease?

A. Andrews *(UK)*

Obviously yes, but we have a very low deathrate. During the 5-year period we had a 1.4% overall mortality, and 0.8% was due to pneumonia. If we had enough mortality, then it is a good idea, but I do try to get them home alive, although not always successfully! As a sideline, we have looked at deaths, and an animal which is treated for a respiratory disease has a greater probability of dying than one which is not treated, regardless of cause. We have several types of cause besides pneumonia. Pneumonia is obviously the largest one, but other causes are bloat, gid and the odd accident. These animals were slaughtered, but all of them happened to have been treated.

N.J.L. Gilmour *(UK)*

When you found respiratory disease, is it upper respiratory disease, lower respiratory disease, or a combination of both? I think it is necessary to define these, and your criteria for ascertaining the necessity for treatment.

A. Andrews

I do not treat all these animals. They are treated by the practitioners at the stations. Our criteria for treatment are dependent on, firstly, dyspnoea or hyperpnoea, secondly, inappetance and, thirdly, pyrexia. Some had a muco-purulent discharge and others did not. Some had an intermittent cough and others did not, but those are things which I take as my criteria for treatment - an animal which is ill.

N.J.L. Gilmour

Would you say they had pneumonia, or not?

A. Andrews

Perhaps not in every case, but I have not seen every case.

In the vast majority of cases, from what I have been able to
establish from the clinicians, they think the animals had pneumonia, and the ones I have seen have also had pneumonia.

L.H. Thomas (UK)

I would like to support Dr. Andrews on this. I think that
is about the best you can do for diagnosing pneumonia on the
hoof.

O.C. Straub

The stations are run by laymen. Do the laymen call the
veterinary surgeons in, or do the laymen take the temperatures
routinely?

A. Andrews

The stations are run by managers who are laymen and they
call the veterinary surgeon in and he does the treatment. The
layman will have taken the temperature but it will have been
checked by the veterinary surgeon himself. I have tried having
routine temperatures taken but we gave it up because I was trying to get a temperature over which the manager could expect
trouble. We went up to a temperature of $41^{\circ}C$ and we still had
animals in that situation which did not need treatment.

O.C. Straub

Those animals must have had an infection.

A. Andrews

Yes, I agree, and this is one of the troubles with my looking at the influence of respiratory disease treatment on liveweight, because I do not know all these animals which have had
respiratory disease. I accept that entirely.

J. Asso (France)

Do you think that it is possible, Dr. Harkness, that animals
could have had some communication between pens for the local
transmission of disease?

J. Harkness *(UK)*

Yes.

J. Asso

So transmission is possible via licks or something like that, as well as by aerosol?

J. Harkness

I should have explained that, although the calves are in individual pens, they are not solid-sided pens, and the animals can on occasion reach over the top or through the slats and touch each other.

R.N. Gourlay

I was wondering whether you took this a bit further and took the calves to autopsy or to slaughter, and then examined the lungs of the various calves at slaughter.

J. Harkness

We obviously did not do that for all the calves which went through this particular study. Before the study, for some eight months we had been paying regular visits, and following crops of calves through to slaughter, and looking at their lungs, so we did see the gross pathology. We did not do any detailed histo-pathology.

O.C. Straub

Did you measure any environmental factors such as ammonia, or H_2S?

J. Harkness

We did a lot of environmental monitoring during this same period I am talking about, before we started this type of recording. We took samples of ammonia and various other gases, but we were not able to find sufficiently reliable or cheap trans-ducers to allow us to monitor the ammonia or other gases over a long period of time.

O.C. Straub

You could measure the humidity, or some factor like that.
Dr. Andrews pointed out that in March, April and May he had the
lowest incidence, whereas you had a fairly high incidence in the
same months, and conditions in general would be the same in the
two months, wouldn't they? Would these months be the lowest
period of humidity in your area?

J. Harkness

No, it would be from June onwards. That is when we start
seeing disease again. The disease is rising when the humidity
is going down, in June and July. Obviously I did not explain
all the environment details. These are controlled environment
animals. The calves have as much free access to ordinary, common
air as possible.

J. Asso

So the date of birth during the year does not play any role.
That means that all the year round we have the same thing. It
has been said that colostrum is not the same in autumn as it is
in spring. We have found exactly the same problem, and at any
age, because we have problems after two or three weeks.

J. Harkness

Anyone who brings animals together has those problems.

A. Wiseman

Did you state that you determine when the calves are going
to be treated, or was it the stockmen?

J. Harkness

The calves are treated under veterinary supervision. I do
not determine it.

I.E. Selman *(UK)*

Just to return to the comments which were made about the
seasonal variation of colostrum antibody in calves, that seasonal
variation was very marked when we looked at calves born to dairy

cattle in the West of Scotland in 1965. In those days, almost
all the calves were born in byres, and the mothers were tied by
the neck. There was no dam/offspring interplay whatsoever. In
the winter, the colostrum was fed artificially in small amounts.
The seasonal variation was never quite so marked south of the
border, and the further south you went, the less the variation,
simply because many of the cows were loose-housed in the winter
time or, in fact, out of doors. We are noticing differences now,
with an increased tendency to loose housing. I would not have
expected much of a seasonal variation in observed antibody in
calves in the Southwest of England.

J. Asso

It is because the animals are housed all the year round.

I.E. Selman

No, it is because the calves are born either to loose-housed
mothers during the wintertime, or else the cows were outdoors
during the winter in the Southwest of England, which is not the
same as the Southwest of Scotland, where we initially did this
seasonal variation study.

J. Asso

Does anyone wish to comment on conditioning or pre-conditioning the animals? I have no experience of the problem and I
think it might be a good idea to compare experiences.

G. Rognoni (Italy)

I can report experiments which have been made by Italian
and French veterinarians. The calves which were exported to
Italy were preconditioned by anthelmintic treatment, by vaccination and by an adaptation to their regime. In Italy the losses
were considerably reduced by these methods. I come back to the
point I made this morning - it appears that the vaccine used
was an inactivated IBR vaccine. One can assume that the French
calves were not infected with IBR when they came to Italy and
that they were sensitive to the IBR virus.

J. Asso

    Is anyone conditioning the calves before sending them?

O.C. Straub

    We condition the calves when we have received them.

J. Asso

    So you condition them in some centre when you receive them. That is not preconditioning, it is postconditioning.

O.C. Straub

    Yes, it is postconditioning.

P. Eyre *(Canada)*

    I have one very small question to ask. What anthelmintic is commonly used in the treatment of calves in various countries, because there is a very definite amount of evidence now that some anthelmintics have quite a measurable effect on the animal's immune system. Organophosphates, for example, are measurably immunosuppressive; Levamisole is measurably immunostimulant. I wondered if this had any influence at all on the prevalence of disease. The various conditions which we have been talking about today could be related to different regimens of anthelmintics. I wondered what the situation was in different countries in different parts of the world. I would think that there may be some relationship to the particular use of certain drugs in pre-treatment. It is something which occurred to me when you were talking about the pre-treatment of animals. I wonder if anyone has any comments?

O.C. Straub

    I can comment on IBR in the US. In the States Professor McKercher has used Levamisole together with IBR vaccination and with other combination preparations. Dr. McKercher says that he did not have a decrease in immunogenic stimulants. In human medicine Levamisole obviously has a very positive effect upon older people. So far we have merely been watching the effects, but in the States, as far as humoral antibodies are concerned,

they think that there is no increase in immunity. I personally
think we should look into it, especially as Levamisole should
act via fibrocytes - that is on the cell mediated immunity. I
think it is good that you brought up this point. Perhaps in the
future we should look a bit further into what Levamisole does.
Workers in Israel have come out in favour of using Levamisole,
although they have used it experimentally only on small animals
such as mice, guinea-pigs and rabbits.

P. Eyre

Levamisole will increase the production of humoral antibodies to some micro-organisms, but not necessarily to all. The
interesting point I was going to make was the organophosphates
are immunosuppressive, and there could be a real difference
between the different drug treatments. I do not know that it
exists - I said there could be a difference.

O.C. Straub

People are aware of it but they have not made up their
minds yet.

P.W. Wells *(UK)*

I would like to make one comment about the immunostimulant
properties of Levamisole. I have heard it said, although I do
not know how much experimental evidence there is to back this,
that Levamisole is only effective as an immunostimulant in
animals which are infected with helminths, and someone has
suggested that it is something to do with the helminth expulsion
process which has the immunostimulant effect.

H.J. Bürger

What you are referring to may be a completely different
thing, because it has been shown in several models that there
is some interference between one helminth and another pathogen.
It may be between one bacterium and a helminth, or one helminth
and another helminth, for example, but as far as I know, this
interference is not always along the same lines. Infection with
a helminth will not necessarily reduce antibody production

towards some other organism. It may reduce it in some cases, and it may enhance it in others. In this case, if you treat animals with Levamisole you will eradicate the population of helminths and then you will change the immunological response, and if the helminths reduce the immunological response you will thus restore it.

A direct answer to Dr. Eyre's question, and I can only speak for Germany, is that the most common drug used in cattle during the last two or three years was Levamisole, and second to it was Pyrantel tartrate with some Thiabendazole. An organophosphate, Coumaphos, was used, especially in housed cattle. Since Fenbendazole came on to the market last year there has been a change and I am not sure of the percentage of cattle which have been treated by Fenbendazole during the last season.

SESSION 3

PNEUMONIA/VIRUSES

Chairman:

O. Straub

Co-ordinator:

J.M. Sharp

ON RESPIRATORY VIRAL INFECTIONS IN CATTLE IN DENMARK

V. Bitsch,
The State Veterinary Serum Laboratory, Bülowsvej 27,
1870 Copenhagen V., Denmark.

ABSTRACT

In a microbiological study of 50 pneumonic calf lungs well-known bovine viruses could be demonstrated in 9 lungs (18%). The viruses isolated were the bovine respiratory syncytial (BRS) virus in 4 cases, bovine virus diarrhoea (BVD) virus in 3 cases, and bovine parainfluenza 3 (PI3) virus in 2 cases. Unidentified cytopathic agents were demonstrated in a few lungs.

In other examinations of material from the respiratory tract of cattle, infectious bovine rhinotracheitis (IBR) virus and Aujeszky's disease virus have also been isolated. Among unidentified isolates are strains that appear to belong to the adenovirus group.

The incidence of some viral infections in cattle herds has been elucidated by examination of 50 sera of heifers aged about 2 years and originating from 50 different herds. The sera were selected at random and examined for antibody to IBR, BVD, BRS, and PI3 virus. Only one sample (2%) was found IBR-positive in a P_{24}^{37} test (preincubation at $37^{\circ}C$ for 24 hours) with a titre of 22. Thirty-six (72%) were BVD-positive in a P_4^{37} test with titres from 5.6 to 720, while the rest had titres <1. Forty-two samples (84%) were BRS-positive with titres from 22 to $\geqslant1440$ in a P_4^{37} test. The remaining 8 sera showed titres $\geqslant11$, but the specificity of these low reactions was considered questionable. All 50 sera were PI3 positive with titres from 22 to $\geqslant1440$.

In conclusion, the results presented have demonstrated that viruses may play a role in the aetiology of respiratory diseases in cattle, and that the incidence of certain viral infections in Danish cattle herds is extremely high.

INTRODUCTION

The complexity of infectious respiratory diseases in cattle was elucidated in a previous paper (Bitsch et al., 1976). A short account of the virological examinations in this report will be given here in addition to results of other personal studies on viral infections of the bovine respiratory tract.

To elucidate not only the prevalence but also to some extent the incidence of certain viral infections in the Danish cattle herds, serum samples from a number of herds have been examined for virus-neutralising antibodies to four different bovine viruses. These serological examinations will be described here in detail.

THE SEROLOGICAL EXAMINATION OF CATTLE SERA.   METHODS AND RESULTS

Material

In all, 50 sera of heifers from 50 different herds in Jutland were selected at random from samples received for other examinations and with no immediate history of disease in the herds of origin. The heifers were pregnant and aged from 2 to 2½ years.

Viruses

The following viruses were used as test antigens: infectious bovine rhinotracheitis (IBR) virus (Da B 69), bovine virus diarrhoea (BVD) virus (VK 549/72), bovine respiratory syncytial (BRS) virus (VK 49 73) and bovine parainfluenza (PI 3) virus (SF 4).

Serological tests

The sera were examined for virus-neutralising antibody (VNA). The virus test dose was 100 $TCID_{50}$ per 0.1 ml in tube tests or 0.025 ml in micro-titre tests. In both tests, virus

suspensions and serum dilutions were mixed in equal amounts.
Titrations were performed with twofold dilutions of test sera
and titres given as 50% endpoint dilution factors. In tube
tests, two tissue culture tubes were inoculated from each
dilution, while in micro-titre titrations only one well was
used for each dilution. Final readings were taken after 6 to
9 days.

IBR: only the tube test - with preincubation at $37^{\circ}C$ for
24 hours (P_{24}^{37} test) - was employed and used with calf kidney
cell cultures at a low passage level.

BVD and PI 3: P_{5}^{37} tube tests with the above cells were
used for screening. Titration was performed with P_{4}^{37} micro-
titre test.

BRS: only the micro-titre test was used with the 30th and
22nd passage of a bovine turbinate cell line (NADC, Ames, Iowa).

RESULTS

One sample was IBR-positive with a titre of 22, while the
rest were negative (P_{24}^{37} titres <1). Thirty-six sera (72%),
which did not give BVD P_{5}^{37} antibody titres <1, had P_{4}^{37} titres
from 5.6 to 720. Five sera had BRS P_{4}^{37} titres of <1 to 1.4,
while the rest had titres from 5.6 to $\geq$1440. All sera were
found PI 3-positive (Figure 1).

DISCUSSION

In the microbiological study of 50 pneumonic calf lungs,
which was referred to above, well-known viruses were isolated
from 9 lungs (18%): BRS virus in 4 cases, BVD virus in 3, and
PI 3 virus in 2 cases. Unidentified cythopathogenic agents
were demonstrated in a few lungs.

214

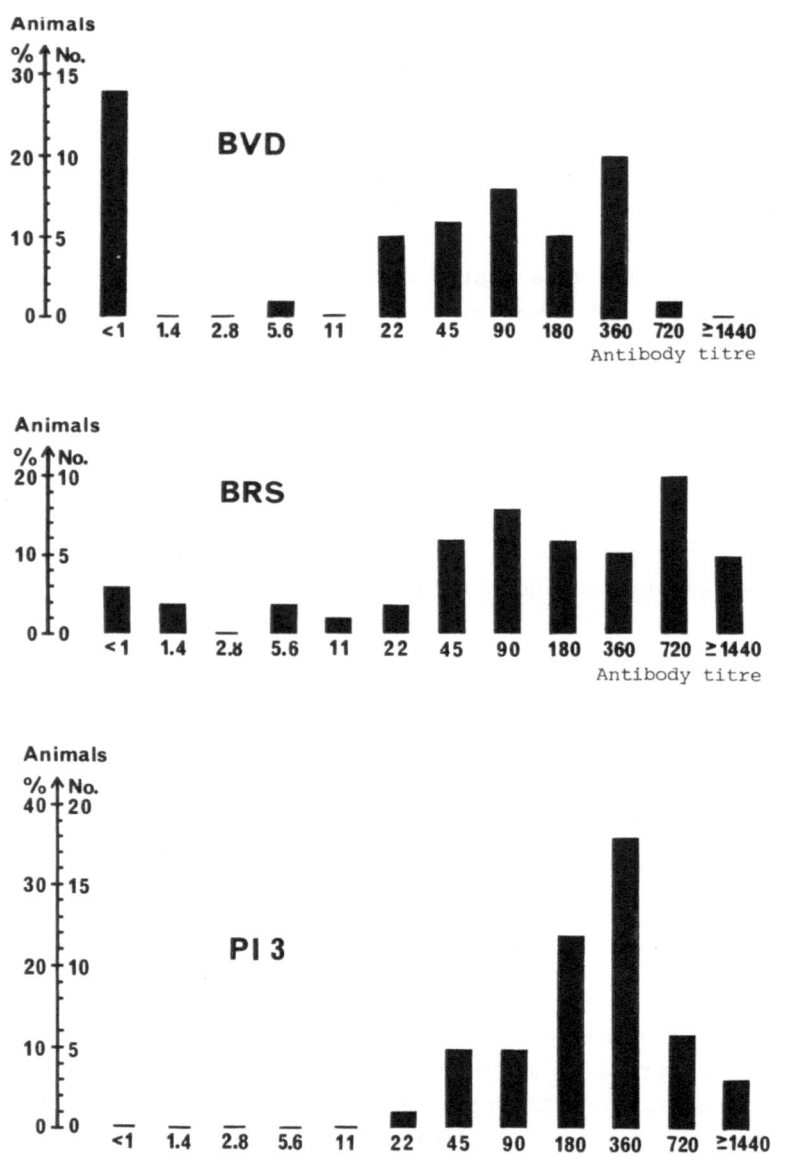

Fig. 1.   Virus-neutralising antibody titres to BVD, BRS and PI 3 viruses in
          sera of 50 heifers representing 50 different herds.

Among viruses found in material from routine diagnostic examinations were also strains of IBR virus, but the IBR infection is not widespread in Denmark (Bitsch, 1975a) and consequently plays only a minor role in the aetiology of respiratory disease. This is in keeping with the finding that only one sample out of 50 in the present study appeared to be IBR-positive.

From the results of the serological examinations the importance of the BVD, BRS, and PI 3 infections is more obvious: during their first two years of life most animals in cattle herds will be exposed to BVD infection and practically all animals to infection with BRS and PI 3 viruses.

The use of relatively high sensitivity in the serological tests was not disadvantageous. On the contrary, in the IBR and BVD tests it obviously facilitated distinction between negative and positive samples. With regard to the BRS test the titre distribution did not seem to favour the notion that the low reactions might be specific.

It is of interest that cattle may be infected with Aujeszky's disease virus by the respiratory route. In many cases from the category of outbreaks with an anterior localisation of pruritis (or virus), for virus has been demonstrated in mucous membranes of the upper respiratory tract and in one case in lung tissues (Bitsch, 1975b).

REFERENCES

Bitsch, V. 1975a . Bull. Off. int. Epizoot. 84, p. 95.
Bitsch, V. 1975b. Acta. vet. Scand. 16, p. 420.
Bitsch, V., Friis, N.F. and Krogh, H.V. 1976. Acta. vet. Scand. 17, p. 32.

BOVINE RESPIRATORY SYNCYTIAL VIRUS INFECTION AND SYMPTOMS OF ATYPICAL INTERSTITIAL PNEUMONIA

C. Holzhauer,

Prov. Gezondheidsdienst voor Dieren in Gelderland,
'Klein Rosendael', Postbus 10, Rosendael, Netherlands.

ABSTRACT

Young cows in the Netherlands are commonly affected with an enzootic bronchopneumonia which is called 'pinkengriep'.

This virus-pneumonia may be recognised in affected animals by the clinical signs. At the outset there is an accelerated respiration accompanied by coughing, conjunctivitis and a soporific demeanour. In some affected animals symptoms similar to those of 'fog-fever' appear during the second stage of the disease.

Some similarity exists with the illness which is seen in young children infected with respiratory syncytial virus, namely bronchiolitis and pneumonia.

In the autumn of 1973 and 1974 a total of 292 animals with 'pinkengriep' were examined serologically for respiratory virus infections. Complement fixation tests showed that there was a significant increase in antibodies to respiratoy syncytial virus (R S virus) in 76% of the animals.

During the early stages of the disease, R S virus was isolated from the nasal secretions of some animals.

Calves which died due to this respiratory disease had an atypical interstitial pneumonia.

These findings suggest an aetiological role for bovine respiratory syncytial virus in such cases of atypical interstitial pneumonia.

INTRODUCTION

In addition to lung-worm infection and enzootic pneumonia
of calves, a disease which affects calves of one or a few months
of age, enzootic respiratory diseases of young calves in the
Netherlands include a form of bronchopneumonia which has a
distinctive character. Stock-owners in the Netherlands refer
to it as 'pinkengriep' (Literally: 'yearling influenza', an
approximation being: bronchopneumonia of yearlings).

The acute onset of respiratory symptoms, such as cough and
rapid respiration in from 80 to 90% of the animals of a particular age group, is characteristic. At an advanced stage of
the disease, some of the animals show expiratory dyspnoea as
in fog fever.

The course, the failure to respond to treatment with antibiotics and the post-mortem findings suggest a virus disease.

In 1972, preliminary serological studies in animals
affected with this condition showed that the animals had had a
bovine syncytial virus infection during the period of disease.

INCIDENCE OF BRONCHOPNEUMONIA OF YEARLINGS

In the Netherlands, bronchopneumonia of yearlings occurs
particularly during the autumn months, the incidence being
highest in October and November. The symptoms are most severe
during the period in which the disease is most common. Cases
of bronchopneumonia of yearlings also occur in the spring but
they are not so common during this period. Young calves are
affected from approximately three months to twelve to fifteen
months of age. In large herds in which the disease recurs
annually, those animals which are still under twelve months of
age are invariably affected.

When an inquiry was conducted on twenty-four fattening bull
farms including a total number of almost 2 500 young animals,

stock owners acquainted with the clinical picture and believing
they could identify it, reported that bronchopneumonia of yearlings occurred on twenty-three farms (96%) during the autumn of
1975. Stock owners on seventeen farms of this group (71%)
described the condition in terms of 'severely sick animals' and
'in very serious trouble'. On the six other farms, the disease
was described as 'being mildly ill'. On the farms on which the
inquiry was conducted, a total number of twenty-six animals
died and eight animals were disposed of prematurely during the
outbreak.

CLINICAL SYMPTOMS AND COURSE

The severity of the symptoms may vary markedly. The
disease usually occurs in herds and the onset is marked by
coughing. Conjunctivitis accompanied by lachrymation is
usually observed during the first stage. Affected animals
develop systemic disease within two to seven days. There is
loss of appetite, activity diminishes and the respiration rate
increases. A number of animals have fever which may vary from
a slight rise in temperature to one of 41°C. The cough also
increases. There is slight serous rhinorrhoea and inspection
shows that the nasal mucosa presents an even red appearance.
Salivation may occur. Increased vesicular respiration is
frequently perceptible on auscultation and bronchial respiration
is heard in a small number of animals, being discernible in the
region of the apical pulmonary lobes in every case.

When the disease runs a favourable course, improvement will
appear within one or two days, the animals become more active,
appetite increases and the respiration rate shows a decrease.
As a rule, the cough persists for a few days. When the course
is not so satisfactory, the clinical picture is marked by
changes such as those associated with fog fever. The respiration
rate may increase to over one hundred. Moreover, moist rales
and occasional crepitation may be heard. Subsequently, expiration
becomes dyspnoeic, in which case the respiration rate decreases
again and respiration assumes an abdominal character. Severely

ill animals extend their necks and show latero-cranial displacement of the shoulders. Expiration may be accompanied by moaning. There is foam about the mouth, with an admixture of blood in some cases. This severe picture terminates in death in a number of cases.

In other patients, improvement occurs within two to five days after the onset of the second stage of the disease. Breathing becomes easier, the appetite increases and the outward appearance shows few peculiar features. Changes such as moist rales, crepitation and bronchial respiration continue to be perceptible on ausculation for a few days. Cough will persist for several days.

In those cases in which housing is unsatisfactory from the point of view of ventilation, a more chronic picture of interstitial pneumonia may develop, which is marked by abdominal respiration. When the house climate has been improved or the animals are at pasture, this lesion will disappear wholly or in part.

Morbidity in herds affected with bronchopneumonia of yearlings ranges from 80 to 100%. Rarely, only a single animal is affected. Mortality varies. It may be confined to a single animal but may be from 10 to 20% of the herd in other cases.

In young calves under approximately four months of age, few, if any, symptoms of fog fever are observed during outbreaks of bronchopneumonia of yearlings. There is some suggestion, however, that when bronchopneumonia occurs in the older calves, there is a relatively higher incidence than usual of pneumonia in young calves. The majority of patients are cases of pleuropneumonia.

Symptoms such as those described in the present paper as occurring in bronchopneumonia of yearlings were also reported by Wellemans and Leunen (1975) in bovine respiratory syncytial virus infection in young cattle. They reported symptoms of fog fever, which may rapidly terminate in death in some cases.

POST-MORTEM FINDINGS

Morbid-anatomical changes are confined to the respiratory tract. The lungs of animals which died during the acute stage, are voluminous and heavy. They collapse completely. The pleurae are smooth and glossy. Subpleural emphysema is occasionally perceptible through the pleurae; it often is evenly distributed but may also appear as bullae. In some cases, it is associated with extensive breakdown of pulmonary tissue. For the rest, the cut surface of the lung tissue shows a variegation of colours ranging from yellowish white to deep red.

Lobar catarrhal bronchopneumonia presenting a greyish red appearance is usually present in the apical and cardiac lobes.

In addition to these lesions, atypical interstitial pneumonia marked by lobular involvement and considerable oedema in the interstitial tissues may be observed in large portions of the bodies of the lungs and other portions of the small lobes.

Inflammatory signs are absent or only slight in the deeper parts of the respiratory tract.

On the other hand, diffuse haemorrhage and, in some cases, slightly foamy contents and blood clots are frequently observed in the trachea and bronchi of animals which have died.

In cases running an acute course, bacteriological studies are invariably negative.

SEROLOGICAL STUDIES

In 1973 and 1974, serological studies for the presence of infection with respiratory viruses were done on a number of farms during outbreaks of bronchopneumonia of yearlings. On

these farms, blood samples were collected from animals of
affected herds during the acute stage as well as three weeks
or longer after. The paired blood samples were examined for
complement-fixing antibodies to a number of viruses believed
to be possible causes of respiratory disease in cattle.

Specifically: bovine respiratory syncytial (BRS) virus,
para-influenza virus 3 (PI3), bovine virus diarrhoea virus
(BVD) as well as bovine adenoviruses serotypes 1 to 3 inclusive
and 4 to 10 inclusive (B Ad V_1 and B Ad V_4 respectively). In
1974, studies were also done for chlamydial infection (Chlam.).

Serological studies for the presence of infectious bovine
rhinotracheitis (IBR) virus were not done as there was no
clinical evidence to suggest that this infection was present
on the farms concerned.

The studies included thirty-three cases of bronchopneumonia
of yearlings, namely twenty-three on dairy farms on which calves
were reared, seven on calf-rearing farms and three on fattening-
bull farms. The diseased animals were from four to eleven
months of age.

Table 1 shows the number of significant increases in titre,
which occurred during the period in which the symptoms also
appeared.

Of the toal group of 292 animals, 76% were positive for BRS
virus infection.

On twenty-eight farms, at least 50% of the animals studied
showed a significant increase in titre, or 211 out of 256
animals. That is 82%.

Of the five other farms, a serological response positive
for BRS was observed in less than 50% of the animals studied,
namely in twelve out of thirty-six animals (33%).

TABLE 1

RESULTS OF SEROLOGICAL EXAMINATIONS ON A NUMBER OF FARMS WITH 'PINKENGRIEP'

Farm	Number of animals examined	BRS	PI3	BVD	BAdV1	BAdV4	CHALAM
1973							
1	17	11*	16	10	5	4	-
2	4	3*	1	1	1	1	-
3	3	2*	O	O	O	2	-
4	4	3*	O	1	O	O	-
5	8	6*	O	O	1	1	-
6	10	4	8	O	1	4	-
7	11	10*	4	O	O	O	-
8	5	5*	2	O	O	O	-
9	6	3*	O	1	1	O	-
10	10	10*	10	O	1	2	-
11	4	2*	O	O	O	1	-
12	12	7*	3	O	1	O	-
13	4	4*	1	O	O	O	-
14	6	6*	O	O	O	O	-
15	4	3*	O	O	O	O	-
16	13	13*	12	3	1	3	-
1974							
17	8	7*	6	1	2	O	O
18	21	11*	13	1	2	3	1+
19	8	7*	O	O	2	2	O
20	10	8*	5	O	3	2	1
21	4	4*	2	O	O	O	O
22	7	3	7	O	O	O	O
23	6	5*	4	O	3	1	O
24	5	1	O	1	O	O	1
25	7	7*	O	O	1	O	O
26	9	7*	O	O	1	1	O
27	6	6*	6	1	O	O	1
28	25	25*	17	10	5	1	6
29	20	18*	2	4	O	O	-
30	13	11*	11	1	1	1	1
31	7	3	1	1	O	O	1
32	7	1	O	1	1	3	2
33	8	7*	8	1	2	O	O
Total	292	223	139	38	35	32	14
in %	100	76	48	13	12	11	10

* Serologically significant reaction detected in at least half of the animals

+ Eight animals were tested for Chlamydia infection on these premises.

A number of animals on these five farms had already shown positive titres in the first sera, namely fourteen out of thirty-six (39%). The samples in question may have been taken when infection had been present for some time.

The virus neutralisation test, performed as a plaque reduction test, is a more sensitive method of detecting anti-bodies to BRS virus than is the complement fixation test. On some farms on which the neutralisation test was also performed, the number of significant increases in titre using this test was larger than that observed when the complement fixation test was used so that the 82 and 76% recorded probably are an unduly low estimate of the actual number of serological responses.

Increases in titre on testing for PI3 virus were also relatively common during outbreaks of bronchopneumonia of yearlings. In fourteen out of thirty-three herds, a significant increase in titre in regard to this virus was observed in at least 50% of the animals, increases in titre being absent on twelve farms. On five of the latter farms, there was no evidence whatever to suggest that PI3 infection was present in the animals studied. That is to say, there were neither increases in titre nor any high initial titres at the time at which the first samples were taken. A number of increases in titre were observed in the animals on the seven other farms, namely in fourteen out of sixty-three animals (22%). Of the total number of 292 animals on the thirty-three farms, 139 (48%) responded with an increase in titre.

Only on a single farm, did more than 50% of the animals show an increase in titre on testing for BVD virus. The total number of animals showing a significant increase in titre to this agent was thirty-eight (13%).

When B Ad V_1 and B Ad V_4 antigens were used, a significant increase in titre was observed in thirty-five and thirty-two cases respectively (12 and 11% respectively). In fourteen cases, there was a significant increase in titre to the two antigens. Of 138 animals tested for antibodies to Chlamydia, fourteen (10%) showed a significant increase in titre.

VIROLOGICAL STUDIES

In 1974, there was an opportunity to try and isolate virus from the nasal secretions and pharyngeal mucus during a number of outbreaks of bronchopneumonia of yearlings.

This was done on farms, 18, 28 and 33 (Table 1). On farm 18, PI3 virus was isolated from the pharyngeal mucus in six out of ten animals from which samples were taken.

On farm 28, samples of pharyngeal mucus were taken from thirteen animals and nasal secretions from twelve animals. PI3 virus was isolated from one sample of pharyngeal mucus and BRS virus from another. Four samples of nasal secretions contained BRS virus on the first day on which symptoms of bronchopneumonia of yearlings were observed in the group.

CONCLUSION

In conclusion we may state: All the young cattle became infected and sometimes a second infection is noticed.

The first infection usually occurs in the autumn when the animals have been more or less adequately housed, and is accompanied by bronchopneumonia . At this time most of the animals are 4 - 12 months old, and these animals are called 'Pinken'. The disease can be indentified clinically only when it takes a particular course. The pneumonias occurring in these animals are atypical interstitial pneumonias.

REFERENCE

Wellemans, G. and Leunen, J. 1975. Annls. med. Vet. 119, p. 359.

EPIDEMIOLOGY OF RESPIRATORY DISEASES IN CALVES IN 1977 IN THE WEST OF FRANCE

C. Le Jan and A. Asso

Station de Recherches de Virologie et d'Immunologie, INRA,
Thiverval-Grignon 78850, France.

ABSTRACT

From 100 nasal swabs obtained from claves with respiratory disease we were able to recover about 10 IBR strains at the first passage in primary cultures of embryo calf kidney.

In a few other cases, nasal swabs from adults were also found with IBR virus. Very often we found in the same swabs, not only specific antibodies neutralising IBR, but also the virus.

In about 50% of the samples there were only antibodies (or neutralising activity) against IBR in the mucus.

In no case did we find antibodies against BVD.

It seems than an animal can harbour virus in the nasal cavities and have a pulmonary disorder from some other origin (intoxication by fungus).

Sometimes we have found by electron microscopic examination not only herpes virus but also small viruses (rhinovirus, togavirus) which may be more difficult to propagate in tissue culture.

From two large cooperatives in the west of France, we have obtained two hundred sera and nasal mucus samples from calves one week to three months old. These two associations obtained over thirty thousand animals which were allocated to two hundred calf rearing establishments. These animals developed respiratory disease with a mortality rate over 10%. Morbidity level was 80%.

Nasal mucus and sera were inactivated at 56°C for thirty minutes and, after dilution (1/5 for nasal mucus, 1/100 for sera) were used to neutralise 100 and 1000 $TCID_{50}$ infectious bovine rhinotracheitis (IBR) virus and bovine virus diarrhoea (BVD) virus. The mixtures were incubated at 37°C: twelve to eighteen hours for IBR virus, one hour for BVD virus. We then looked for residual virus on MDBK cells.

Before inactivation we also looked for presence of viruses in nasal swabs on calf kidney cells.

RESULTS FOR PRESENCE OF ANTIBODIES IN SERUM

A fortnight after the first serum sample, we usually received a second sample from the same animals.

In the first samples, colostral antibodies against IBR virus were very often high; in the second sample, we observed an increase of the neutralising activity in about 70% of animals. In these cooperatives we have not observed seroconversion or nasal antibodies against BVD virus.

MUCUS SAMPLES

Before inactivation these were inoculated to monolayers of calf kidney cells. Cytopathic effect was observed several times, and in ten samples, IBR virus was identified by electron microscopy and neutralisation.

In these mucus samples, after heating, we found neutralising activity against IBR virus. So, antibodies and virus coexist together in nasal mucus and exposure to 56°C is enough to inactivate the virus.

Recent infection is manifested in nasal mucus by the presence of local antibodies. There is a good correlation between seroconversion and local antibodies, but with nasal mucus, one sample is enough for diagnosis, whereas paired serum samples are necessary to make a diagnosis.

The results of examinations on four different farms are summarised in Table 1.

We can say that the presence of local antibodies in the first sample is sufficient to indicate a recent infection by IBR virus. This conclusion is supported by results of experimental infection of calves with IBR virus by nasal route: local antibodies appear at day four, and disappear at day fourteen.

When we have observed the cultures inoculated with nasal mucus samples by electron microscopy, very often we saw not only the large and easy to identify IBR virus, but also many other particles, which could have been rhinoviruses, enteroviruses, BVD virus. From time to time we found paramyxoviruses. In these circumstances it is difficult to decide which is the important agent. When we tested different pairs of sera against several pathogenic agents like IBR virus, BVD virus, reoviruses, adenoviruses, respiratory syncytial virus, parainfluenza 3 virus, chlamydia, very often a seroconversion against several agents occurred simultaneously.

The choice of agents used for diagnostic tests limits the number of possible answers, and it is impossible to look for all viruses, bacteria and mycoplasma which are involved in this kind of respiratory trouble.

TABLE 1

	Number of samples	Isolation of IBR virus	Neutralising antibodies in the first sample	Neutralising antibodies in the second sample	Conclusions (diagnosis)
1st Farm	6	On two calves	Nasal antibodies > 100 Serum antibodies 10 to 100	Nasal antibodies 0 to 10 Serum antibodies > 100	Infection by IBR virus
2nd Farm	6	0̅	Nasal antibodies > 100 Serum antibodies 0 to 100	Nasal antibodies 0 to 10 Serum antibodies > 100	Infection by IBR virus
3rd Farm	6	0̅	Nasal antibodies > 100 Serum antibodies 0 to 10	Nasal antibodies 0 to 10 Serum antibodies > 100	Infection by IBR virus
4th Farm	6	0̅	Nasal antibodies 0 to 10 Serum antibodies 0 to >100	Nasal antibodies 0 to 10 Serum antibodies 0 to 10	No infection by IBR virus

As soon as a sample is cultivated, there is some kind of selection which favours the virus which is the most able to grow in vitro and, maybe, eliminates the true pathogen. There are also some problems associated with direct examination of nasal swabs, such as the small amount of virus in some samples.

THE ROLE OF VIRUSES IN ACUTE RESPIRATORY DISEASE OF CATTLE

E. J. Stott, L.H. Thomas, A.P. Collins,
S. Hamilton, J. Jebbett and P.D. Luther.
Agricultural Research Council, Institute for Research on
Animal Diseases, Compton, Newbury, England.

ABSTRACT

*During a three year survey of respiratory disease in young cattle on
a large beef farm, 539 virus infections were diagnosed. Parainfluenza-virus
type 3 (PI3) accounted for 135 infections, respiratory syncytial virus
(RSV) for 78, rhinovirus type 1 for 102, mucosal disease virus for 49,
adenoviruses for 29, reoviruses for 53, enteroviruses for 88 and unidentified
viruses for 5. Six outbreaks of respiratory disease occurred during the
survey. Only RSV, PI3 and, to a lesser degree, rhinovirus infections
were significantly associated with disease.*

*Fifteen calves were experimentally infected with PI3 and 15 with RSV
but clinical signs were not detected and the mean disease score of infected
animals was similar to that of 36 control animals held under the same
conditions.*

*An inactivated vaccine was prepared in order to determine whether the
association between PI3 and disease was a causal one. Small trials on 61
animals showed that this vaccine protected 70% to 100% of calves against
experimental PI3 infection. This vaccine was then used during two winters
on the same large beef farm. A total of 267 animals were vaccinated and
320 calves remained as unvaccinated controls. Respiratory disease was
detected in 15.4% of the vaccinated animals and in 9.1% of the controls.
Thus, a vaccine which reduced the incidence of PI3 infection did not reduce
the incidence of disease.*

*These results suggest that, although PI3 infection occurs during out-
breaks of disease, it may not be an important cause of that disease. The
role of RSV remains to be assessed.*

INTRODUCTION

Viruses were first isolated from the respiratory tract of cattle in the late 1950's (Madin et al., 1956; Reisinger et al., 1959; Klein et al., 1959). Despite almost 20 years of investigation the basic question of whether or not these viruses are the major cause of respiratory disease in the field remains largely unanswered.

If viruses are an important cause of bovine respiratory disease it should be possible to show that:

1) In epidemiological surveys, virus infections are detected significantly more often during outbreaks of disease than at other times.

2) In experimental studies, viruses which are significantly associated with disease reproduce that disease when inoculated into susceptible animals under appropriate conditions.

3) Vaccines which protect against such virus infections significantly reduce the incidence of disease in the field.

This paper presents recent data on these three aspects of the role of viruses in respiratory disease.

EPIDEMIOLOGICAL SURVEY

A survey was carried out on a large beef progeny testing farm between October, 1972 and September, 1975. Calves under 10 days old were collected from farms all over England and reared in groups of 80 - 100 animals until slaughter 12 to 18 months later. Detailed records were kept of their health and performance. Eight animals in each group were studied virologically. Nasopharyngeal swabs and blood were collected from the same eight animals every three weeks until they were eight months old. The swabs were examined for viruses by inoculation into cell cultures of calf kidney and calf testis. Sera were tested for antibodies to parainfluenzavirus type 3 (PI3),

respiratory syncytial virus (RSV), mucosal disease (MDV),
rhinovirus type 1 (RV) and reovirus type 1 (REO). Whenever
possible ·swabs were also collected from animals treated for
respiratory disease.

The results of the survey indicated that 1 590 calves
entered the farm, 354 (22.2%) required treatment for respiratory
disease and 41 (2.5%) died with extensive pneumonia. Most of
the respiratory disease (66%) occurred in the first four months
of life; only 2.5% was seen in calves over nine months of age.
Over 90% of all respiratory disease was detected during six
outbreaks in November 1972, April and October 1973, February
and December 1974 and March 1975.

Virus infections were diagnosed either by isolation of virus
or by demonstration of a fourfold or greater rise in antibody
titre in consecutive sera. The animals sampled routinely
yielded 194 viruses from 958 swabs and 326 infections were
diagnosed serologically from 1 058 serum samples (Table 1).

TABLE 1

VIRUS INFECTIONS DIAGNOSED - OCTOBER, 1972 - SEPTEMBER, 1975

Number samples examined	Routine animals			Treated Animals Swabs 185	Total
	Swabs 958	Sera 1058	Both 2016		
No. positive for indicated virus.					
PI3	61	72	108*	27	135
RSV	5	69	74	4	78
RV	18	83	96+	6	102
MDV	0	49	49	0	49
AD	22	ND	22	7	29
REO	0	53	53	0	53
ENT	83	ND	83	5	88
Untyped	5	ND	5	0	5
All viruses	194	326	490	49	539

AD = Adenovirus (1 strain was type 2, the remainder were type 3)

ENT = Enterovirus

* Includes 25 infections diagnosed from both swabs and sera

+ Includes 5 infections diagnosed from both swabs and sera.

There were 30 calves in which infection was diagnosed
both by virus isolation and serology. Therefore, a total of
490 separate virus infections were diagnosed by routine sampling.
A further 49 viruses were isolated from 185 swabs collected
from animals being treated for respiratory disease. Infections
most commonly diagnosed were PI3 (135), RV (102), enterovirus
(88) and RSV (78). Infectious bovine rhinotracheitis virus
was not isolated.

The significance of these virus infections in relation to
disease was assessed by comparing the number of infections
diagnosed during months in which the six outbreaks of disease
occurred with those diagnosed during the remainder of the survey
(Table 2).

TABLE 2

SIGNIFICANCE OF VIRUS INFECTIONS IN RESPIRATORY DISEASE.

	Number during survey	Number during outbreaks	% during outbreaks	Probability
Investigations	847	181	21.4	–
Virus infections diagnosed				
PI3	108	41	38.0	< 0.001
RSV	74	43	58.1	< 0.001
RV	96	29	30.2	< 0.05
MD	49	9	18.4	> 0.5
AD	22	5	22.7	> 0.98
REO	53	15	28.3	> 0.2
ENT	83	14	16.9	> 0.2

Treated animals were excluded from this comparison because
no serology was available. The routine survey comprised 847
investigations of calves for virus infections, 181 (21.4%) of
these were during outbreaks of respiratory disease.

If, therefore, virus infections occurred at random and were
unrelated to respiratory disease, 21.4% of them would be
expected to occur during outbreaks of disease. The observations
in Table 2 show that the percentages of MDV, AD, REO and ENT

infections which occurred during outbreaks of disease were not
statistically significantly different from the expected value
of 21.4%. In contrast, 38.0% of PI3 infections and 58.1% of
RSV infections were detected during outbreaks and the difference
between these values and the expected 21.4 was highly significant
at the 0.1% level. Rhinovirus infections were also found
significantly more often during outbreaks than expected but at a
higher probability (P <0.05).

This survey, therefore, indicated that PI3, RSV and, to
a lesser extent, RV infections are significantly associated
with outbreaks of respiratory disease. The survey did not,
and was not intended to, prove that these viruses cause disease;
such infections may result from disease. The survey did, however, indicate those viruses which deserved further investigation and on this basis PI3 and RSV were selected for
experimental inoculation into calves.

EXPERIMENTAL INFECTION

Experimental infections were carried out in a series of
carefully controlled trials based on methods developed at the
Common Cold Unit, Salisbury, for work on respiratory viruses of
man (Tyrrell, 1963; Thomas et al., 1977). Calves aged between
two and six months were isolated in groups of three in pens
10 metres apart. The isolation conditions reduced the
introduction of extraneous infections from outside the trial
and eliminated cross-infection between calves within the trial.
The animals were examined daily, before and for 21 days after
inoculation, by a clinician who was unaware which animals were
given virus and which were uninfected controls. Clinical signs
were scored and calculations, based on observations before and
after infection, gave an illness score and grade for each
animal.

A strain of PI3 which was isolated during an outbreak of
respiratory disease and passed only in organ cultures of bovine
foetal trachea to prevent attenuation was inoculated

intranasally into 15 calves. All these animals showed a
significant antibody response to PI3 and virus was recovered
from their nasopharynx, often in high titre (up to 10^7 p.f.u/ml).
There was no evidence of PI3 infection in 9 control animals in
the same trial. Serological studies during the trial revealed
no evidence of infection by either RSV or MDV in any of the
calves.

Clinically, the infected animals remained healthy throughout the trial (Table 3). The mean illness score of the
infected calves was 14.9 which was not significantly different
from the score of 10.9 for the control animals. None of the
24 calves had any clinical reaction since all were graded as
subclinical.

TABLE 3

EXPERIMENTAL INFECTION OF CALVES WITH PARAINFLUENZAVIRUS TYPE 3

Infection	Number of calves	Illness			Mean score
		Grade			
		Subclinical	Mild	Moderate	
PI3	15	15	0	0	14.9
None	9	9	0	0	10.9
Total	24	24	0	0	-

Respiratory syncytial virus was used in two similar trials
involving 42 calves. Fifteen animals were infected as judged
by recovery of virus from their nasopharynx, detection of a
significant antibody response, or both. There were no antibody
responses to either PI3 or MDV during these two trials,
indicating that these viruses were absent.

Clinically, there was no evidence that RSV infection
produced disease (Table 4). The mean illness score of 9.6 for
infected animals was not significantly different from the 9.1
for control calves. The only significant clinical response was
in one control animal which was graded as a mild reaction.

TABLE 4

EXPERIMENTAL INFECTION OF CALVES WITH RESPIRATORY SYNCYTIAL VIRUS

Infection	Number of calves	Illness			
		Grade			Mean score
		Subclinical	Mild	Moderate	
RSV	15	15	0	0	9.6
None	27	26	1	0	9.3
Total	42	41	1	0	-

Despite the significant association between the occurrence of PI3 and RSV infections and respiratory disease in the field, there was no evidence that experimental infection reproduced that disease. In order to resolve these apparently conflicting results, a vaccine which protected calves against PI3 infection was developed and used in the field to assess its effect on the incidence of disease.

VACCINE TRIALS

The experimental PI3 infection described above was used as a challenge to assess the protection induced by an inactivated vaccine. Trials on 61 animals showed that this vaccine produced high antibody levels and, depending on the immunisation schedule, protected 70% to 100% of calves against PI3 infection (Probert et al., 1978).

A field trial of this vaccine was then conducted on the same farm on which the epidemiological survey had been conducted. Three groups of animals aged 1 to 5½ months were vaccinated twice during September, 1975. Serum samples collected before, and three weeks after, the second vaccination indicated that 98% of the oldest animals and 40% of the youngest groups responded to the vaccine (Table 5). After vaccination all three groups had a mean single radial haemolysis zone area of greater than 50 mm^2. Only one control animal had an antibody response to PI3 indicating that natural infections with this virus were rare during the period of vaccination. In September, 1976 a further three groups of animals were vaccinated in a similar manner; but serum samples were only collected from the oldest group. These showed that 98% of calves had responded to the vaccine. However, the finding that 19% of the control animals also had a significant increase in antibody to PI3 indicated that natural infections had occurred on the farm before vaccination was completed (Table 5).

TABLE 5

RESPONSE TO PARAINFLUENZAVIRUS TYPE 3 VACCINATION

Group	Age in months	Number of calves	Mean Area* Pre	Mean Area* Post	Number with+ antibody rise
1975					
1 Vacc		45	2.7	59.3	44 (98%)
Con	5½	53	1.4	O	O
2 Vacc		36	18.9	50.9	28 (78%)
Con	3	42	19.5	7.2	1
3 Vacc		48	55.8	55.5	19 (40%)
Con	1	55	57.4	35.7	O
1976					
4 Vacc		46	24.8	108.8	45 (98%)
Con	5½	52	24.7	27.3	10 (19%)
5 Vacc		48	ND		ND
Con	3	57			
6 Vacc		44			
Con	1	59	ND		ND

* Single radial haemolysis (SRH) zone area in mm^2 before (pre) and three weeks after (post) vaccination.

+ An increase in SRH zone area of $\geq 10mm^2$ indicated a significant antibody response.

The history of the animals during the winter after vaccination in September, 1975 indicates that the incidence of PI3 infections was reduced from 78% in control calves to 42.6% in vaccinated animals (Table 6). However, there was no corresponding decrease in the incidence of respiratory disease. Although the incidence of PI3 infection in 1976-77 winter was not determined, there was again no evidence that vaccination against PI3 reduced the occurrence of respiratory disease.

TABLE 6

HISTORY OF CALVES AFTER PARAINFLUENZAVIRUS TYPE 3 VACCINATION

Group	Number of calves	PI3 infections		Treatments+	
		Number	%	Number	%
1975-76					
Vacc	129	55	42.6	21 (1)*	16.3
Con	150	117	78.0	15 (3)	10.0
1976-77					
Vacc	138	ND		20 (0)	14.5
Con	168	ND		14 (2)	8.3

+ Treatments were for respiratory disease

* Figures in parenthesis indicate deaths from pneumonia.

DISCUSSION AND CONCLUSIONS

The isolation of PI3 and, more recently, RSV from cattle
during outbreaks of respiratory disease has been reported on
many occasions (see review by Phillip and Darbyshire, 1971;
Paccaud and Jacquier, 1970; Wellemans et al., 1970; Jacobs and
Edington, 1971). However, the significance of these observations
was difficult to assess because the distribution of these viruses
in healthly animals was not known. The survey described above
has shown that, although infections with PI3 and RSV were
detected in the absence of disease, there was a statistically
significant correlation between the occurrence of these viruses
and outbreaks of respiratory disease.

Experimental infection of calves with either PI3 or RSV
have given variable results. In some experiments animals
developed pyrexia, leukopenia and pneumonia, whereas in others
disease was mild or absent (Frank and Marshall, 1973; Jacobs
and Edington, 1975: Mohanty et al., 1975). There may be many
reasons for these variable results: the bias of the clinical
observer, the age and immune status of the calf, the route of

inoculation, the history and titre of the virus, or simultaneous infection of the calf with other agents. The latter is a particular problem when inocula are grown in bovine tissue cultures which are frequently infected with non-cytopathic mucosal disease virus (Nuttall et al., 1977). The problem of reproducing disease experimentally is that the causative agent may only produce symptoms 'under appropriate conditions' and until the pathogenesis of the disease is fully understood the 'appropriate conditions' are unknown. Thus, our failure to produce disease in animals infected with either PI3 or RSV is disappointing but is not strong evidence against their causal role in respiratory disease.

Vaccines containing PI3 antigen have been in use for many years. However, controlled field trials of monovalent PI3 vaccines in Britain have rarely been described. The vaccine trial described above clearly shows that a significant reduction of PI3 infection was not accompanied by a reduction in disease. This observation indicates that PI3 was not the major cause of the disease.

In conclusion, our field survey provided no evidence that mucosal disease virus, adenoviruses or reoviruses were sign-ificantly associated with respiratory disease. Furthermore, the vaccine trial suggested that, although PI3 was associated with disease, it was not a major cause. In the light of these findings, the value of incorporating these viral antigens into bovine respiratory vaccines must be questioned. Further research with vaccines against RSV is required to define the role of this virus in respiratory disease of cattle.

ACKNOWLDEGEMENTS

We thank the staff of the Milk Marketing Board's beef progeny testing station at Warren Farm for their co-operation. We are also grateful to Dr. M. Probert and Wellcome Research Laboratories for help with the vaccine trials.

REFERENCES

Frank, G.H. and Marshall, R.G. 1973. J. Am. vet. med. Ass. 163, p. 858.

Jacobs, J.W. and Edington, N. 1971. Vet. Rec. 88, p. 694.

Jacobs, J.W. and Edington, N. 1975. Res. vet. Sci. 18, p. 299.

Klein, N., Earley, E. and Zellat, J. 1959. Proc. Soc. exp. Biol. Med. 102 p.1.

Madin, S.H., York, C.J. and McKercher, D.G. 1956. Science 124, p. 721.

Mohanty, S.B., Ingling, A.L. and Lillie, M.G. 1975. Am. J. vet. Res. 36, p. 417.

Nuttall, P.A., Luther, P.D. and Stott, E.J. 1977. Nature 266, p. 835.

Paccaud, M.F. and Jacquier, Cl. 1970. Arch. ges. Virusforsch. 30, p. 327.

Phillip, J.I.H and Darbyshire, J.H. 1971. Ad. vet. Sci. comp. Med. 15 p. 159.

Probert, M., Stott, E.J., Thomas, L.H. Collins, A.P. and Jebbett, J. 1978. Res. vet. Sci. (In press).

Reisinger, R.C., Heddleston, K.L. and Manthei, C.A. 1959. J. Am. vet. Med. Ass. 135, p. 147.

Thomas, L.H., Stott, E.J., Collins, A.P., Jebbett, N.J. and Stark, A.J. 1977. Res. Vet. Sci. 23, p. 157.

Tyrrell, D.A.J. 1963. Am. Rev. resp. Dis 88, Supplement, p. 128.

Wellemans, G., Leunen, J. and Luchsinger, E. 1970. Annls, Med. Vet. 114, p. 89.

THE ROLE OF VIRUSES AS AETIOLOGIC AGENTS FOR RESPIRATORY DISEASES IN CATTLE

O.C. Straub*

Federal Research Institute for Animal Virus Diseases.
D 7400 Tübingen, Germany.

ABSTRACT

In connection with respiratory diseases in cattle numerous viral agents were found to be involved, mainly IBR-, RSV, BVD-MD-, PI2, PI3, Adeno, Reo-, and Rhinoviruses. From those only IBR-virus, however, will regularly cause disease following an experimental inoculation. BVD-MD-virus inoculations are usually followed by a mild disease occurring only in a proportion of animals. The other viruses - except RSV perhaps - seem to act as precursors since they, in general, do not cause sickness after inoculation. Fungi, yeasts, mycoplasmas, chlamydiae and many bacterial agents act as secondary or synergistic agents. Any combination of agents seems to be possible. In spite of this it is possible to lower the incidence of diseases other than IBR- or BVD-MD by prophylactic treatments with live or attenuated vaccines. Numerous mono-and multivalent preparations are available. After the outbreak of disease, however, besides treatment with conventional drugs, only the application of live vaccines or interferon inducers is possible.

* Part of this work has been conducted in collaboration with Prof. Dr. H. Woernle, Stuttgart, and Dr. H. Geilhausen, Cologne.

INTRODUCTION

During acute outbreaks of respiratory disease in cattle
numerous viral agents have been isolated. The distribution of
these agents seems to be different in the various countries of
the European Community. Respiratory syncytial virus, for
example, is obviously widespread in some countries and not
present in others. Lately, outbreaks of infectious bovine
rhinotracheitis have more frequently occurred in the Federal
Republic of Germany than in the past. In the following this
disease is not included since it can be separated from the
disease complex called enzootic bronchopneumonia of cattle
('Rindergrippe'). The symptoms of infectious bovine rhinotracheitis are striking and inoculation of susceptible cattle
with recovered agents always leads to disease, whereas cattle
inoculated with the other agents recovered from cases of
bronchopneumonia hardly show any clinical symptoms. A seroconversion is in general the only proof of a successful
infection.

In the studies reported it was tried to identify besides
viruses other agents present at the time of illness in the
respiratory tract and subsequently a number of animal experiments
were conducted.

MATERIALS AND METHODS

On 37 occasions samples from 198 sick animals belonging to
15 herds located in 4 States were taken. Nasal swabs were
collected from all animals, paired blood samples from a
substantial number (see Tables). Swabs and serum were tested
using conventional methods. For the tissue culture studies
calf kidney and calf testicle cells incubated at 37 and 32°C
were used. In the serological evaluation increasing antibody
titres were taken as evidence for a recent infection with the
specific agent, decreasing ones as colostral antibodies.

RESULTS

No viruses were recovered from the swabs. The indirect proof by serological methods is demonstrated in Table 1.

TABLE 1

RESULTS OF SEROLOGICAL EXAMINATIONS:

1.1. Increasing titres			
Virus	No. of samples	Positive	Percentage
REO I	35	7	20
REO III	35	O	O
MD/VD	60	19	32
ADENO (Types 4 and 8)	60	8	13
PI2	60	11	18
PI3	60	2	3
RSV	35	O	O
1.2. Decreasing titres			
Virus	No. of samples	Positive	Percentage
REO I	38	8	21
REO III	35	O	O
MD/VD	70	3	4
ADENO (Types 4 and 8)	70	4	5
PI2	60	11	18
PI3	52	42	80
RSV	35	O	O
(IBR-IPV	62	12	19)

An active antibody production against chlamydiae was found in 1 of 35 samples (3%), colostral antibodies had 6 from 70 samples (8%).

Mycoplasmas were isolated in 36 from 144 swabs checked (25%). A differentiation was not performed. The result of the bacterial test is summarised in Table 2.

244

TABLE 2

RESULTS OF BACTERIAL EXAMINATIONS

Agent	No. of samples	Positive	Percentage
Pasteurella	86	35	40
Streptococci	56	26	46
Staphylococci	56	3	5
Achromobacter	56	1	2
E. coli	56	3	5
Polybacterial growth	29	16	55

Fourteen swabs were also checked for the presence of yeasts and fungi. In 13 (93%) one or more of them were found: 5 x aspergillums, 1 x mucor, 2 x aspergillums plus mucor, 1 x aspergillums plus penicilliums, 1 x penicilliums plus mucor; 1 x penicillium, and 2 x aspergillums plus candida albicans.

In Table 3 a summary of the combinations of the various agents found in individual animals except fungi and yeasts is presented.

EXPERIMENTAL WORK

Eight animals were intranasally inoculated with a field strain of PI3 virus. All of them shed virus. The maximum was 7 days. They also showed a slight temperature elevation, but unless checked the animals would have been considered as normals. The same happened in three animals after inoculation with rhinovirus. This virus has been neglected in the serological studies reported above. If rhinovirus was, however, inoculated into the mammary gland, a mastitis developed.

Then 8 animals were inoculated (intranasally plus intravenously) with Mucosal Disease / Virus Diarrhoea virus. Virus could be reisolated until Day 14, a double rise in temperature (average 5th and 10th day p.i.) and a drop in the number of leukocytes was observed. But those animals would also have been considered as normals without a careful checkup.

TABLE 3

COMBINATIONS OF AGENTS FOUND IN CASES OF ENZOOTIC BRONCHOPNEUMONIA

	Viruses			Other agents		
REO I	Mucosal disease			Bacteria		Mycoplasmas
	Mucosal disease	PI2		Bacteria		Mycoplasmas
		PI2	PI3	Bacteria		Mycoplasmas
				Bacteria		Mycoplasmas
	Mucosal disease	PI2				Mycoplasmas
		PI2	PI3			Mycoplasmas
		PI2				Mycoplasmas
			PI3			Mycoplasmas
	Mucosal disease			Bacteria	Chlamydiae	
REO I	Mucosal disease			Bacteria		
REO I		PI2		Bacteria		
REO I			PI3	Bacteria		
REO I			Adeno	Bacteria		
	Mucosal disease		Adeno	Bacteria		
	Mucosal disease			Bacteria		
			Adeno	Bacteria		

THERAPEUTIC MEASURES

When clincial symptoms have been observed in a herd it is too late to administer inactivated vaccines. The latter are available in two different compositions. If outbreaks occur in spite of prophylactic vaccination a number of treatments have been carried out lately. Attenuated or avirulent PI3 vaccines are supposed to give satisfying results when applied after the first appearance of clinical symptoms. Injections of irradiated avian poxviruses are being tested lately. They are also given to sick animals.

Our own developments have led to an interferon inducer. This is an avirulent IPV virus which has lost its immunogenicity for IBR-IPV- in other words - animals treated with the inducer do not develop an immunity against the disease caused by the group of IBR-IPV viruses. It is administered intranasally to sick or exposed animals. Maximum interferon levels are generally detected on days 3 - 6 p.i. Until now some 30 000 animals have been treated. The animals should receive additional treatment with conventional drugs until the interferon levels have reached their maximum. Experiments have shown that in comparison to controls, animals pretreated with the interferon inducer shed less than 1% of FMD virus.

DISCUSSION

From our experimental work it can clearly be stated that many agents play an obviously important role as precursors for enzootic bronchopneumonia. There can also hardly be any doubt that no matter which vaccine is applied there will not be a 100% success. Therefore the environmental factors should be emphasised. This includes the building of quarantine and hospital sheds, proper hygienic and nutritional measures.

As to details reported the role of the PI2 virus is not understood yet. The low incidence of active antibody production against PI3 virus is due to the high incidence of positive adults. When PI3 vaccines are, in spite of this fact, of some value in treating sick animals it will be due to the interference phenomenon. Humoral antibodies do not completely inhibit virus multiplication in the superficial cell layers of the respiratory tract.

A pleasing answer cannot be given as to the role the mycoplasma organisms play. There are certainly some strains, like M. dispar, which may by themselves cause disease but the majority of strains requires also some disorders which then cause an explosion where nothing else can be found anymore but mycoplasmas.

After the recovery of the animals the 'normal' composition of microbiological agents including mycoplasmas is found. As far as Mucosal Disease virus is concerned it is surprising in how many cases of respiratory disease it is involved. Those animals never showed any symptoms of digestive disorders. The

low percentage of *E. coli* found supports this observation.
Therefore this virus should be incorporated in prophylactic
measures. The same is true for pasteurellas. The role of
these agents is also not fully understood. Their behaviour
resembles that of mycoplasmas.

Animal experiments with REO I, Adeno-, and PI2 virus have
not been conducted, but from other publications it is known
that at least Adeno- and REO-viruses do in general also not
lead to disease after inoculation. The application of
inactivated vaccines containing these antigens have led to a
decrease in incidence and severity of enzootic bronchopneumonia.
Therefore it seeems justified to further promote and perhaps
improve those vaccines, although it will always be difficult to
demonstrate their efficacy in experimental trials.

THE RESPIRATORY TROUBLES OF CATTLE IN BELGIUM

G. Wellemans, R. Strobbe and E. van Opdenbosch

Institut National de Recherches Vétérinaire,
Groeselenberg 99, 1180 Bruxelles, Belgium.

ASBTRACT

Paired sera of cattle from 500 herds, in which severe respiratory troubles had been observed, were examined.

As a result of this survey, four types of respiratory disease were distinguished:

1. The autumn respiratory disorders in which the RSB (Bovine Respiratory Syncytial virus) was present in more than half of the cases.

2. The springtime and summertime respiratory diseases in which no virus, except possibly IBR virus (Infectious Bovine Rhinotracheitis), seemed to play an important role.

3. The respiratory diseases due to transport (Shipping fever). In this complex, IBR is the principal agent and other viruses seemed to have no significant role.

4. The respiratory disorders of young beef cattle at 5 to 6 weeks of age. These troubles seemed to have a non-viral cause.

The two important cases (IBR and RSB) are succinctly described.

INTRODUCTION

Respiratory diseases of cattle are a growing problem in all those countries where beef production is increased by the selection of cattle breeds with higher production rates.

The respiratory diseases of cattle have become more and more important since 1964. The disorders are the consequence of the orientation of the Belgium White Blue (BWB) cattle to a beef type and as a result also of the increasing production rates.

In an attempt to elucidate the causes of this pulmonary disorder we examined paired sera from diseased animals in more than 500 farms over a period of 10 years.

CAUSATIVE VIRUSES

Each series of sera, taken from an average of 3 cows per herd, was tested for the following viruses: infectious bovine rhinotracheitis (IBR), parainfluenza 3 (PI3) adenovirus types A and B, bovine viral diarrhoea (BVD), reovirus 1 and 2 and bovine respiratory syncytial virus (BRSV). For each virus, we used at least two serological tests. These tests have been published already in former reports. For the reoviruses, the haemagglutination-inhibition test was the only test used.

The comparison of the results obtained by different tests enables a diagnosis to be made and gives information about the viral aetiology. When one of the tests gave an uncertain result, a third method was used for confirmation (Table 1).

To consider a virus as a cause of the disease observed in a herd, we have to detect a seroconversion against that virus in all, or at least in most, of the tested animals. Indeed, it happens for unknown reasons, that some animals react in a different serological way to their neighbours or that they are not affected by the viral infection.

TABLE 1

VIRUS STRAINS AND SEROLOGICAL TESTS

Virus	Strain	Serological test
IBR	Belgian: 3760	CF, IIF (SNp24 Bitscn, 1973)*
PI3	Belgian: 52/5	HI, CF (IIF)*
Adenovirus type A	WBRI (Darbyshire et al., 1965)	CF, ID
Adenovirus type B	MINK (Bartha et al., 1970)	CF, ID
BVD	$C_{24}V$ (Gillespie et al., 1960)	CF, ID (IIF, SN)*
RSV	Belgian: POUM 2	CF, ID (IIF, SN)*
Reovirus 1 and 2	(Rosen, 1960)	

Key to abbreviations:

CF : Complement fixation
HI : Haemagglutination inhibition
IIF : Indirect immunofluorescence
ID : Immunodiffusion
SN_{P24} : Seroneutralisation Bitsch
* : Alternative test.

CLINICAL ASPECT

The study of the results obtained over more than 10 years, shows that the respiratory diseases may be grouped in four classes:

1. Pneumonias of autumn.

2. Pneumonias from March to October.

3. Pneumonias of transport and assembling (shipping fever).

4. Pneumonias of beef calves, 5 to 6 weeks old.

1. The respiratory troubles of Autumn

These are responsible for most of the mortalities and economic losses especially in the forced beef cattle, 5 to 6 months old.

Table 2 shows that the BRS virus plays the most important aetiological role. Its high prevalence in the country makes it the main respiratory virus. The BRSV infection is lethal in some cases, especially in the beef type herd. This myxovirus is the aetiological agent in more than 50% of the herds where animals have respiratory troubles in autumn. This important percentage is comparable to the percentage found by Holzhauer and van Nieuwstadt in the Netherlands (1976).

TABLE 2

RESULTS OF THE EXAMINATION FOR CAUSATIVE VIRUSES IN PNEUMONIAS OF AUTUMN

Season	Number of cases	Negatives	PI3	Adeno 3	BVD	BRSV	Reo 1 and 2	IBR
65 - 66	8	4	2	1	–	4	–	–
66 - 67	6	3	0	2	0	2	0	0
67 - 68	40	9	11	7	3	19	5	0
68 - 69	19	11	0	4	1	5	1	1
69 - 70	14	4	3	2	3	7	0	0
70 - 71	19	4	0	2	4	12	0	0
71 - 72	22	5	4	2	4	10	1	0
72 - 73	39	10	0	2	7	21	1	0
73 - 74	50	11	4	4	5	29	2	11
74 - 75	25	7	4	2	2	13	2	4
75 - 76	52	10	10	5	3	31	1	0
76 - 77	53	18	6	5	6	31	6	4
Total	347	96	44	38	38	184	19	20
Percentage total		27.6	12.7	10.9	10.9	53	5.4	5.7

The symptoms of this disease may be summarised as follows: all the cattle on the affected farm, especially 'late calves' at weights between 100 and 300 kg, are simultaneously found to have a body temperature of about 40°C. Apparently as a result of the effect of antibiotic treatment against secondary bacterial infection, there is then a rapid drop in the body temperature, together with very marked improvement in the general state of health.

About two or three days later, when everything seems to be satisfactory again, the animals suddenly present difficulty in breathing, accompanied by bouts of dry coughing. The body temperature when these latter symptoms are first manifested, is close to normal. The breathing of the sick calves becomes

increasingly rapid and shallow and the condition is aggravated
by bouts of coughing. There is little or no discharge from
the nostrils. Frequently there is frothing at the commissure
of the lips. Constipation is a commonly occurring symptom and
there is complete loss of appetite. The animals can neither
lie down nor eat and they make desperate efforts to breathe
through an open mouth. On auscultation, some harshness in the
breathing can be detected but rales are not often heard, and
towards the end of the disease state, the classic signs of
emphysema begin to appear. There can be up to 30% mortality
in the herd and farms specialising in late calves tend to have
the highest losses.

On opening of the thoracic cavity, the necropsy reveals
widespread pulmonary emphysema and distended air spaces. In
some cases the pleurae are broken, so that pneumothorax results.

The presence of tracheitis or rhinitis is comparatively
rare.

The next virus in order of importance as the causative
agent of respiratory diseases is PI3 virus with 12.5% of the
cases. Up till the last 3 years we had noted a cyclic two
yearly appearance without any detectable cause, but this
peculiarity has now disappeared.

The viruses of the adenovirus group are classified in two
sub-groups, based on their growing capacities on bovine foetal
kidney (BFK) cells. The A sub-group includes the types 1, 2
and 3 growing easily on BFK cells. The B sub-group includes
the types 4 to 8. This last group does not multiply on BFK cells
but will on bovine testicle (BT) cell cultures. The members of
the B sub-group play an important role in respiratory diseases
of Belgian cattle. Although anti-A sub-group antibodies were
frequently found in the examined sera, the viruses of this
sub-group could not be considered to cause these respiratory
diseases because no seroconversions were shown.

The symptomatology of the BVD virus was in the past limited to the digestive tract. Since 1969 (Wellemans, 1969) we have observed a tropism for the respiratory system, even without digestive symptoms.

At present we consider BVD virus as a rather important (10.8%) aetiological agent of respiratory disorders.

The role of reovirus 1 and 2 seems to be of minor importance (4.4%). The low percentage of IBR virus does not point to a limited incidence of this virus, but is the consequence of the fact that this virus was not tested by the paired sera method. Indeed the isolation of IBR virus is fast and sure enough to make serological testing unnecessary. Second sera were rarely taken by the practitioners in IBR affected herds.

The total of seroconversions presented in Table 2 is greater than the total of tested sera. This apparent anomaly results from the fact that in many cases seroconversion was observed for two or even three different viruses simultaneously in a single herd. This combined action is not rare and often concerns both PI3 and BRSV. Less frequently, we have also observed combined action of BVD, adeno and reoviruses.

2. Pneumonias from March to October

These respiratory diseases are not as severe as those observed in autumn. Nevertheless, the economic losses are often important in springtime, and not negligible in summer.

During past years we have paid attention to this type of disease and the results of our findings are presented in Table 3.

Viruses play only a small part in this disorder except some cases of IBR virus infections appearing from time to time throughout the year. We only noted one case of PI3, in September 1976, and one case due to adenovirus in October 1975. This low percentage of diseases due to a viral infection

for this period of the year justifies the conclusion that
viruses, at least the presently known ones, play little or no
role in the pneumonias from March to October.

TABLE 3

INCIDENCE OF VIRUSES IN THE RESPIRATORY DISEASES FROM MARCH TO OCTOBER

Year	Number of cases	IBR	Other viruses	Negative
1973	8	1	0	7
1974	7	1	0	6
1975	50	2	1 (Adeno)	47
1976	35	0	1 (PI3)	34
Total	100	4	2	94

3. Respiratory disease due to transport and gathering

Though only a few cases have been examined, some conclusions
may be drawn:

The principal pathogenic viral agent of this disorder is
IBR virus. The symptoms appear a few days after gathering.
The animals show the typical symptomatology of this herpesvirus:
an important hyperthermia reaching and even exceeding $42^{\circ}C$,
conjunctivitis, ptyalism, rhinitis, tracheitis, etc.

When this virus was introduced into Belgium, we recommended
intranasal vaccination with an apathogenic strain on the day of
arrival of the animals at the fattening farm. As a consequence
of this vaccination, the IBR cases in these farms decreased
very significantly.

Nevertheless, all the respiratory disease did not disappear
and the serological examinations for viruses, we realised, were
negative in those cases. To this date, no other viruses with
pulmonary tropism, like PI3, can be incriminated, in con-
tradiction with the American investigators. Bacterial inter-
vention seems to be a principal cause of this disease of
transport. Injection of animals with γ-globulins on arrival
at the farm is tentatively used to reduce or suppress

the troubles. The limited number of injected animals until now does not allow us to confirm that we have solved this economic problem.

TABLE 4

PNEUMONIAS AFTER GATHERING (SHIPPING FEVER)

Total of examinations	IBR	Other viruses	Negative
49	20	O	29

4. Respiratory disorders of young beef cattle

We have only examined twenty cases in this group. The few results are not significant. Nevertheless, in these few cases only seldom was a virus isolated or a clear seroconversion to the usual viruses found.

In ten cases, the service of bacteriology of the Institute isolated *Salmonella dublin*. Not all the sick animals presented digestive symptoms, as the bacteriological examination would suggest. In only one case did we note rising antibody titres for BRSV.

TABLE 5

RESPIRATORY DISEASES OF CALVES 5 TO 6 WEEKS OLD

Total of cases	Negatives	BRSV	Isolation of *Salmonella dublin*
20	19	1	10

CONCLUSIONS

The survey of about 500 herds with severe respiratory diseases of cattle allows us to incriminate a viral agent in the pneumonias of autumn. In fact, we noted about 80% positive seroconversions in these cases. In contrast a viral aetiology seems less certain for the other types of respiratory disease. Indeed, only 2% of the examined cases of respiratory disease from March to October show positive seroconversion.

The pneumonias of transport and gathering of animals (shipping fever) do not seem to be due to a viral infection, unless it is one of the often severe consequences of IBR virus infections.

Only once was a virus (BRSV) detected in young cattle 5 to 6 weeks old. The limited number of observed cases makes a valuable conclusion impossible.

REFERENCES

Bartha, A., Mathe, S. and Aldasy, P. 1970. Acta. physiol. hung. 20, p. 399.

Bitsch, V. 1973. Acta. vet. scand. 14, p. 767.

Darbyshire, J.H., Dawson, P.S., Lawson, P.H., Ostler, D.C. and Pereira, H.G.
        1965. J. comp. Path. 75, p. 327.

Gillespie, J.H., Baker, J.A. and McEntee, K. 1960. Cornell Vet. 50, p. 73.

Holzhauer, C. and van Nieuwstadt, A. 1976. Tijdschr. Diergeneesk. 101, p. 1023.

Rosen, L. and Abinanti, E.R. 1960. Am. J. Hyg. 71, p 250.

Wellemans, G. 1969. Annl. Med. vet. 1, p. 47.

DISCUSSION

J.B. McFerran *(UK)*

Dr. Bitsch, could I ask you about your best reaction time of your virus-serum mixtures. Do you ever get sera, which have been negative on a standard neutralisation test at 1 or 2 hours at 37°C, becoming positive after a 24-hour incubation period?

V. Bitsch *(Denmark)*

If we take the IBR neutralisation test as an example, I can say that about 50% of the animals which we find positive in a 24-hour test will not be found positive in a 1-hour test if you use a serum dilution of 1/2. If you use undiluted serum at an incubation of 1 hour at 37°C, you will not detect 25% of antibody carriers. That refers to Danish conditions.

J.B. McFerran

That has certainly not been our experience. We have turned out quite a lot of sera and we have run them at 37°C for 1 hour, 2 hours and 24 hours and I agree that it certainly increases the titre but we have not found that it turns a negative animal into a positive animal.

V. Bitsch

As I said before, we have had many examples of that.

O.C. Straub *(West Germany)*

How many units of the tissue culture infective doses do the two of you use in your studies?

J.N. McFerran

One hundred.

V. Bitsch

One hundred.

O.C. Straub

What happens if you decrease the $TCID_{50}$?

V. Bitsch

Examine, if you will, $10^{1.5}$, $10^{2.5}$, $10^{3.5}$ and so forth, and you will see that an increase of the virus dose by a factor of 10 will lower the titre of the serum by about twofold.

O.C. Straub

Do you think it will go the same way if you go below $10^{1.5}$ which is already 30 $TCID_{50}$? Can you go down as low as 10 $TCID_{50}$?

V. Bitsch

We cannot go much further down.

O.C. Straub

Not in the microsystem, but in other systems you can go down to 10 easily.

V. Bitsch

Yes, exactly, but it is important that we follow the same way. There is no reason to doubt that.

J.B. McFerran

It is hardly affecting the test. If we run it at 10 $TCID_{50}$ every week we will be getting into trouble.

V. Bitsch

Yes, and you probably cannot get much more sensitivity by lowering from 100 units to 10 units. Almost nothing.

H.M. Pirie (UK)

I am interested in the four pneumonic lungs from which you isolated bovine respiratory syncytial virus. Can you tell me if they were all from the same farm, how old the calves were, and at what time of the year?

V. Bitsch

They were from four different herds. I do not have the data about what time of the year we examined the lungs, but I think they were received in the autumn.

O.C. Straub

I think we should add a few words about Aujeszky's disease
virus for those of you who are not too familiar with virology.
Aujeszky's disease virus is a herpes virus, just as IBR, and
bovine pneumonitis virus, but in the classification it belongs
to the porcine herpes viruses and the porcine species are the
natural carriers of it. Cattle always die from the disease. In
general we do not have transmission from cow to cow, but only
from pig to pig, and then when it comes into contact with cattle
the cattle always die.

I think that Dr. Bitsch's work, demonstrating the posterior
and anterior cases in Denmark, is remarkable. It can be seen in
his publications. There is also a case from Belgium, where they
demonstrate that a whole herd of calves died after they had been
bought in a market. Some 40 calves all died of Aujeszky's disease. So if you have a case like this where just about everything dies then you should think of Aujeszky's disease but keep
in mind that it is a porcine virus which kills the calves.

J.B. McFerran

This is the situation as you described it up until the
present. We have the classical European strains which grow in
the pig, are excreted by the pig in the upper respiratory secretions, and are not excreted in the faeces. This has markedly
changed. In certain areas of the world Aujeszky's virus is now
excreted in the faeces of the pig, and the Americans say that
they are now getting direct calf to calf transfer of virus.
This is a tremendous change. Aujeszky's disease in these last
two or three years has been turned upside down and is almost
worth a symposium to itself!

O.C. Straub

We must be aware of this: it could happen in Europe.

V. Bitsch

I feel that we still have the original form of the disease
in Denmark. The first cases observed in Denmark were in 1931,

and these were two outbreaks with anterior localisation of
pruritis. I also have to add that practically all the cases
from the 1940s up until about 1964 were cases with posterior
pruritis. But we did have anterior pruritis earlier.

J.B. McFerran

I am not questioning that at all. The cow is equally infectious at either end, but we now have a new dimension. As the
virus has come into the faeces, obviously when one starts to
spread slurry on to the ground beside cattle, one has the opportunity for widespread dissemination in the bovine. This is
a very worrying thought.

V. Bitsch

How long does it stay viable in the slurry?

J.B. McFerran

I do not know, but certainly the Americans are claiming
that they are getting a spread on fomites, straw and this sort
of thing over quite a long time.

V. Bitsch

How long is that - is it weeks or days or months or even
years?

J.B. McFerran

Certainly days, and possibly weeks. Once again, this work
is very new, and there are no hard facts. There is more evidence
on epidemiology, but I think there have been some very large
changes.

O.C. Straub

I think we have to be aware of the problem. We hope that
the Americans keep those strains to themselves!

L.H. Thomas (UK)

I was rather struck by the similarity between pinkengriep
and the acute respiratory distress syndrome which my Glasgow

colleagues are more than familiar with. I do not want to pursue that particular one, however.

I would like to make an observation on biological findings. I would be more convinced of the association of viruses with pinkengriep if it had been shown that these viruses were not present in the healthy animal, and I am sure that many people who were listening to Dr. Bitsch's presentation will have observed that he has found these viruses in healthy heifers also. I wonder, Dr. Holzhauer, whether you have looked at the healthy animal in comparison with the pinkengriep animal?

C. Holzhauer *(Netherlands)*

Yes, we did, and we found serological evidence of infections in animals which did not show any symptoms at all. Sometimes we have found infections when the cattle are housed in well-ventilated houses or stalls, or when they are on pasture. We have looked at many animals when they were brought into stables, and the animals which had antibodies in the serum at that time did not subsequently develop symptoms. Animals in the group in which there were no antibodies at all developed symptoms of the disease - not all to the same degree. Sometimes the illness was marked and sometimes it was not. Not every infection will give symptoms but I think this is true with all other virus infections. We have monitored one farm for five years, as Dr. van Nieuwstadt told you yesterday. During the five years there, 211 animals have been examined, and all of them have had infections with BRS virus, with parainfluenza virus, with BVD virus, with adenoviruses. When IBR infection started on this farm, all the animals that became infected had, after some time, developed antibodies, very often without showing any symptoms. But when the infection is by BRS, and is in the autumn, then there are serious symptoms. When the infections are in spring or summer, not every animal becomes ill.

J.B. McFerran

Dr. le Jan, could I ask you about your technique for the direct examination of the nasal secretions by electron microscopy when you are looking for viruses in the nasal secretions.

C. le Jan *(France)*

It is difficult to pick out the cells from the nasal swabs. We have to culture the nasal swabs on cells and observe them under the electron microscope afterwards. So we cannot directly observe the virus in the nasal secretions.

O.C. Straub

It would be very difficult to take a virus right from the nasal swab. Sometimes, though, the concentrations are as high as 10^{10} per ml, but I think it would be difficult to do it right from a nasal swab. What I think is remarkable in your studies is that you find nasal antibodies on day 4 after infection. What kind are they, and how did you identify them?

C. le Jan

In the neutralisation test.

O.C. Straub

But you would not know whether they are IgA or IgG or IgM. You did not separate them and try them?

C. le Jan

We did not do that with IBR.

O.C. Straub

What is your opinion on that, Dr. McKercher - have you seen antibodies as early as the fourth day?

D.G. McKercher *(USA)*

I have seen them at 4 or 5 days. That is reasonable.

O.C. Straub

I suppose that is true with IgA.

C. le Jan

If you have a sensitive technique like radioimmunoassay you would certainly find it. It depends upon the sensitivity of the technique.

O.C. Straub

Perhaps IgA is always there. You can tell us next time that you have found IgA.

J.M. Sharp *(UK)*

I have three questions for Dr. Stott, although the first two are really linked together. How did maternal antibody and the age of the calf affect the response to your PI3 vaccine on your farm in terms of the antibody response?

Linked with this, have you compared the incidence of PI3 infections and disease with presumably good responders to the vaccine, and poor responders? I am assuming that the maternal antibody has interfered with the response to your vaccine.

The third question is, did your vaccination have any effect on the incidence of other viral infections?

E.J. Stott *(UK)*

Yes, of course, maternal antibody does affect the response to the vaccine, and if you look at Table 5 of the paper you will see that, in the first 1975 winter, the third group, which comprised the youngest animals, with an age of 1 month, and which had the highest antibody levels before vaccination, were the group in which only 40% responded to the vaccine. In the oldest group which were virtually sero-negative at the beginning of the vaccination 98% responded to the vaccine. The answer to the first question is, yes, the maternal antibody, as everyone has shown, significantly affects the response to the vaccine.

In answer to the second question, whether the response to the vaccine affected the disease outcome, or the subsequent history when the disease hit the farm, the incidence of disease

in the younger group was higher than it was in the older group.
We are now getting down to very small figures because the amount
of treatments in these two groups was quite small. As far as we
were able to tell, there was no higher incidence in non-responders
than there was in responders. The reason for this would be that
the non-responders in general were the ones with the highest
maternal antibody and may well have been protected for that
reason. It becomes very difficult to interpret the data when
you have high levels of maternal antibody. It is a difficult
question to answer, but as far as we could tell, the reason why
the animals failed to respond was not the reason why they required treatment subsequently.

P.W. Wells (UK)

Do you think that the animals which did not respond to the
initial vaccination may have been primed, even though you did
not see any obvious antibody response? Have you any evidence
that might support that?

E.J. Stott

I think that you might have better evidence in sheep than
we have. We have not specifically looked at that and so I cannot
answer that question. We specifically chose animals which we
had kept until their maternal levels were low, in our vaccine
tests, in order that we could accurately see what the vaccine
was doing.

J.M. Sharp

The third part of my question was whether your vaccination
with the PI3 vaccine affected other viral infections.

E.J. Stott

No, there was no evidence for that. In fact, the survey I
showed, and the survey data, went up to September 1975, which
was just before we started this vaccination. Obviously, vaccination would have affected the results if we had continued the
survey. We did continue that survey through the first winter
of the vaccine trial, and there was no evidence that the incidence

of other virus infections was any different. The only infection
which was at all reduced was PI3.

A. van Nieuwstadt *(Netherlands)*
 Can you tell us something more about your system of
evaluating the severity of respiratory disease symptoms, in the
clinical trials?

E.J. Stott *(UK)*
 I think that, as Dr. Thomas was the clinician who made the
assessments, he should answer the question. I did the inoculations so that he would not know what had happened.

L.H. Thomas *(UK)*
 This system has been published in "Research in Veterinary
Science" recently, if you wish to pursue it. The method includes
daily clinical examinations. As you heard, I am not aware of
what animals have been infected, and each animal has a score
sheet on which I record a number of different parameters involving principally the respiratory tract, but also taking other
parts of the animal into account. This is continued for the
three weeks of the trial. At the end of the trial we tot up
the scores for each individual animal and produce a score, and
then I go along to Dr. Stott, and we then allot my scores to
the infected and the control groups.

A. van Nieuwstadt
 I am interested in your system of evaluation. I hope it
is useful in the field as well.

E.J. Stott
 It is not possible in the field.

A. van Nieuwstadt
 What kind of symptoms are you looking at - are you looking
at the number of days on which the animals had fever?

L.H. Thomas

Are you talking about the field disease or the experimental set-up?

A. van Nieuwstadt

Both of them. I need a system to evaluate the symptoms in the field.

L.H. Thomas

I am afraid that this evaluation of the experimental disease is too detailed to apply to the field situation. In the field you can only rely on an assessment at the time at which disease is identified. We make no disease score of the field disease. This would be impracticable.

A. van Nieuwstadt

You need a system because the symptoms are not reproducible in isolated conditions. The symptoms in an experimental infection are always less serious than those seen in the field. You need a system to evaluate a vaccine in the field situation, and you need a system to evaluate the seriousness of the respiratory disease symptoms in the field.

E.J. Stott

We do need a system but the fact is that Nature serves up what is there, and it does not appear to be practical to have a system of the sort of detail which is needed. I do not think it can be done, even though it is to be greatly desired.

J.B. McFerran

Dr. Stott, you made two assumptions there on which I would like you to elaborate. The first is that PI3 vaccines should not be used on the basis of this work. Are you sure that all strains of PI3 behave in a similar fashion on all farms, or are you dealing here with a special case?

The second thing is: you said that we have to use dead vaccines in this country. I do not think that this is true.

There is a possibility of using live vaccines, if the evidence
for them is good enough.

E.J. Stott

I did not say that PI3 vaccine should not be used. What
I said was that I think we should seriously question its use.
That is different. I think that the running has been too much
in favour of the vaccine manufacturers and the vaccine advert-
isers, who have sold the vaccine on data which in my opinion is
seriously questionable. I want seriously to question it, and I
would like other people to do the same. I think we need a lot
more data. I accept entirely that this is based on one farm in
the south of England. I should add that I think it is a very
representative farm. It collects calves from all over the South
of England, but nevertheless it is only one farm.

The second question is not my decision but, as I understand
the current attitude of the Ministry, and perhaps I can be put
right on this, in this country live respiratory virus vaccines
are at least discouraged if not prohibited.

J.B. McFerran

I can tell you that it has been discussed and if a good
enough case is made out for a live vaccine, I am sure that it
would be considered.

B. Morein *(Sweden)*

You got a reduction of PI3 infections from 78% in controls
to 43% in vaccinates. Was it due to the antibody rise, or what?
If you already had an antibody response it might be very difficult to find an antibody rise following an infection.

E.J. Stott

Certainly, and I accept the point, but it might have been
even better in some senses. We looked at both isolation and
serology. Isolations were very few, but we never isolated
virus from any vaccinated animal. The same difficulty arises

if you have a high antibody level... but this is all we can do. There is no doubt that there was a significant reduction.

B. Morein

If you had a local infection you might have it without finding any antibody rise in the serum, particularly if the IgA antibody response was going down. It sometimes does after vaccination.

E.J. Stott

In fact these levels seem to hold up quite well, certainly throughout the winter.

B. Morein

Then again, we know that it is quite easy to infect calves with, for instance, quite high antibody titres in the serum if you choose the right strain of virus.

E.J. Stott

That has not been our experience.

B. Morein

We can do it. The second thing is: are you going to try this respiratory syncytial virus in field work? It has been used in children with disastrous effects. It has not given any beneficial results.

E.J. Stott

Absolutely. This is a problem. We have done a trial. I am using killed vaccines - not because I think they are the best but because I think under our present circumstances this is the most likely vaccine we are ever going to be able to use. I am aware of the situation in children. However, we have absolutely no data to support the idea that the same thing arises in cattle. There has been one paper published, but I do not think that the data presented there is adequate. It suggests that cattle which had been vaccinated had more respiratory disease, based on about two or three animals. We have had

no evidence, during our vaccine trial, that the vaccinated
animals were more severely ill when challenged than unvaccinated
animals. I think the question about the use of an inactivated
vaccine may depend very much upon the way you inactivate it.
This has been clearly shown in measles virus, where, if you inactivate with formalin, you destroy the haemolysin antigen,
and this is probably the explanation as to why, after the use
of inactivated measles you get bizarre pneumonias. I think that
if you inactivate the virus in a different way, probably using
detergent, you may not have this problem. This is something
we shall have to look at.

H.M. Pirie

I would like to ask you if you foresee any problems in
vaccinating against the virus, apart from the hypersensitivity.
From your answer to Dr. Morein, I had always assumed that this
was a peculiarity of the situation in children with the syncytial
virus, but you seem to have evidence that it can occur with
.other viruses like human measles.

E.J. Stott

Certainly with measles there is very good evidence that
inactivated vaccine can cause a lot of respiratory problems,
with very bizarre results.

P.W. Wells *(UK)*

My question is to Dr. McFerran. He is arguing in favour
of live vaccines, yet the data which Dr. Stott has presented
would suggest that inactivated PI3 vaccine given on two occasions subcutaneously seemed to be very effective. Is there
any reason why you would argue in favour of live vaccines in
the face of this sort of evidence?

J.B. McFerran

On this particular thing today, I am not arguing in favour
of live vaccines, but I would hate us to turn aside from live
vaccines on non-scientific grounds. This would be entirely
wrong. I think that, if the scientific evidence is good enough,

we could have live vaccines if they are required. Certainly I have been an advocate of live vaccines from my experience in poultry. I must admit that the evidence that we have seen today on the PI3 looks very good.

O.C. Straub

I think that we could discuss live and killed vaccines for many hours. Sometimes one side is up and the other side down. Generally speaking I think it is wrong to be dogmatic about one argument or the other. I think we should always go to the specific agent with which we are dealing. For example, in Marek's disease in the avian field, or whether we deal with the PI3 in the bovine or in the sheep, it is different according to the animal or species you are dealing with.

G. Dannacher *(France)*

I would like to ask if you have some evaluation of the percentage of virus reactors in British cattle. Is infection widespread or not?

E.J. Stott

Yes, but we have not looked at British cattle in a large sense. We have in addition to this survey looked at a number of animals from other farms, and BRS virus is common. I cannot give you a figure, but it is common.

H. Ernø *(Denmark)*

I would like to put a question to Professor Straub. Would it be possible for you to identify some of the many mycoplasmas which you isolated? I am especially interested to know whether you isolated *Mycoplasma dispar* or any of the explosive ones you were talking about. As you realise, if you say that you are cultivating mycoplasmas, that is just the same as saying that you are cultivating viruses. I am sure that you would appreciate the difference between IBR and BRS infection.

O.C. Straub

We identified *M. dispar* four times. It was the British

work especially which showed that *M. dispar* was causing the deep pneumonias, if I remember correctly. I would consider that *M. dispar* is one of those agents which one should look into. If you could tell me who does differentiation work on mycoplasmas I would be glad to send them material.

H. Ernø

If you will differentiate your strains a little I will be happy to identify, let us say, ten strains for you.

O.C. Straub

That is a good offer. Would anyone like to identify another ten...?

A. Andrews *(UK)*

Dr. Opdenbosch, I am interested in pneumonias occurring from March to October. Are these in housed animals or are they outside, and what kind of mortality are you getting with them? Have you any idea of the aetiology?

E. van Opdenbosch *(Belgium)*

As I have shown, we do not have much mortality from March to October - only 2 or 3% due to viral causes. Normally they are held at pasture day and night. They do not come inside. There are two situations in Belgium. We have the Ardennes, where we have the meat production, and then we have the milk production in Flanders. We see most of the respiratory troubles in the meat type of herd.

E.J. Stott

Dr. van Nieuwstadt has said that he thought that the Belgian Blue-White breed was particularly susceptible to BRS virus. Do you have any data comparing this breed with another breed for its sensitivity to the virus?

E. van Opdenbosch

I do not have that data with me because I am not a specialist in this matter, but I know that we tried to infect

Friesian-Holstein cows with the wild strain, and after a natural infection they did not show any symptoms. When we did the same with the Belgian Blue-White cattle, as you have seen, 50% of them died, after the natural infection. It is a highly sensitive type of cattle.

A. van Nieuwstadt

How many animals were used in the experimental infections you are talking about?

E. van Opdenbosch

I will have to look up the papers.

B. Martin

I wonder if Dr. Opdenbosch could say a little more about the fluorescent antibody test he was using. I gather he said it was a direct test, and I wonder if you would say a little more about it. How did you produce your anti-serum, for instance?

Secondly, during which period of illness do you find antigen in the lungs? How long do you find antigen present in the lungs?

E. van Opdenbosch

The antiserum is taken from calves which we have previously tested with the indirect immunofluorescence test. If they have no antibodies against the normally occurring respiratory viruses such as IBR and others, then they are infected with the wild strain. After a few days we take the blood and test it for the presence of antibody with other tests such as the complement fixation, to see if we have produced immune serum. The serum is then directly stained with fluorescein isothiocyanate, and it is with this conjugate that we stain our sections of the lung. It is only when the animals die very quickly after the beginning of the disease that we can find the antigen. In animals which survive for several weeks after the beginning of the disease, the antigen can no longer be detected.

H.M. Pirie *(UK)*

Would you say a little more about the microscopic appearance of the lungs which are positive. For instance, do you see multi-nucleated syncytia in them which I believe have been described by some people?

E. van Opdenbosch

We do not carry out histology on the lungs so I cannot answer that question.

O.C. Straub

Does anyone else present have any experience? Would anyone like to answer the question?

C. Holzhauer *(Netherlands)*

We always see a few syncytia, but most of the cells are round lymphocytes.

H.M. Pirie

Could I also ask this: in the animals which die, apart from the interstitial emphysema, do they have hyaline membranes and oedema?

C. Holzhauer

When you talk about the condition of emphysema, I call it the third stage of illness. I think that after vaccination you can get the first symptoms such as catarrhal symptoms and a high temperature. As to what we see in those animals which die from this infection, they have oedema and emphysema in the interstitia, just like parasitic bronchitis.

E. van Opdenbosch

Are you talking about the symptoms after vaccination?

C. Holzhauer

No, I am talking about the natural infection. After vaccination we did not see animals with emphysema as well, just as in Belgium.

May I ask you about the slide of the animal with IBR? I
would have said that it was BVD. We have had animals with an
IBR infection and they get mucosal disease, or BVD, as well.
They have diarrhoea. We have had cows for three or four years
and then they have died. They had symptoms of BVD infection,
but we could isolate IBR, and other animals in the group had
IBR symptoms.

I would like to ask you if you detected a serum antibody
response to all infections, such as PI3 virus and other infections on the mucus: in trials they always gave us a serum response. I think there will always be a serum antibody response
when a virus comes into the area, and this is a local infection.
Do you think that these local infections always give a seroconversion, just like IBR or BVD?

E. van Opdenbosch

I think we are talking a different language. When we
have a good seroconversion against PI3 we can draw the conclusion
that there was a PI3 infection.

C. Holzhauer

You may be right, but you do not find seroconversions in
summer, and perhaps the infection has only given a local response.
I would think that could be possible.

E. van Opdenbosch

We did not detect local antibodies.

O.C. Straub

I think the question about IBR and BVD is very important.
Dr. McKercher, have you any evidence that IBR has caused symptoms
such as this?

D.G. McKercher

They have isolated the virus from the intestinal tract of
calves, but I think it possibly got there simply by being carried

there in the saliva. I do not believe there were any pathologic changes. My personal feeling is that IBR virus does not cause any enteric problems.

O.C. Straub

In our experience it can be carried anywhere by leukocytes, but it does not go through the digestive tract unless you have changes in the abomasum. Usually the abomasum has a pH of 1.8 to 2.5, and the IBR virus will not pass through that. On the other hand, if you take leukocytes and you have some intestinal trouble where the permeability of the digestive tract is changed, you can very easily have the IBR virus transported to the membranes via the leukocytes. This is probably the way in which the IBR virus gets to the uterus, for example. That also happens, as you know from the States. Belgium certainly has a unique situation in Europe as far as the digestive trouble is concerned. As far as mouth lesions are concerned, I have never seen anything like it. As Dr. Holzhauer mentioned, it might be a combination of both of them.

H.J. Bürger

May I ask whether this was possibly a field case of a cow which had been outside on pasture, and may have picked up some Ostertagia infection, which produced these alterations in the abomasum as you described them.

F. Lomba

It was a very young calf coming from the same farm as the heifer, born by caesarian section. When the caesarian was performed many calves on this farm became ill with IBR. They had never been on pasture - they were very young calves.

H.J. Bürger

The lesions were rather the same as the erosions of the mucosa and the front part of the alimentary tract in the housed calves which were shown on the slide.

SESSION 4A

MYCOPLASMAS

Chairman:

J.M. Rutter

Co-ordinator:

G.E. Jones

MYCOPLASMAS INVOLVED IN BOVINE PNEUMONIA

H. Ernø

FAO/WHO Collaborating Centre for Animal Mycoplasmas,
Institute of Medical Microbiology, Bartholin Building,
University of Aarhus, Denmark.

ABSTRACT

At least 20 mycoplasma species or serogroups have been isolated from cattle, viz: Mycoplasma bovirhinis, M. dispar, M. mycoides subsp. mycoides, M. alkalescens, M. arginini, M. bovis, M. bovigenitalium, Acholeplasma laidlawii, A. modicum, A. axanthum, Ureaplasma sp., Leach's Group 7, M. gallinarum, M. gateae, M. bovoculi, M. verecundum, M. canadense, M. alvi, and two Anaeroplasma spp. The first 12 listed have been recovered from the respiratory tract of cattle; of these, M. dispar, M. bovirhinis and ureaplasmas have been reported in many countries and would appear to be the most commonly occurring species. Some of these mycoplasmas have been shown to be pathogenic for the bovine mammary gland, but their roles in pneumonia cannot be directly inferred, nor is much known about the pathogenic mechanisms of mycoplasmas. However, experimental studies in gnotobiotic calves have shown that M. bovis is pathogenic and M. dispar and ureaplasmas potentially pathogenic for the respiratory tract. In addition, evidence of pathogenicity for the respiratory tract has been claimed for M. arginini, M. bovirhinis, M. bovigenitalium and acholeplasmas, but more conclusive proof involving the experimental infection of gnotobiotic as well as conventional animals is needed. Determination of the importance of the different species in natural infections requires the development of appropriate techniques: cultivation alone, even when quantified, is not of much diagnostic value, but a combination of the complement fixation test and some modification of the passive haemagglutination test may provide greater understanding of the role of mycoplasmas in bovine pneumonia.

I have assumed by major task at this seminar to be that of
introductory speaker on the subject of mycoplasmal involvement
in bovine pneumonia. The views expressed will be my own -
though based, of course, on work performed by many workers in
several countries. From my viewpoint as a laboratory diagnostician, I shall attempt to outline those experiments and
investigations which I consider are urgently required before
the importance of mycoplasmas in calf pneumonia can be
adequately assessed - and it hardly needs to be said that such
assessments are essential before the spending of time and money
on diagnosis and control are considered.

First, I shall mention those species or serogroups that
have been isolated from cattle. The cultivation and identification of mycoplasmas present no greater problems than are
encountered with bacteria or viruses. At the present moment,
at least 20 spp or serogroups have been recovered from cattle,
namely: *Mycoplasma bovirhinis*, *M. dispar*, *M. mycoides* subsp. *mycoides*,
M. alkalescens, *M. arginini*, *M. bovis*, *M. bovigenitalium*, *Acholeplasma
laidlawii*, *A. modicum*, *A. axanthum*, *Ureaplasma* sp., Leach's group 7,
M. gallinarum, *M. gateae*, *M. bovoculi*, *M. verecundum*, *M. canadense*, *M. alvi*,
and 2 *Anaeroplasma* spp. The first 12 listed have been recovered
from the respiratory tract of cattle; of these *M. dispar*,
M. bovirhinis and ureaplasmas have been reported in many countries
and would appear to be the most commonly occurring species.
It is particulalry interesting to note geographic differences
in occurrence. For example, neither *M. bovis* nor *M. arginini*
have been isolated in Denmark, although the occurrence of
M. arginini in many countries has been known for some time, and
M. bovis - after the first isolations in the USA - has subsequently been identified in many European countries. Since,
as mentioned earlier, our knowledge concerning isolation and
identification techniques is satisfactory, it would be desirable
to have an up-to-date summary of those mycoplasma species
occurring in the 9 EEC countries.

Some of the mycoplasma species mentioned have been shown
to be pathogenic for the bovine mammary gland, but their roles

in pneumonia cannot be directly inferred from this. However, experimental studies in gnotobiotic calves have shown that *M. bovis* is pathogenic, and *M. dispar* and ureaplasmas potentially pathogenic for the respiratory tract. These investigations will be discussed by Dr. Gourlay. I should also mention that other mycoplasma species have been incriminated in the calf pneumonia complex - in particular *M. bovirhinis*, *M. arginini* and *M. bovigenitalium*. It appears to me, however, that the evidence for the pathogenicity of these organisms is weak, and further experiments in both conventional and gnotobiotic calves is necessary, not only to confirm or invalidate earlier work but also to provide better understanding of the pathogenesis, immunopathology and serological responses involved. As an example, except for *M. mycoides* subsp. *mycoides*, which does not occur in Europe, only *M. bovis* has been shown to produce a toxin, probably a polysaccharide. In the mammary gland and oviduct the toxin of *M. bovis* provokes a histological response which is characterised, in the acute phase, by eosinophilic infiltration. Does the same response occur in the lungs? Do other mycoplasmas produce toxins or does pathogenicity depend on some other factor, perhaps hypersensitivity? Does macrophage suppression play a role? It seems to me that research into basic questions such as these is vital for a better understanding both of the host-mycoplasma relationship and the interactions that may occur between mycoplasmas and other microorganisms.

Such investigations have a further value, enabling the selection, development and evaluation of serological methods which ultimately may be used as routine diagnostic methods. It will always be difficult to interpret antibody responses to potentially pathogenic microorganisms unless very clear changes in titre are observed. By this I mean that even a 4-fold change in antibody titre cannot be regarded as conclusive evidence for the causal involvement of a specific mycoplasma in the pneumonia investigated. A relatively weak antibody response may arise simply from a general stimulation of the immune apparatus, or from secondary invasion of pre-existing lesions.

The interpretation of antibody responses to mycoplasmas must always depend on which test is employed. For experimental pathogenicity studies the work performed with mycoplasmas in other animals and the sparse knowledge available from investigations into bovine mycoplasmosis in general suggest that the most suitable methods are the passive haemagglutination (PHA), complement fixation (CF) or immunofluorescence tests.

For sero-epidemiological investigations, selection of the most suitable test is made easier in that maximum sensitivity is required, a condition fulfilled by the PHA test. Several modifications of the test, including the use of fresh or aldehyde-treated sheep erythrocytes are commonly employed. An alternative test which has been used with success in sero-epidemiological surveys has been the latex agglutination test. However, the degree of cross-reaction which may occur in these tests between mycoplasma species or between mycoplasmas and other microorganisms, for example bacteria, is difficult to say at present and requires further study.

We already know that common antigens can be demonstrated for some of the bovine mycoplasmas by the double immuno-diffusion test. Whether the same cross-reactions will occur in PHA and CF tests may depend on the methods used for the production of serologic antigens. This problem may be particularly important when serologic tests are applied to the diagnosis of disease induced by known mycoplasma pathogens, and one cannot assume that the successful application of a specific sero-logical test for this purpose in one animal species will mean that the same test will be of value in other animal hosts infected by their specific mycoplasma pathogens. For example, the known mycoplasma pathogens of man, *M. pneumoniae*, and of pigs, *M. suipneumoniae*, do not share common antigens with the other mycoplasmas occurring within their hosts. Thus the CF test is highly successful in its application to these 2 organisms, but this need not necessarily be the case with bovine mycoplasmas.

It is therefore obvious that much work needs to be done before we can answer the question: do mycoplasmas play an important role in calf pneumonia, and if so, can diagnosis readily and reliably be performed!

RESPIRATORY DISEASE AND THE INCIDENCE OF PULMONARY MYCOPLASMOSIS IN INTENSIVELY-REARED CALVES IN ITALY

P. Pignatelli

Vetem, Via B. Crespi; 27, 20159 Milano, Italy.

ABSTRACT

During 1975, 1976 and the first 4 months of 1977, the pulmonary incidence of mycoplasma spp. in veal calves was surveyed in 42 Italian farms rearing a total of more than 100 000 calves per year. Mycoplasmas were recovered from 392 of the 534 specimens collected (73.40%), of which 277 isolates were identified as comprising Mycoplasma agalactiae subsp. bovis (54.21%); M. bovigenitalium (7.45%), M. arginini (3.98%), M. alkalescens (1.87%), M. bovirhinis (0.8%), Leach's Group 7 (0.8%), and Acholeplasma laidlawii (0.8%): 115 isolates could not be identified.

The highest mycoplasma recovery rate was in young lean calves (milk substitute fed) and veal calves (concentrate fed). The isolation rate was not significantly different between healthy calves and sick, culled or dead calves. The highest incidence of mycoplasmas occurred in family-managed farms, and the lowest in the large, highly specialised farms.

The economic losses due to respiratory disease, assessed for the years 1975 and 1976, varied from 3.1% to 7.5% of the average value of lean calves, 4.1% to 7.0% of weaning calves and 1.4% to 2.4% of fattening calves. Extrapolation of these figures to the Italian calf rearing industry as a whole indicate that losses due to respiratory disease in calves amount to an estimated 100 billion lire per year.

INTRODUCTION

Virtually all intensively reared veal calves in Italy are
imported from abroad. The Italian Institute of Statistics
gives the calf importation figures for the last 3 years as
1 765 555 (1974), 2 236 287 (1975) and 2 273 680 (1976). A
variety of factors may therefore influence the performance of
these calves in veal producing units, in particular:

1. The country of origin, breed and ages of the imported
animals.

2. Stress due to transportation, and changes in environment, feeding, climate and treatment.

3. Lack of history and preconditioning.

4. Inadequate housing conditions, including lack of
microclimate control, overcrowding and poor sanitation.

5. No 'all-in all-out' policy for calf batches.

6. Non- or insufficient vaccination of calves against the
major bacterial and viral diseases.

7. High infection rates with viral and bacterial
respiratory micro-organisms due to the constant presence
of carriers.

The overall analysis of these factors is given in Table
1, together with the incidence of two major diseases affecting
veal calves. Gastro-intestinal diseases are most common in
lean calves (milk substitute fed), in which they generally occur
concomitantly with respiratory disease; on the other hand, veal
calves (concentrate fed) suffer more frequently from respiratory
than gastro-intestinal diseases.

The aim of this study was to investigate the extent of
mycoplasmal involvement in diseases of veal calves in Italy,
with particular regard to the respiratory tract. We have
looked at a) the recovery rate and identity of mycoplasmas from
calves with respiratory disease during 1975, 1976 and the first
4 months of 1977, and b) attempted to assess the economic

losses incurred due to all forms of respiratory disease
(mycoplasmosis included) in intensively-reared veal calves.

TABLE 1

MAIN CHARACTERISTICS OF INTENSIVE REARING OF VEAL CALVES IN ITALY

Characteristics	Lean calves	Veal calves	
		Weaning	Fattening
Stalling	Cage battery Chain battery	Cage Box	Chain Box
Animal type	Dairy	Beef	Beef
Admission age	8 - 10 days	10 - 15 days	3 - 4 months
Admission weight (kg)	35 - 50	55 - 85	130 - 150
Ratio females/males	1 : 1	1 : 4	1 : 4
Rearing period	1974: approx. 100 days 1977: 125 - 135 days	90 - 100 days	10 - 12 months
Slaughter weight (kg)	1974: approx. 120 1977: 180 - 200	-	550 - 600
Gastroenteric diseases	60 - 80%	30 - 60%	10 - 20%
Respiratory disease	30 - 100%	50 - 100%	75 - 100%

MATERIAL AND METHODS

1. Animals

The animals involved were lean and veal calves of various
breeds, nearly all of which were imported at ages ranging from
2 weeks to 10 months. The calves were maintained on 42 farms,
33 in Northern Italy and 9 in Central Southern Italy.
Fourteen of the farms specialised in producing lean calves,
85.71% of which were reared in batteries: 28 farms specialised
in producing veal calves, 10 for weaning and 18 for fattening.
The mean calf numbers involved in each cycle were 820 head
(range 250 - 3000) in farms producing lean calves, 148 head
(range 100 - 480) in farms producing weaning calves, and 320
head (range 250 - 1800) in farms producing fattening calves.

2. Prophylactic and therapeutic treatment of calves

Most calves were vaccinated against parainfluenza 3 (PI3),
infectious bovine rhinotracheitis (IBR) viruses and pasteurellae
on their arrival at the farm. At the same time antibiotics
(tetracyclines and macrolides), nitrofurans, sulfa-drugs,
vitamins and oligoelements were administered orally for 5 - 7
days on a group basis. The most stressed animals were also
treated with a single parenteral injection of cortisone
combined with cardiotonic drugs. Calves suffering from
respiratory disease were treated with the same antibiotics,
chemotherapeutics and vitamins, on both a group and an
individual basis.

3. Materials examined

Specimens were taken from 326 calves suffering from
respiratory diseases associated with a variety of respiratory
micro-organisms, including viruses (PI3 and IBR, both singly
and in combination) and bacteria (pasteurellae, streptococci,
haemophili, chlamydiae, etc). Of the 534 specimens examined,
432 (80.89%) were from the nasopharynx, 17 (3.18%) from joints
and 85 (15.92%) from lungs.

4. Mycoplasmology

The reference mycoplasma strains and isolation and
identification techniques have been described previously
(Nicolet and De Meuron, 1970a; Nicolet and De Meuron, 1970b;
Pignattelli and Galassi, 1971, 1972 and 1973).

5. Economic losses

Economic losses due to all forms of respiratory disease
were assessed from the records of the 42 farms involved in the
survey.

RESULTS AND DISCUSSION

Different prevalences of respiratory disease in the calves
were noted according to their breed and country of origin. The
highest incidence appeared in the animals imported from France,

followed by those from Belgium, Holland and Germany: the least
affected animals came from Britain and Eastern Europe. Several
factors account for this variation in the incidence of respiratory
disease, in particular the sanitary conditions and methods of
collecting the animals at the originating source, the methods
of transportation and the hygienic conditions at the destination
rearing farm.

Mycoplasmas were recovered from 392 of the 534 specimens
examined (73.40%). The analysis of recoveries according to
specimen examined and the type of animal sampled is given in
the following table.

	*NF	SF	L	Total
Lean calves	163	9	48	220
Weaning veal calves	106	4	16	126
Fattening veal calves	40	1	5	46
Isolated mycoplasma total	309	14	69	392

(*NF = nasopharyngeal swabs; SF = synovial fluid; L = lungs)

Identification, performed on 376 of the mycoplasma isolates,
largely supported previous findings (Pignattelli and Galassi,
1972); these results are shown in Table 2. *M. agalactiae* var *bovis*
was the most frequently recovered mycoplasma (53.72%) followed
by *M. bovigenitalium* (7.45%), *M. arginini* (3.98%), *M. alkalescens*
(1.8%) and *M. bovirhinis, A. laidlawii* and *M.* serotype 7 (all 0.80%);
A. modicum was not recovered. The number of mycoplasmas not
identified (30.58%) with the 8 reference immune sera appeared
to be very high. It is interesting to note that in fattening
calves (< 4 months old) a higher frequency of *M. bovigenitalium*
(15.55%) and *M. arginini* (6.66%) coincided with a lower incidence
of *M. agalactiae* var *bovis* (46.66%). *M.* serotype 7 and *A. laidlawii*
were each recovered from 3 samples.

The recovery rates of mycoplasma spp. from calves affected
by respiratory disease are shown in Table 3. It is apparent

that higher isolation rates were obtained from young animals
(lean and veal calves) but there were no significant differences
in recovery rates from sick, culled or dead calves. In fattening
calves the isolation percentage is 10 - 15% lower than in
younger calves.

TABLE 2

IDENTIFICATION OF MYCOPLASMAS ISOLATED IN 42 VEAL-CALF REARING FARMS IN
YEARS 1975-1976 AND FIRST 4 MONTHS OF 1977

Serotypes	Lean calves		Veal calves weaning		fattening		Total	
	No.	%	No.	%	No.	%	No.	%
M. *agalactiae var. bovis*	115	54.50	66	55.00	21.	46.66	202	53.72
M. *bovigenitalium*	15	7.10	6	5.00	7	15.55	28	7.45
M. *arginini*	7	3.31	5	4.17	3	6.66	15	3.98
M. *bovirhinis*	-		2	1.67	1	2.23	3	0.80
A. *modicum*	-		-		-		-	-
M. serotype 7	-		2	1.67	1	2.23	3	0.80
M. *alkalescens*	3	1.42	3	2.50	1	2.23	7	1.87
A. *laidlawii*	1	0.47	1	0.82	1	2.23	3	0.80
Unidentified mycoplasmas	70	33.20	35	29.17	10	22.21	115	30.58
Total	211	100	120	100	45	100	376	100

Table 4 indicates the mycoplasma isolation rates according
to the type and size of rearing unit. These results, all
obtained during the same period of observation, indicate that
higher recovery rates were obtained in the smaller, family-
managed farms than in the large and highly specialised units.
This apparent anomaly - one might normally expect higher recovery
rates to be obtained in the large units rearing greater numbers
of animals - can be explained by the better prophylactic
measures, treatment, housing systems and feeding adopted by the
specialised units, which also practise an all-in all-out system
for lean calves and, in some cases, veal calves.

TABLE 3

INCIDENCE (%) OF MYCOPLASMOSIS (POSITIVE ISOLATION OF MYCOPLASMA) IN RESPIRATORY SYNDROMES OF INTENSIVELY REARED VEAL-PRODUCING CALVES (AVERAGE OF SURVEYS OF YEARS 1975 and 1976).

Type of Breeding	Rearing units No.	Head No.(+)	A) Morbidity % (*) R.S.	Myc.	B) Mortality % (*) R.S.	Myc.	C) Discard % (*) R.S.	Myc.	Totals B + C R.S.%	Myc.
Lean calves	14	29 360	30 - 100	50 - 80	0.6 - 1.3	50 - 65	1.0 - 30	60 - 75	1.6 - 4.3	=
Veal calves:										
Weaning	10	13 680	50 - 100	57 - 85	0.7 - 2.5	50 - 80	1.6 - 2.5	55 - 85	2.7 - 3.5	=
Fattening	18	11 680	75 - 100	35 - 70	0.3 - 0.2	40 - 70	0.7 - 1.2	42 - 73	1.2 - 2.0	=

R.S. = Incidence (%) of respiratory syndrome of various aetiologies.

Myc. = Incidence (%) of mycoplasmosis (positive isolation of mycoplasma) in animals affected by respiratory disease

(*) = Full range of incidence

(+) = Average number per year.

TABLE 4

ISOLATION PERCENTAGES OF MYCOPLASMA SPP. FROM RESPIRATORY SYNDROMES IN THE DIFFERENT TYPES OF REARING UNITS

Type of farm	Domestic Head No (*)	Domestic Isolation Mycop.%	Specialised (semi-industrial) Head No. (*)	Specialised (semi-industrial) Isolation Mycop.%	Highly specialised (industrial) Head No. (*)	Highly specialised (industrial) Isolation Mycop.%
Lean calves — weaning only	180- 230	65 – 90	250 – 1000	50 – 80	1000 – 10000	30 – 75
weaning only	30 – 100	65 – 90	100 – 350	65 – 90	350 – 1000	40 – 75
Veal calves — weaning plus fattening	10 – 70	65 – 90	100 – 350	60 – 85	350 – 2500	35 – 70
calves — fattening	5 – 10	30 – 70	50 – 500	40 – 70	500 – 6500	30 – 60

(*) = number of animals per rearing cycle.

The economic losses due to respiratory mycoplasmosis are very high; the exact amount cannot be evaluated, but an assessment was made of the losses due to all forms of respiratory disease by examination of the records maintained by the 42 survey farms. These estimated losses are shown in Table 5: the expenses incurred by therapeutic treatments, vaccinations, disinfection and sanitation measures are given in column 1: mortality losses in column 2; and the culling and estimated growth losses in column 3. The fourth column, showing totals and means, indicates loss due to respiratory disease to be 3.1 - 7.5% in lean calves, 4.1 - 7.0% in weaning calves and 1.4 - 2.4% in fattening calves.

TABLE 5

ECONOMIC LOSSES (IN LIRA PER HEAD) DUE TO RESPIRATORY DISEASE IN INTENSIVELY REARED VEAL CALVES (*).

Type of calves produced	Costs due to: Treatments	Deaths	Culls and estimated growth losses	Totals
	lira	lira	lira	lira
Lean calves	1000 - 5000	1200 - 2600	3000 - 7500	5200 - 15100
Veal {weaning calves{	5000 - 7000	2500 - 8750	7000 - 9000	14500 - 24750
{fattening	1500 - 1800	2000 - 4800	5300 - 8200	8800 - 14800

(*) - from data obtained in years 1975 and 1976 from records of 42 concerns of different management and type, for a total of 113 628 veal producing calves.

Considering that more than 3 million calves (domestic and imported) valued at more than 2000 milliards are intensively reared for veal production every year in Italy, the losses due to respiratory disease alone, calculated from the above figures, probably exceed 100 milliards. It should be borne in mind that the farms included in this survey were of a good standard of management.

The contribution of respiratory mycoplasmosis to these calculated losses, which are little different from those of other authors (Bertocchi, 1977a, Bertocchi, 1977b; Mondini, 1977), can only be guessed at from the mycoplasma isolation rates already reported. In any case, some 5 - 6 milliards are spend annually on treatment of respiratory disease, and at least 50% of these expenses concern drugs which are active against mycoplasmas. The high cost of respiratory mycoplasmosis to the veal production industry in Italy can therefore be imagined.

CONCLUSIONS

At present, it is practically impossible to define the role of mycoplasmas in respiratory diseases of intensively-reared veal calves. The only certain element is the constancy of mycoplasma isolation from calves affected by respiratory syndromes, even where other viral or bacterial agents may also be recovered (Galassi, 1974; Galassi, 1975; Mondini, 1977; Nicolet and De Meuron, 1970a; Nicolet and De Meuron, 1970b; Pignattelli and Galassi, 1971; Pignattelli and Galassi, 1972).

The results obtained have demonstrated the high frequency (68.61%) of some mycoplasma serotypes regarded as pathogenic for cattle. On a practical level we have to consider that the massive and timely use of macrolide antibiotics, singly or in combination with other drugs aids more than 90% of animals affected by pneumonia to recover (Pignattelli and Galassi, 1973).

These facts tend to confirm indirectly the importance of mycoplasmas as pathogens, even if they are considered to be minor and/or opportunist agents in respiratory diseases of fattening calves (Galassi, 1974; Galassi, 1975; Pignattelli and Galassi, 1973).

REFERENCES

Bertocchi, D. 1977. ll Giornale degli Allevatori, 27. (4), p. 27.

Bertocchi, D. 1977. Atti Soc. Ital. Buiatria (In press).

Galassi, D. 1974. Proc. VIII Intern. Conference on Diseases of Cattle: Milano,
      September, p. 42.

Galassi, D. 1975. Vet. ital. 15, p. 19.

Mondini, S. 1977. Inftore. zootec. 24, (11), p. 6.

Nicolet, J. and De Meuron, P.A. 1970a. Cha. Med. Vet. 39, p. 13.

Nicolet, J. and De Meuron, P.A. 1970b. Zbl. Vet. Med. 17, p. 1031.

Pignattelli, P. and Galassi, D. 1971. Atti. Soc. It. Buiatria, 3, p. 544.

Pignattelli, P. and Galassi, D. 1972. Atti. Soc. It. Sci. Vet. 24, p. 599.

Pignattelli, P. and Galassi, D. 1973. Riv. Zoot. Vet. 1, p. 157.

ISOLATION AND PATHOGENICITY OF MYCOPLASMAS
FROM THE RESPIRATORY TRACT OF CALVES

R.N. Gourlay and C.J. Howard
Agricultural Research Council, Institute for Research
on Animal Diseases, Compton, Newbury, Berkshire, England.

ABSTRACT

   Convincing evidence of pathogenicity has been obtained with only eight of the twelve species of mycoplasma which have hitherto been recovered from the respiratory tract of cattle. Mycoplasma mycoides subsp. mycoides is the causal agent of contagious bovine pleuropneumonia and is relatively unimportant in Europe, except for occasional outbreaks on the Iberian peninsula. M. alkalescens, M. bovigenitalium and Leach's Group 7 mycoplasmas have been rarely isolated from the respiratory tract: they are, however, capable of causing experimental mastitis in cattle but Koch's postulates have not yet been fulfilled in respect of their aetiological role in pneumonia.

   M. bovirhinis, M. bovis, M. dispar and Ureaplasma sp. are the mycoplasma species most frequently isolated from the respiratory tract of pneumonic calves. All are capable of producing experimental mastitis in cattle, although the mastitis induced by M. bovirhinis is only subclinical. M. bovis, M. dispar and Ureaplasma sp. are also capable of producing pneumonia when pure cultures are inoculated into gnotobiotic calves.

There is no doubt that mycoplasmas on their own can produce pneumonia in man and animals. Examples of this are atypical pneumonia in man due to *Mycoplasma pneumoniae*, contagious bovine pleuropneumonia caused by *M. mycoides* subsp.*mycoides* and pneumonia in mice and rats due to *M. pulmonis*.

At Compton our aim has been to determine whether mycoplasmas play a role, and if so what role, in pneumonia of calves, particularly those reared under intensive conditions of husbandry.

MYCOPLASMA ISOLATIONS

In an earier study (Gourlay et al., 1970) we reported the isolation of mycoplasmas from 75% of 65 pneumonic lungs of calves in South-West England. These comprised *Ureaplasma* sp. from 58% of lungs, *M. dispar* (a hitherto unknown species) from 51% and *M. bovirhinis* from 23%. Although we failed to isolate *Acholeplasma laidlawii* from the pneumonic lungs in this study, this organism has been isolated, usually from the upper respiratory tract, both by us and other workers.

M. bovirhinis has been recognised for many years (Harbourne, et al., 1965) and has been reported from many different countries. It appears to be the species most commonly isolated from the bovine respiratory tract probably because of its ubiquity and undemanding growth requirements.

Since 1970, ureaplasmas have been been isolated from pneumonic bovine lungs in Canada from 1 out of 8 lungs (12%), USA (5/7 lungs, 71%), Japan (15/22, 68%), Scotland (8/12, 66%) and Denmark (31/50, 52%) (Ruhnke and van Dreumel, 1972; Livingston, 1972; Shimizu et al., 1975; Pirie and Allan, 1975; Bitsch et al., 1976). *M. dispar* has been isolated from Australia (11/37, 30%), USA (3/11, 27%), Scotland (6/12, 50%) and Denmark (31/50, 62%) (St. George et al., 1973; Ose and Muenster, 1975; Pirie and Allan, 1975; Bitsch et al., 1976).

Isolation of these two mycoplasmas have usually been from pneumonic lungs, but *M. disapar* and *Ureaplasma* sp. have also been isolated from the respiratory tract of non-pneumonic animals (Gourlay and Thomas, 1970; Thomas and Smith, 1972). Recent studies indicate that *M. dispar* is probably the most common microbial species in the respiratory tract of calves in the Compton area. This species has been isolated from naso-pharyngeal swabs from 38 out of 41 (93%) 1½ to 8 weeks old Ayrshire calves between March and May this year.

M. bovis has been isolated from many countries in North America and Europe; however, it was not known to be present in the United Kingdom until 1975 (Thomas et al., 1975) when it was isolated from an outbreak of pneumonia. Since then it has been isolated from many pneumonic lungs and from some outbreaks of mastitis.

PATHOGENICITY STUDIES

The association of a micro-organism with a diseased tissue does not necessarily imply a causal relationship. It is, therefore, important to distingish between the mycoplasmas that play a significant role in the disease, whether as a primary or secondary agent, and those that are saprophytes or commensals. It is, of course, quite possible that an organism that plays a secondary role may be as important in the disease situation as the primary agent.

To prove a causal relationship between a micro-organism and a disease, it has sufficed in the past to fulfil Koch's postulates in conventionally reared animals. This was perfectly acceptable when the micro-organism concerned was highly pathogenic and capable of causing serious disease or even death of the host, and when the resident microflora played an insignificant part in the disease process. However, fulfilment of Koch's postulates in conventionally reared animals becomes less meaningful when the organism concerned is less pathogenic and especially when its significance may only be expressed

fully in association with some other organism or organisms.
Most pathogenic mycoplasmas fall into this category. In this
case, to determine the exact role of a mycoplasma in the
disease process, it is necessary to employ 'SPF', gnotobiotic
or germ free animals. This is additionally important in
studies on calf pneumonia as many apparently normal calves
suffer from subclinical pneumonia.

Apart from the fulfilment of Koch's postulates, other
evidence of pathogenicity or pathogenic potential may be of
value in assessing the role of a mycoplasma in a disease
situation. Such evidence can be the ability to cause damage
to any tissue, either in vivo or in vitro; such as damage after
inoculation into another anatomical site like the mammary
gland, or the inoculation of tissue or organ cultures. Certain
biophysical or biochemical characteristics of the mycoplasma
may be suggestive of pathogenic potential such as the production
of a toxin or hydrogen peroxide, the presence of a capsule, or
a terminal attachment structure. Incidentally, production of
antibody by an animal inoculated with a particular organism
does not necessarily imply aetiological significance, the
organism may simply be multiplying in the diseased tissue.

M. dispar and Ureaplasma sp.

These two mycoplasmas are frequently isolated from the
same pneumonic lung. They both possess extra-membraneous
material; in the case of M. dispar this is in the form of a
'capsule' (Howard and Gourlay, 1974). Both these organisms
multiply in tracheal organ cultures but only M. dispar produces
any cytopathic effect (Thomas and Howard, 1974). Both M. dispar
and Ureaplasma sp. produce clinical mastitis when inoculated into
the bovine mammary gland. However, some isolates of both these
species are apparently avirulent (Gourlay et al., 1972; Howard
et al., 1973; Brownlie et al., 1976).

In 1969 we inoculated both M. dispar and Ureaplasma sp.
endobronchially into conventionally reared calves and reported

that they were capable of producing pneumonia (Gourlay and
Thomas, 1969). Further experiments were reported using
ureaplasmas (Gourlay and Thomas, 1970). It was only when more
detailed studies were made with M. *dispar* that we became aware
of the disadvantages of using conventionally reared calves for
this type of work. The disadvantages were that all calves had
bacteria (many of them pathogenic species) in their respiratory
tracts, many calves had M. *dispar* or other mycoplasma species in
their respiratory tracts, and worst of all, many calves were
suffering from sublcinical pneumonia before inoculation.
Respiratory virus infections were also common during the
experiments. For these reasons we were cautious in ascribing
the pneumonic lesions produced to the mycoplasmas inoculated.
Similar uncertainties apply to the results of St. George et al.
(1973) in Australia who inoculated three 1 - 2 day old
caesarian-derived or colostrum-deprived calves with M. *dispar*
culture material intratracheally and killed them 2 - 8 days
later. Atelectasis was observed in the lungs of all 3 calves
and M. *dispar* and coliform bacterial were isolated from two of
them. Histologically the lesions observed were a proliferative
interstital pneumonia. Two control calves revealed no
macroscopic lesions.

Inoculation of M. *dispar* and *Ureaplasma* sp. into gnotobiotic
calves by the endobronchial route (Howard et al., 1976) showed
that both mycoplasmas were capable of causing macroscopic but
subclinical pneumonia. Even in these animals, certain non-
pathogenic species of bacteria were isolated from most of
the experimental and control calves. In this work inoculation
of ureaplasmas produced histological cuffing pneumonia in both
calves inoculated, but only one out of three calves inoculated
with M. *dispar* revealed cuffing pneumonia histologically. Since
then, a further 10 gnotobiotic calves have been inoculated once
intratracheally with a culture of the GRI 226 strain of M. *dispar*
and the results (Table 1) reveal that macroscopic pneumonia
involving 1% to 17% of the lung tissue was produced in 8 of the
calves (Gourlay et al., unpublished observation). Histologically
the lesions produced were of interstitial alveolitis centred

around the bronchioles.   Peribronchiolar cuffing was not observed.

TABLE 1

EXTENT OF PNEUMONIA, NUMBER OF MICRO-ORGANISMS AND HISTOPATHOLOGICAL LESIONS IN LUNGS OF GNOTOBIOTIC CALVES INOCULATED INTRATRACHEALLY WITH 10^8 or 10^9 *Mycoplasma dispar* STRAIN GRI 226

Calf No.	Breed‡	%P*	Log$_{10}$ number[+] of organisms		Histopathology**				
			M. dispar	bacteria	RCI	C	CB	AL	A
K67	F	O	5	5	-	-	-	±	-
K78	A/AAF	2	5	4	+	-	-	+	+
K106	AA	6	5	<1	±	-	-	+	+
K114	AA/F	7	6	2	-	-	-	+	+
K186	F	17	6	3	+	±	-	++	+
K195	F	6	5	4	+	-	+	++	+
L16	AA/SF	<1	4	4	-	-	-	+	-
L25	AA/H	3	6	4	+	-	+	+	+
L80	J	1	4	<1	+	-	-	+	-
L132	J	7	5	5	+	-	++	++	+

%P* = Area of lung with macroscopic lesions

+   = Number of organisms per ml. lung homogenate

‡   = A = Ayrshire: AA = Aberdeen Angus: F = Friesian: H = Hereford: J = Jersey: S = Sussex

**   = RCI = round cell infiltration: C = cuffing: CB = catarrhal bronchiolitis: AL = alveolitis: A = atelectasis.

The demonstration that *M. dispar* and *Ureaplasma* sp. are capable of producing pneumonia is interesting but does not answer the important question as to what part they play in the disease that occurs in calves in the field. A recent study in conventionally reared calves (Gourlay et al., 1976) attempted to shed some light on this question. Experimental pneumonia was produced in 45 Channel Island calves by the endobronchial inoculation of lung homogenates from an outbreak of pneumonia. Inoculation of irradiated homogenate produced minimal pneumonia, ampicillin treatment of the homogenate and calves reduced the extent of pneumonia, and treatment with tylosin tartrate prevented the experimental pneumonia. These results suggest that the total pneumonia was due to organisms susceptible to tylosin tartrate and the residual pneumonia remaining after ampicillin treatment was due to organisms susceptible to tylosin tartrate but not to ampicillin. Of the organisms isolated from the lungs of the calves, the ones in this category most likely to be responsible were *M. dispar* and *Ureaplasma* sp.

M. bovis

M. bovis has long been incriminated in outbreaks of clinical mastitis and polyarthritis, particularly in the USA and Canada, and it is undoubtedly of aetiological significance in these conditions. Although this mycoplasma has been isolated from the bovine respiratory tract in many parts of the world, its role in respiratory disease is not clear. Onoviran, in 1972, inoculated a culture of *M. bovis* intranasally into seven 3 year old conventionally reared Zebu bulls. They were killed 3 - 8 weeks later and three had areas of lung consolidation from which the organisms were reisolated. The remaining animals and 3 controls had no pneumonic lesions. We inoculated a culture of a cloned strain of *M. bovis* into 4 gnotobiotic calves by the endobronchial or intratracheal routes. The calves were killed 2 weeks later and the results indicated that *M. bovis* is capable of producing macroscopic but subclinical cuffing pneumonia (Gourlay et al., 1976). In two of these calves, clinical signs of lameness were also observed. *M. bovis* was reisolated from the lungs of all the calves and from the joint of one calf that was still lame at the time of slaughter.

M. bovirhinis

This mycoplasma established and multiplied in bovine tracheal organ cultures but did not produce any cytopathic effects (Thomas and Howard, 1974). However, four strains of *M. bovirhinis* caused subclinical mastitis when inoculated into the bovine mammary gland (Brownlie et al., 1976) indicating that this organism was mildly pathogenic.

Two cloned strains of *M. bovirhinis*, L866 (freshly isolated from a pneumonic lung) and C155 were inoculated intratracheally and intraocularly into one and two gnotobiotic calves respectively, at titres of 10^{10} organisms (Howard et al.,unpublished observations). Signs of respiratory disease or eye infection were not observed during the 3 weeks before slaughter. At autopsy, the lungs of two calves revealed no significant macroscopic lesions while the lungs of the third calf had 6% pneumonic consolidation (Table 2). However, the lungs of the latter calf possessed high titres of four different bacterial species (*Klebsiella, Pseudomonas, Alkaligenes* and *Chromobacterium*) whereas the lungs of the other two calves were bacteriologically sterile. *M. bovirhinis* was not reisolated from the lungs of the two calves with insignificant lesions and only at low titre from the other calf. However, this organism was reisolated from nasopharyngeal swabs of all calves 14 days after inoculation.

TABLE 2

EXTENT OF PNEUMONIA, NUMBER OF MICRO-ORGANISMS AND HISTOPATHOLOGICAL LESIONS IN LUNGS OF GNOTOBIOTIC CALVES INOCULATED INTRATRACHEALLY WITH 10^{10}
Mycoplasma bovirhinis

Calf No.	Inoculum strain	Breed‡	%P*	Log 10 number[+] of organisms	
				M. bovirhinis	Bacteria
L150	C155	F/FA	6	2	6
L192	L866	F/AAF	<1	0	<1
L196	C155	F/SF	0	0	<1

%P* = Area of lung with macroscopic lesions

+ = Number of organisms per ml. lung homogenate

‡ = A = Ayrshire: AA = Aberdeen Angus: F = Friesian: S = Sussex

A. laidlawii

It is generally agreed that *A. laidlawii* is non-pathogenic. Certainly our evidence from bovine tracheal organ culture and bovine mammary gland inoculations support this view. This organism established and multiplied in the organ cultures but did not produce any cytopathic effects (Thomas and Howard, 1974) and the inoculation of four strains of *A laidlawii* into the bovine mammary gland failed to produce mastitis (Brownlie et al., 1976). In view of these results we have not inoculated this organism into gnotobiotic calves.

CONCLUSIONS

The species of mycoplasma isolated at Compton from pneumonic lungs of calves, in the order of frequency, are *M. dispar, Ureaplasma* sp. *M. bovirhinis, M. bovis* and *A. laidlawii*.

Strains of *M. bovis, M. dispar* and *Ureaplasma* sp. are pathogenic and are capable on their own of producing pneumonia in gnotobiotic calves.

It appears to us that under field conditions, mycoplasmas can produce a pneumonia which is predominantly sub-clinical but economically important and which, in a few animals in certain circumstances and with the involvement of other micro-organisms, can lead to clinical disease and even death.

REFERENCES

Bitsch, V., Friis, N.F. and Krogh, H.V. 1976. Acta Vet. scand. 17, p. 32.

Brownlie, J., Howard, C.J. and Gourlay, R.N. 1976. Res. Vet. Sci. 20 p. 261.

Gourlay, R.N., Howard, C.J. and Brownlie, J. 1972. J. Hyg. 70, p. 511.

Gourlay, R.N., Howard, C.J., Thomas, L.H. and Stott, E.J. 1976. Res. vet.
    Sci. 20, p. 167.

Gourlay, R.N., Mackenzie, A. and Cooper, J.E. 1970. J. comp. Path. 80, p. 575.

Gourlay, R.N. and Thomas, L.H. 1969. Vet. Rec. 85, p. 583.

Gourlay, R.N. and Thomas, L.H. 1970. J. comp. Path. 80, p. 585.

Gourlay, R.N., Thomas, L.H. and Howard, C.J. 1976. Vet. Rec. 98, p. 506.

Harbourne, J.F., Hunter, G. and Leach, R.H. 1965. Res. vet. Sci. 6, p. 178.

Howard, C.J. and Gourlay, R.N. 1974. J. gen. Microbiol. 83, p. 393.

Howard, C.J., Gourlay, R.N. and Brownlie, J. 1973. J. Hyg. 71, p. 163.

Howard, C.J., Gourlay, R.N., Thomas, L.H., and Stott, E.J. 1976. Res. vet.
    Sci, 21, p. 227.

Livingstone, C.W. 1972. Am. J. vet. Res. 33, p. 1925.

Onoviran, O. 1972. Bull. epizoot. Dis. Afr. 20, p. 275.

Ose, E.E. and Muenster, O.A. 1975. Vet. Rec. 97, p. 97.

Pirie, H.M. and Allan, E.M. 1975. Vet. Rec. 97, p. 345.

Ruhnke, H.L. and van Dreumel, A.A. 1972. Can. J. comp. Med. 36, p. 317.

Shimizu, T., Nosaka, D. and Nakamura, N. 1975. Jap. J. vet. Sci. 37, p. 121.

St. George, T.D., Horsfall, N. and Sullivan, N.D. 1973. Aust. vet. J. 49
    p. 580.

Thomas, L.H. and Howard, C.J. 1974. J. comp. Path 84, p. 193.

Thomas, L.H., Howard, C.J. and Gourlay, R.N. 1975. Vet. Rec. 97, p. 55.

Thomas, L.H. and Smith, G.S. 1972. J. comp. Path. 82, p. 1.

SOME FEATURES OF PULMONARY MYCOPLASMOSIS IN GROUPS OF NATURALLY INFECTED CALVES

E.M. Allan

Department of Veterinary Pathology, University of Glasgow
Veterinary School, Bearsden Road, Bearsden, Glasgow, Scotland.

ABSTRACT

Several species of bacteria and mycoplasma were isolated from groups of conventional calves housed together for specific periods of time, during which respiratory disease was observed in some animals. The cumulative results suggested that Mycoplasma dispar was closely associated with lesions of cuffing pneumonia amongst naturally infected calves. Mycoplasma bovirhinis, Acholeplasma laidlawii and Ureaplasma sp. were also recovered, but isolations were as frequent from non-pneumonic as pneumonic tissue.

M. dispar is not readily isolated by direct lung culture and a 50% recovery rate from lesions of cuffing pneumonia may be expected. Mycoplasmas can be detected indirectly by immunofluorescence and electron microscopy.

In cuffing pneumonia, as in pulmonary mycoplasmosis in other hosts, there is a massive infiltration of lymphocytes around the airways forming cuffs of cells which do not appear to be antibody producing. Another characteristic of cuffing pneumonia is a marked increase in mucus production and an alteration in its composition.

In many calves mycoplasmas were detected by electron microscope in the bronchial epithelium but were seldom identified in alveolar tissue. The organisms were always extracellular and formed a close association with the cilia and microvilli of the epithelium. Mycoplasmas with extracellular capsules were recognised in pulmonary tissue treated with ruthenium red — a feature associated with M. dispar.

Changes in the ultrastructure of the bronchial epithelial cells were apparent in some cases; many cells lost their cilia and the cytoplasm of the epithelial cells protruded into the lumen. The mitochondria were often distended and disrupted and vacuoles were recognised in the cytoplasm.

Pneumonia is widespread in housed calves in the west of
Scotland. The lesion commonly seen in these animals has been
described as cuffing pneumonia (Jarrett, 1956), a bronchopulmonary change that, in other species, has been attributed to
mycoplasma infection. In Great Britain *Acholeplasma laidlawii*,
Mycoplasma bovirhinis, *Ureaplasma* sp., *M. dispar* and *M. bovis* have been
isolated from the bovine respiratory tract (Harbourne et al.,
1965; Davies, 1967; Gourlay, 1968 and 1969; Gourlay and Leach,
1970; Gourlay et al., 1970; Thomas and Smith, 1972; Pirie and
Allan, 1975; Thomas et al., 1975; Allan et al., 1976). *M. dispar*,
Ureaplasma sp. and *M. bovis* have been shown experimentally to
produce pneumonia in gnotobiotic calves, the resultant lesions
in some experiments having several of the characteristics of
cuffing pneumonia (Gourlay and Thomas, 1969 and 1970; Gourlay
et al., 1976; Howard et al., 1976). A close association between
M. dispar and *Ureaplasma* sp. and naturally occurring cuffing
pneumonia was demonstrated in a group of calves (Pirie and Allan,
1975) and further studies have implicated *M. dispar* as the more
important organism (Allan et al., 1976). In addition, mycoplasmas
have been seen in the respiratory tracts of calves with pneumonia
(Allan and Pirie, 1977).

This paper will review some of the data previously reported
and present additional findings relative to the natural infection
with mycoplasmas in calves.

MATERIALS AND METHODS

The studies involved examination of the lungs of five groups
of calves. Microbiological examination was for mycoplasmas,
bacteria and, in some cases, viruses. The pathological studies
involved macroscopic examination, histological, histochemical
and electronmicroscopical examinations; in addition, pulmonary
tissue was studied by the indirect immunofluorescence technique
for the presence of *M. dispar*. The methods involved in the
study have been described in previous reports (Pirie and Allan,
1975; Allan et al., 1976; Allan and Pirie, 1977; Allan et al.,
1977).

TABLE 1

FREQUENCY OF ISOLATION OF M. *dispar*, *Ureaplasma* sp., M. *bovirhinis* AND A. *laidlawii* FROM FIVE GROUPS OF CALVES. THE CALVES RANGED FROM ONE MONTH TO SIX MONTHS OLD AND SOME FROM EACH GROUP WERE AFFECTED WITH MACROSCOPIC PNEUMONIA

Group	Age (months)	Mycoplasma isolations from pneumonic calves					Mycoplasma isolations from non-pneumonic calves				
		No. calves with pneumonia	M. *dispar*	*Ureaplasma* sp.	M. *bovirhinis*	A. *laidlawii*	No. calves without pneumonia	M. *dispar*	*Ureaplasma* sp.	M. *bovirhinis*	A. *laidlawii*
1a	6	6	3	0	0	3	3	0	0	0	1
1b	6	12	6	8	3	9	8	0	1	1	5
2	3	12	7	0	1	4	0	–	–	–	–
3	2	4	3	1	1	2	0	–	–	–	–
4	1	6	0	0	2	1	5	0	0	3	0
Total		40	19	9	7	19	16	0	1	4	6

RESULTS

The 56 calves within the five groups were 1 - 6 months old.
Forty had moderate to severe macroscopic lung lesions at
post-mortem examination. The isolation frequency of mycoplamas
from pneumonic and non-pneumonic calves within each group is
shown in the table.

Four mycoplasma sp. were isolated from the calves, namely
M. dispar, *Ureaplasma sp.*, *M. bovirhinis* and *A. laidlawii* .

M. dispar was recovered from 19 of the 40 calves with
pneumonia (approximately 50%); no isolations were made from
the lung tissue of the younger calves. *M. dispar* was not
isolated for any of the 16 non-pneumonic calves. Although the
isolation frequency of *Ureaplasma* sp. was high from the
pneumonic calves within one group, the recovery rate was
inconsistent since these organisms were not found in another
similar six months old group. One six months old non-pneumonic
calf yielded *Ureaplasma* sp. from its lung tissue. *M. bovirhinis*
and *A. laidlawii* were recovered from some calves in most groups.
The four species of mycoplasmas were isolated at low titres
from the lung tissue of most calves.

More than one species of mycoplasma was isolated from the
lung tissue of some calves and only four of the 19 animals
positive on culture for *M. dispar* yielded this organism only.
Bacteria were isolated with *M. dispar* from the lung tissue of
some cases, particularly the three months old calves, while
bacteria, mycoplasmas and *M. dispar* were cultured from the
older calves.

The pneumonia present in most of these calves was cuffing
pneumonia or, in the younger animals of two or three months old,
the lesion considered to develop into cuffing pneumonia.
Macroscopically the lesions were most severe in the anterior lobes
of the lungs; the lesions were smooth and red-purple in
appearance. Histologically, the cuffing pneumonia was characterised by the presence of bronchitis and bronchiolitis with most

of the smaller airways surrounded by follicular accumulations
of lymphocytes which frequently ensheathed the bronchiole and
extended down its length. Infiltrating lymphocytes, which
extended into the lamina propria, obliterated the muscularis of
many airways. Germinal centres were seen in many of the
accumulations. Alveolitis with neutrophils, macrophages and
occasional plasma cells and giant cells was evident in some
cases, while others had alveolar collapse. Similar lesions
were recognised in the younger animals although the lymphocytic
aggregates formed a diffuse layer around the airway with only
a few follicular arrangements.

Histochemical examination of the lung tissue of the
pneumonic calves indicated an increase in the number of goblet
cells in the bronchial epithelium which extended down to the
small bronchi and bronchioles - a position not normally
occupied by goblet cells. Hypertrophy of the bronchial submucosal glands, with dilation, was observed in the pneumonic
animals. Specific staining of formalin-fixed tissue enabled
recognition of an alteration in the composition of pulmonary
mucus. Sulphomucins and a small amount of sialomucins were
produced by the goblet cells of the pneumonic animals, unlike
the goblet cells of non-pneumonic animals which produced
sulphomucins exclusively. The glands of non-pneumonic animals
produced approximately equal proportions of neutralmucin,
sulphomucin and sialomucins, whereas an increase in the
proportions of sulphomucins and sialomucins was detected in
the glands of pneumonic animals.

Pulmonary tissue from some calves was studied by indirect
immunofluorescence for the presence of M. dispar. The organisms
fluoresced bright yellow-green and were positioned in the
region of the cilia in the bronchial epithelium. This technique,
however, was not totally satisfactory as culturally positive
material was not necessarily positive by immunofluorescence.
Antibody producing cells, also detected by the indirect
immunofluorescent techniques, were found in the pulmonary
tissue of a number of calves. A few IgG producing cells were

detected but most cells were IgA producing; these were mostly located in the lamina propria. IgM producing cells were infrequent. Antibody producing cells did not appear to be present in the cuffs of lymphocytes around the airways found in many of the pneumonic animals.

Mycoplasmas were observed by the electron microscope in the pulmonary tissue from 16 of 28 calves; the organisms were always present on the bronchial epithelium. In two cases a few mycoplasma cells were seen in the alveolar air spaces, usually as individual organisms.

In the bronchial epithelium the mycoplasmas were found on and between the cilia, often organised in two or three layers of cells, giving the appearance of a micro-colony on the surface of the bronchial epithelium. Most of the mycoplasma cells were oval or round in shape, although cells penetrating between the cilia appeared elongated, as if they had squeezed between these structures. The organisms were never seen within the cytoplasm of the epithelial cells. The mycoplasmas had cellular characteristics typical of the *Mycoplasmatales*; a triple layered unit membrane enclosed the cell which contained densely stained ribosomes lying at the cell periphery and aggregates of nuclear material were found in the clear central area of the cell with electron-dense strands stretching towards the periphery. Amorphous material could be detected around some organisms giving an almost beaded appearance to the surface of the cell.

Mycoplasmas with extracellular capsules were recognised in pulmonary tissue fixed by the ruthenium red technique (Howard and Gourlay, 1974). Dark-staining material was seen around the mycoplasma cells. Further staining of ultra-thin sections fixed in ruthenium red with uranyl acetate and lead citrate enabled visualisation of the fine structure of the mycoplasmas and bronchial epithelial cells. An extra-cellular capsule around *M. dispar* has been demonstrated when pure cultures were examined ultrastructurally after fixation in solutions containing ruthenium red (Howard and Gourlay, 1974);

this suggests that the capsulated organisms recognised in the pulmonary tissue of these calves were probably M. *dispar*. Additionally, comparison of the detection rate of mycoplasmas by electron microscopy with the cultural data indicates that the organisms recognised by electron microscopy were likely to be M. *dispar*.

Ultrastructural changes in the pulmonary tissue were evident, most of the changes being found in the bronchial epithelium. Loss of cilia was common, leaving only basal bodies at the apex of the ciliated cells. The most obvious cytological feature in these cases was the protrusion of the apical cytoplasm of bronchial cells into the lumen. Some of these structures contained very little cytoplasmic material and consisted of granular material in which the rudiments of cilia could be recognised. In bronchial epithelial cells many of the mitochondria were distended, with loss of cristae and total organelle destruction in some cells. Cytoplasmic vacuolisation was a typical feature of the bronchial cells examined.

Neutrophils packed with electron-dense granules were frequently seen passing through the epithelium towards the bronchial lumen. An increase in the number of goblet cells was also a common feature in the pneumonic calves. The goblet cells were tightly packed with mucinogen granules which were often seen spilling into the bronchial lumen.

DISCUSSION

In these studies M. *dispar*, Ureaplasma sp., M. *bovirhinis* and A. *laidlawii* were isolated from the lungs of calves. The overall recovery rate of M. *dispar* from pneumonic lungs was approximately 50%; this is similar to the 60% rate recorded by Gourlay et al. (1970) from 45 randomly collected pneumonic calves of three months old. M. *dispar* is a fastidious and slow-growing organism which may account for its being recovered from only 50% of pneumonic lungs. In the present studies M. *dispar* was most

frequently isolated from older calves (three to six months),
particularly those with lesions of cuffing pneumonia. The
pathogenicity of *M. dispar* has been proven experimentally in
gnotobiotic calves (Gourlay and Thomas, 1969; Gourlay et al.,
1976; Howard et al., 1976), and in tracheal organ cultures the
organism causes progressive sloughing of cells and patchy
flattening of the epithelial layer (Thomas and Howard, 1974).

Experimental infections of mice and pigs with *M. pulmonis*
and *M. suipneumoniae* respectively have been reported (Lutsky and
Organick, 1966; Hodges et al., 1969; Livingston et al., 1972;
Whittlestone, 1972; Lindsey and Cassell, 1973), in which the
development of histological lesions was followed during the
course of the disease. The lesions seen in the acute stage
of the murine and early in the porcine infections were similar
to the pneumonia described in the younger calves in this
study and were characterised by the organisation of lymphocytes
into the peribronchiolar area and the packing of alveolar air
spaces with neutrophils and varying numbers of macrophages.
The cuffing lesions, particularly those with a follicular
pattern and germinal centres (analagous to the lesions in the
six months old calves), developed after the infection had been
established for several weeks. This means that, assuming these
bovine mycoplasmas are pathogens, the peribronchiolar cuffing
will only be present in chronic cases and not in those suffering
the acute phase of the disease.

Histochemical examination of the pulmonary tissue from
pneumonic and non-pneumonic calves indicated an alteration in
the composition of the mucus; there appeared to be an increase
in sialomucin production in the goblet cells and sialomucin
and sulphomucin production in the glands. Alterations in mucus
composition associated with bronchitis have been noted in other
species (de Haller and Reid, 1965; Reid, 1965; Lamb and Reid,
1969; Wheeldon et al., 1976). In these pneumonic cases the
goblet cells increased in number in the bronchial epithelium
and extended peripherally down the airways to the small bronchi
and bronchioles. Goblet cells are considered to proliferate and

increase their rate of secretion following irritation of the bronchial epithelium (Thurlbeck et al., 1961; Jones et al., 1973). Extension of goblet cells into the small bronchi and bronchioles is another feature of epithelial irritation (Reid, 1958; de Haller and Reid, 1965), and the massive goblet cell proliferation seen in the calves suggests the presence of a severe irritant in cuffing pneumonia.

The changes in the composition of the mucus in the pneumonic calves studied were not considered specific for cuffing pneumonia but probably represented a non-specific response by the mucosa to a locally acting stimulus.

The association of mycoplasmas with bronchial epithelium seen in these studies is similar to that described for pathogenic mycoplasmas of other animals, both in experimental infections of the host (Organick et al., 1966; Kohn, 1971; Baskerville, 1972) and in tracheal organ culture studies (Collier and Clyde, 1971; Collier and Baseman, 1973; Hu et al., 1975; Muse et al., 1976). Intracellular organisms were never seen, although Organick et al. (1966) and Kohn (1971) observed *M. pulmonis* in the intracellular spaces and within intracytoplasmic vacuoles in mouse and rat bronchial epithelia respectively. Mycoplasmas were seldom present in the alveolor tissue of the calf and this may have been due to their rapid removal by neutrophils and macrophages. Experimental infections with *M. pulmonis* have demonstrated their rapid removal from alveolar tissue after one week due to speady phagocytosis and destruction by neutrophils and macrophages (Organick et al., 1966).

An extracellular capsule has been detected on *M. dispar* in pure broth culture stained by the ruthenium red technique (Howard and Gourlay, 1974). *M. mycoides* var. *mycoides* is the only other bovine mycoplasma known to have an extracellular capsule and the recognition of the capsulated organisms in the pneumonic tissue examined here suggests that *M. dispar* is the mycoplasma involved in these conditions.

Ultrastructural changes were evident in the bronchial epithelium of calves in which mycoplasmas were detected. Similar ultrastructural changes have been recorded in experimental mycoplasma infections in other species and also in mycoplasma-infected tracheal organ cultures (Organick et al., 1966; Kohn, 1971; Baskerville, 1972; Collier and Baseman, 1973) However, many of these alterations have been reported in diseased respiratory tissues of non-mycoplasmal aetiology (Frasca et al., 1968a; and b) and so the lesions presented here are not pathognomonic.

REFERENCES

Allan, E.M. and Pirie, H.M. 1977. J. med. Microbiol. 10, p. 469.

Allan, E.M., Pirie, H.M. and Selman, I.E. 1976. 9th International Congress on Diseases of Cattle, Paris, p. 381.

Allan, E.M., Pirie, H.M. and Wheeldon, E.B. 1977. Folia. vet. Lat. (In press).

Baskerville, A. 1972. Res. vet. Sci. 13, p. 570.

Collier, A.M. and Baseman, J.B. 1973. Ann. N.Y. Acad. Sci. 225, p. 277.

Collier, A.M. and Clyde, W.A. 1971. Infect. Immun. 3, p. 694.

Davies, G. 1967. J. comp. Path. 77, p. 353.

Frasca, J.M., Auerbach, O., Parks, V.R. and Jamieson, J.D. 1968a. Exp. mol. Pathol. 9, p. 363.

Frasca, J.M., Auerbach, O., Parks, V.R. and Jamieson, J.D. 1968b. Exp. mol. Pathol. 9, p. 380.

Gourlay, R.N. 1968. Res. vet. Sci. 9. p. 376.

Gourlay, R.N. 1969. Vet. Rec. 84, p. 229.

Gourlay, R.N., Howard, C.J., Thomas, L.H. and Stott, E.J. 1976. Res. vet. Sci. 20, p. 167.

Gourlay, R.N. and Leach, R.H. 1970. J. med. Microbiol. 3, p. 111.

Gourlay, R.N., Mackenzie, A. and Cooper, J.E. 1970. J. comp. Path. 80, p. 575.

Gourlay, R.N. and Thomas, L.H. 1969. Vet. Rec. 85, p. 583.

Gourlay, R.N. and Thomas, L.H. 1970. J. comp. Path. 80, p. 585.

Haller, R. de and Reid, L. 1965. Med. thoracalis, 22, p. 549.

Harbourne, J.F., Hunter, D. and Leach, R.H. 1965. Res. vet. Sci. 6, p. 178.

Hodges, R.T., Betts, A.O. and Jennings, A.R. 1969. Vet. Rec. 84, p. 268.

Howard, C.J. and Gourlay, R.N. 1974. J. gen. Microbiol. 83, p. 393.

Howard, C.J., Gourlay, R.N., Thomas, L.H. and Stott, E.J. 1976. Res. vet. Sci. 21, p. 227.

Hu, P.C., Collier, A.M. and Baseman, J.B. 1975. Infect. Immun. 11, p. 704.

Jarrett, W.F.H. 1956. Br. vet. J. 112, p. 431.

Jones, R., Bolduc, P. and Reid, L. 1973. Br. J. exp. Path. 54, p. 229.

Kohn, D.F. 1971. Lab. anim. Sci. 21, p. 856.

Lamb, D. and Reid, L. 1969. J. Path. 98, p. 213.

Lindsey, J.R. and Cassell, G.H. 1973. Am. J. Path. 72, p. 63.

Livingston, C.W., Stair, E.L., Underdahl, N.R. and Mebus, C.A. 1972. Am. J. vet. Res. 33, p. 2249.

Lutsky, I.I. and Organick, A.B. 1966. J. Bact. 92, p. 1154.

Muse, K.E., Powell, D.A. and Collier, A.M. 1976. Infect. Immun. 13, p. 229.

Organick, A.B., Siegesmund, K.A. and Lutsky, I.I. 1966. J. Bact. 22, p. 1164.

Pirie, H.M. and Allan, E.M. 1975. Vet. Rec. 97, p. 345.

Reid, L. 1958. Lect. Sci. Basis Med. 8, p.235.

Reid, L. 1965. Med. thoracalis. 22, p. 61.

Thomas, L.H. and Howard, C.J. 1974. J. comp. Path. 84, p. 193.

Thomas, L.H., Howard, C.J. and Gourlay, R.N. 1975. Vet. Rec. 97, p. 55.

Thomas, L.H. and Smith, G.S. 1972. J. comp. Path. 82, p. 1.

Thurlbeck, W.H., Benjamin, B. and Reid, L. 1961. Br. J. Dis. Chest. 55, p. 54.

Wheeldon, E.B., Pirie, H.M. and Breeze, R.G. 1976. Folia vet. Lat. 6, p. 45.

Whittlestone, P. 1972. In 'Pathogenic Mycoplasmas', Associated Scientific
        Publishers, Amsterdam, p. 263.

DEFENCE MECHANISMS IN CALVES
AGAINST RESPIRATORY INFECTIONS WITH MYCOPLASMAS

C.J. Howard, R.N. Gourlay and G. Taylor
ARC Institute for Research on Animal Diseases,
Compton, Newbury, Berkshire, England.

ABSTRACT

Mycoplasma dispar, M. bovis and Ureaplasma sp are probably the most important mycoplasmas associated with respiratory disease in calves in the UK. Although there seems to be a basic similarity amongst different animal species in the way the lung reacts to mycoplasma infections, each of these three species presents a different problem when methods of immunisation are being considered. The ureaplasmas are serologically heterogeneous and absence of cross protection between serologically distinct strains has been observed in the bovine mammary gland. Calves become infected very early in life with M. dispar, perhaps the most common micro-organism in the calf respiratory tract, and in this situation the problem may be to remove an existing infection. M. bovis seems to occur more sporadically and to infect more transiently than M. dispar and is thus more amenable to investigation.

Experiments with inactivated M. bovis indicate that local administration of antigen is required in order to induce immunity in the lung. Thus it may be inferred that local mechanisms are of prime importance. It is also worth noting that local immunity to M. dispar has been demonstrated in the bovine mammary gland.

Certain antibody mediated effects which are potential defence mechanisms have been demonstrated and these include prevention of mycoplasma attachment, direct killing or stasis of mycoplasma growth with or without complement and immune phagocytosis.

NON-SPECIFIC FACTORS

One of the first host defence systems encountered by an invading organism is probably the various inhibitory substances present in many of the body fluids. A heat stable, dialysable fraction of bovine nasal secretions and whey kills a variety of mycoplasma species (Howard et al., 1975a). Pathogenic and non-pathogenic species are killed as well as virulent and avirulent strains of the same species. These factors may be effective against small numbers of invading organisms.

EVIDENCE FOR A LOCAL IMMUNE RESPONSE IN MYCOPLASMA INFECTIONS

Natural and experimentally-induced respiratory infections with mycoplasmas in a variety of animal species appear to have certain common features. The most notable is perhaps the infiltration of mononuclear cells in the lung (Whittlestone, 1976). This response has been studied in detail in mice and hamsters infected with *Mycoplasma pulmonis* and *M. pneumoniae*. Certain of the infiltrating cells are lymphocytes synthesising specific antibody and it has been suggested that the lung and draining lymph nodes are the main sites of antibody production in respiratory mycoplasmosis. This antibody may be transported or diffuse from these sites into the serum and respiratory secretions (Cassell et al., 1974: Fernald and Clyde, 1974).

No such detailed examination has been made in calves. However, the association of mycoplasmas with cuffing pneumonia in calves has been reported (Gourlay et al., 1970; Pirie and Allan, 1975) and peribronchiolar and perivascular infiltration by mononuclear cells in the lungs of gnotobiotic calves inoculated with *M. dispar, M. bovis* or *Ureaplasma* sp. has been described (Howard et al., 1976a; Gourlay et al., 1976). Also, plasma cells synthesising all classes of bovine immunoglobulin have been observed in the lungs of conventionally reared calves (Bradley, 1974). The similarity between respiratory mycoplasma infections of calves and other animal species makes it likely that the cuffing pneumonia associated with mycoplasma

infections in calves is the result of the animal's immune
response to the mycoplasma. This local response is probably
involved in the control and/or resolution of the infection.

PROBLEMS OF IMMUNISATION WITH THE VARIOUS MYCOPLASMA SPECIES

Immunisation against respiratory mycoplasma infections in
calves may be a means of controlling the disease. However, no
single mycoplasma species has been associated with pneumonia in
calves. In the UK *M. dispar*, *Ureaplasma* sp. and *M. bovis* are probably
the most important mycoplasma species involved in calf pneumonia
(Gourlay and Howard, 1977). Immunisation against each of these
mycoplasma species presents different problems.

UREAPLASMAS

Cows that have been infected in the mammary gland with one
ureaplasma strain, although immune to subsequent infection with
the same strain, are still susceptible to infection with a serologically distinct ureaplasma strain (Howard et al., 1974).
Thus, one approach might be to determine how many serotypes are
associated with calf respiratory disease. If only a few serotypes were associated with disease, immunisation with these might
be considered.

However, studies on the serology of bovine ureaplasmas
indicate that strains do not fall into a few neat circumscribed
serotypes and 8 strains were proposed as possible representatives
of the serological diversity of the group (Howard et al., 1975b)
A further study has been made of 80 fresh isolates to determine
how many of these showed cross reactions with the previously
described 8 strains. Antisera to the 8 representative strains
showed cross reactions in the growth inhibition test with all
but 5 of the fresh isolates. Several of the fresh isolates
reacted with sera to 4 or more of the representative strains.
Thus a current view of the serological structure of bovine
ureaplasmas would seem to be that a range of antigenic determinants exist which are detectable by the growth-inhibition

test. A particular isolate may express various combinations of these determinants. To establish the significance of the above for immunity cross protection in cattle needs to be examined.

Mycoplasma dispar

M. *dispar* is one of the most commonly occurring micro-organisms in the respiratory tract of calves (Gourlay and Howard, 1977). It is, serologically, a fairly homogenous species; thus there is not the problem of serological diversity as seen with the ureaplasmas. However, calves become colonised with this mycoplasma very early in life (Thomas and Smith, 1972). The problem therefore is either to prevent colonisation within a few days of birth or to clear an established infection.

Mycoplasma bovis

This species, which has been isolated recently from severe outbreaks of respiratory disease in the UK, appears to be far less widespread than M. *dispar*. Like M. *dispar* it appears to be serologically fairly homogenous. Thus it may prove possible to immunise against M. *bovis,* and prevent its becoming established in a herd.

METHODS OF IMMUNISING CALVES

In a previously reported study (Howard et al., 1977) it was found that an intramuscular inoculation of formalin-inactivated M. *bovis* in Freunds incomplete adjuvant followed by an intra-tracheal inoculation of inactivated organisms protected calves against subsequent intratracheal challenge with M. *bovis* (Table 1). If the second (booster) inoculation of inactived mycoplasmas was intramuscular no protection could be demonstrated. In these experiments susceptibility to infection was estimated by determining the number of mycoplasmas isolated from the lungs of calves 3 weeks after challenge. Thus there were significantly less M. *bovis* isolated from the lungs of intratracheally boosted animals (P< 0.01, Students' t test) compared with control calves or intramuscularly boosted animals. A reduction in the number of mycoplasmas in lungs following immunisation with inactivated mycoplasma appears to be more difficult to demonstrate than reduction in the extent of pneumonia (Atobe and Ogata, 1977). At the time of challenge the serum antibody levels, as determined by a single radial haemolysis technique, were significantly higher in animals given the intramuscular booster inoculation than in animals boosted intratracheally.

TABLE 1

EFFECT OF INOCULATING CALVES WITH INACTIVATED *M. bovis* ON SUBSEQENT SUSCEPTIBILITY TO INTRATRACHEAL CHALLENGE. COMPARISON OF INTRAMUSCULAR (i.m.) OR INTRATRACHEAL (i.t.) BOOSTING.

Treatment on indicated day			No. of *M. bovis* isolated from lungs day 42
0	14	21	
Freunds incomplete adjuvant i.m.	none		$5.2 \pm 2.60*$
Inactivated *M. bovis* + adjuvant i.m.	inactiviated *M. bovis* i.m.	10^9 *M. bovis* i.t.	3.6 ± 2.32
Inactivated *M. bovis* + adjuvant i.m.	inactivated *M. bovis* i.t.		0.6 ± 1.18

* Log_{10} geometric mean of the number of colour changes units per ml lung homogenate $\pm$ standard deviation.

Subsequent experiments were made to determine whether the priming injection needed to be intramuscular. The results of two experiments are summarised in Table 2. Each group consisted of 8 calves with the exception of the group immunised twice intratracheally, which consisted of 4 animals. Significantly less *M. bovis* (P <0.05) were found in the lungs of animals inoculated with formalinised mycoplasma intramuscularly and then intratracheally compared with animals in the other three groups.

The lack of correlation between serum antibody and immunity together with the apparent necessity to present antigen locally

in order to induce immunity suggests the importance of local
immune mechanisms in the induction of resistance to *M. bovis* in
calves.

TABLE 2

EFFECT OF INOCULATING CALVES WITH INACTIVATED *M. bovis* ON SUBSEQUENT
SUSCEPTIBILITY TO INTRATRACHEAL CHALLENGE. COMPARISON OF INTRAMUSCULAR
(i.m.) AND INTRATRACHEAL (i.t.) PRIMING.

Treatment on indicated day			No. of *M. bovis* isolated from lungs day 42
0	14	21	
Freunds complete adjuvant i.m.	none		4.8 ± 1.83*
Inactivated *M. bovis* + adjuvant i.m.	inactivated *M. bovis* i.t.	10^9 *M. bovis* i.t.	3.4 ± 2.14
Inactivated *M. bovis* i.t.	inactivated *M. bovis* i.t.		5.8 ± 1.16
none	inactivated *M. bovis* i.t.		5.1 ± 2.08

* As colony forming units $\pm$ standard deviation.

Experiments in animals other than cattle have also indicated the superiority of inoculating inactivated mycoplasmas into
the respiratory tract over inoculation by a systemic route.
These include experiments with *M. gallisepticum* in chickens
(Hayatsu et al., 1974), *M. pulmonis* in mice (Taylor et al., 1977;
Atobe and Ogata, 1977) and *M. pneumoniae* in hamsters (Greenberg
et al., 1977).

The inoculation of live organisms systemically has also
been reported to induce immunity to respiratory infection eg
in cattle with *M. mycoides* subsp. *mycoides* (Hudson, 1971), and
mice with *M. pulmonis* (Taylor et al., 1977). The mechanism is
difficult to elicit in this situation since it is possible that
live organisms may reach the lung and induce an immune response
in the respiratory tract, as demonstrated in mice.

Work is now in progress to determine the mechanism of
immunity induced by vaccination. Preliminary results have

shown that antibody to M. *bovis* can be demonstrated in lung
washings taken from calves inoculated intramuscularly and
intratracheally with inactivated organisms. However, antibody
is also present in animals inoculated twice intramuscularly.
Further work is needed to compare levels of antibody or classes
of antibody in the two groups of animals.

Unsuccessful attempts have been made to induce immunity
to M. *dispar* in gnotobiotic calves by the same regime used for
M. *bovis* in conventionally reared calves. Possibly the important
antigens on M. *dispar* are altered by formalin treatment.
Alternatively M. *dispar* may utilise different pathogenic mechanisms
from M. *bovis* and resistance of calves to M. *dispar* may be different
from that to M. *bovis*. It is worth noting that in cows immunity
to reinfection of the udder with M. *dispar* seems to be related to
some local mechanism (Gourlay et al., 1975).

In general the results indicate the importance of local
immune systems in inducing resistance to respiratory mycoplasma
infections in calves. Since cells synthesising all classes
of bovine antibody have been found in calf lungs such local
immunity need not necessarily be mediated by IgA.

POSSIBLE MECHANISMS OF IMMUNITY

There are a variety of ways in which antibody present in
the lung might prevent a mycoplasma infection. Antibody has
been shown to inhibit the attachment of mycoplasmas to cells
(Manchee and Taylor-Robinson, 1968). Thus antibody present in
respiratory secretions may prevent attachment of the mycoplasmas
to ciliated epithelium and therefore prevent the initiation of
infection. Specific antibody inhibits the growth of mycoplasmas
(Edward and Fitzgerald, 1954). Also, mycoplasmas, since they
lack a cell wall, are particularly susceptible to killing by
antibody and complement (Brunner et al., 1972). Although only
small levels of complement are found in respiratory secretions
compared with levels in serum under normal conditions, this may
be sufficent to kill mycoplasmas, and during inflamation higher

levels would be present in secretions. Thus antibody of IgM
and certain IgG sub-classes might be expected to promote
complement-mediated killing. IgA would not be expected to
cause complement-mediated killing of mycoplasmas by the classical
pathway but possibly this immunoglobulin could mediate killing
by the alternate pathway. It is also possible that the alternate pathway could be activated by mycoplasmas in the absence
of specific antibody (Bredt and Bitter-Suermann, 1975).

The most abundant phagocytic cell in the non-inflamed
respiratory tract is the macrophage. However, polymorphs are
found in large numbers in lung washings following infection
with mycoplasma. Experiments with bovine phagocytic cells -
alveolar macrophages and lacteal polymorphs - have shown that
these cells are capable of killing *M. bovis* and *M. dispar* in the
presence of bovine antibody (Howard et al., 1976b). In addition
there are other reports of mycoplasmas being seen inside
phagocytic cells. Thus this may be an important defence
mechanism operating in mycoplasma infections.

The possible involvement of cell mediated immunity has been
investigated in various mycoplasma infections (reviewed by
Whittlestone, 1976) and delayed type hypersensitivity reactions
have been reported in cattle infected with *M. mycoides* subsp.
mycoides. However, as a result of investigations in man, hamsters
and mice (Fernald and Clyde, 1974; Taylor and Taylor-Robinson,
1976) it seems that cell mediated immunity is likely to be of
less importance than (local) antibody synthesis.

REFERENCES

Atobe, H. and Ogata, H. 1977. Jap. J. vet. Sci. <u>39</u>, p. 39.

Bradley, P.A. 1974. MSc. Thesis, University of Bristol.

Bredt, W. and Bitter-Suermann. 1975. Infect. Immun. <u>11</u>, p. 497.

Brunner, H., James, W.D., Horswood, R.L. and Chanock, R.M. 1972. J. Immun. <u>108</u>, p. 1491.

Cassell, G.H., Lindsey, J.R. and Baker, H.J. 1974. J. Immun. <u>112</u>, p. 124.

Edward, D. G.ff. and Fitzgerald, W.A. 1954. J. Path. Bact. <u>68</u>, p. 23.

Fernald, G.W. and Clyde, W.A. 1974. Inserm. <u>33</u>, p. 421.

Gourlay, R.N. and Howard, C.J. 1977. This publication.

Gourlay, R.N., Howard, C.J. and Brownlie, J. 1975. Infect. Immun. <u>12</u>, p. 947.

Gourlay, R.N., Mackenzie, A. and Cooper, J.E. 1970. J. comp. Path. <u>80</u>, p. 575.

Gourlay, R.N., Thomas, L.H. and Howard, C.J. 1976. Vet.Rec. <u>98</u>, p. 506.

Greenberg,H., Helms, C.M., Grizzard, M.B., James, W.D., Horswood, R.L. and Chanock, R.M. 1977. Infect. Immun. <u>16</u>, p. 88.

Hayatsu, E., Sugiyama, H., Kawakubo, Y., Kimura, M. and Yoshioka, M. 1974. Jap. J. vet. Sci. <u>36</u>, p. 311.

Howard, C.J., Brownlie, J. and Gourlay, R.N. 1975a. Proc. Soc. Gen. Microbiol. <u>2</u>, p. 74.

Howard, C.J., Gourlay, R.N. and Brownlie, J. 1974. Infect. Immun. <u>9</u>, p. 400.

Howard, C.J., Gourlay, R.N. and Collins, J. 1975b. Int. J. syst. Bact. <u>25</u>, p. 155.

Howard, C.J., Gourlay, R.N. and Taylor, G. 1977. Vet. Microbiol. <u>2</u>, (In press).

Howard, C.J., Gourlay, R.N., Thomas, L.H. and Stott, E.J. 1976a. Res. vet. Sci. <u>21</u>, p. 227.

Howard, C.J., Taylor, G., Collings, J. and Gourlay, R.N. 1976b. Infect. Immun. <u>14</u>, p. 11.

Hudson, J.R. 1971. FAO Agric. Studies. No. 86.

Manchee, R.J. and Taylor-Robinson, D. 1968. J. Gen. Microbiol. <u>50</u>, p. 465.

Pirie, H.M. and Allan, E.M. 1975. Vet. Rec. <u>97</u>, p. 345.

Taylor, G., Howard, C.J. and Gourlay, R.N. 1977. Infect. Immun. <u>16</u>, p. 422.

Taylor, G. and Taylor-Robinson, D. 1976. Immunology, <u>30</u>, p. 611.

Thomas, L.H. and Smith, G.S. 1972. J. comp. Path. <u>82</u>, p. 1.

Whittlestone, P. 1976. Adv. vet. Sci. comp. Med. <u>20</u>, p. 277.

J.M. Rutter *(UK)*

Thank you, Dr. Ernø, for your very interesting and provocative opener to this session. You have certainly left us
with two very important questions at the end of your paper.
You have also indicated the kind of criteria which you think
are necessary regarding the diagnosis and study of mycoplasma
infections: presumably you would ask the people who have been
working on *Mycoplasma bovirhinis, M. arginini* and *M. bovigenitalium*,
about whose work you were being rather critical, to take note
of this and apply it in the future.

C. Howard *(UK)*

You were suggesting that mycoplasmal infection might make
animals more susceptible to secondary infections by affecting
the macrophages. We have attempted some experiments with *M.
pulmonis*, an organism which can produce a severe pneumonia in
mice. We found that mice infected with *M. pulmonis* were no more
susceptible to a second bacterial infection than are normal
control mice. I think this is good evidence that mycoplasmas
do not play the same sort of role as do viruses in this respect.

H. Ernø *(Denmark)*

As I mentioned, some of my colleagues at the Institute
have been working along these lines. Their preliminary studies
show that leukocytes drawn from a rat which has been inoculated
with *M. arthritidis* have lost their capacity to phagocytose
Escherischia coli to a very high degree - from 10^7 to 10^5 compared
to a control - a hundred-fold decrease. This goes along very
well with your lung experimental infection.

C. Howard

It is just the opposite, is it not? You say there is a
decrease.

H. Ernø

Yes, there is a decrease in the leukocyte phagocytosis.

C. Howard

I am saying that there was no increase in susceptibility.

H. Ernø

It was not the same mycoplasma. This was with *Mycoplasma arthritidis* in rats.

J.M. Rutter

You mentioned the need for further work on hypersensitivity and possibly macrophage suppression. As a diagnostician, do you see any future for tests based on that kind of approach?

H. Ernø

No, not from delayed hypersensitivity tests - but Dr. Gourlay might know more about that.

J.M. Rutter

Dr. Gourlay is indicating "No".

H. Ernø

Dr. Pignatelli, I am interested in the geographical distribution, occurrence and spread of the different species of mycoplasma. Were there any differences in the mycoplasmas isolated from animals from different countries and, more specifically, since it is the most important one, did you isolate *Mycoplasma bovis* from calves obtained from all supplying countries, or only from France and Italy?

I would also like to ask a general question. Does anyone know how *Mycoplasma bovis* came to France? I thought that it came from Canada. I wonder whether the French workers know anything about these rumours...

P. Pignatelli *(Italy)*

75% of the beef producing cattle farms are in the North of Italy, especially in the area around Piemonte and Venice. The highest concentration is around Verona, where individual farms are very close to each other. About 20% of these farms are in

the centre of Italy, and the remaining 10% are in the Southern
and the highland areas.

In Italy the farms are built in very different ways; for
this reason, it is very difficult to say if one type of rearing
unit is more infective than others. We say that the French
calves are the most infected, but this may be because they are
the most numerous. In any case, the percentage of isolation of
M. bovis was virtually the same from all breeds involved. The
only factor of importance in the differences noted was the type
of farm. Family-run farms, where hygiene is poor and no all-in
all-out policy practised, showed a particularly high infection
rate. They buy the calves at different times and ages from
various importers. I think that respiratory disease is always
present at all times of the year, irrespective of the season.

R.N. Gourlay (UK)

I notice that you do not have M. dispar on your list, nor
the ureaplasmas. I am wondering whether your media would have
detected these two mycoplasmas, or whether in fact they do not
exist there.

P. Pignatelli

My research position in this was not very easy because, as
the Chairman explained, for the last three years I have worked
for a small company and I did not have a lot of money for my
research. Thus I was able to produce only 8 hyperimmune sera.
However, I have since moved to a different company and, with the
better resources now at my disposal, I hope to identify the 115
unidentified strains, which were lyophilised at the time, at
some point in the future.

H.M. Pirie (UK)

You recorded a high isolation for M. bovis. I wondered if,
in any of the outbreaks of respiratory disease which you had,
did any of the calves have arthritis as well?

P. Pignatelli

Over the last two or three years the characteristics of mycoplasmal infection of cattle have changed completely. In the past I found pneumonia and arthritis combined, and in these cases I isolated *M. bovis* from the joints. Recently however joint lesions have fallen in incidence. I think this is due to improvement in the design and hygiene of farm buildings.

J.M. Rutter

Dr. Gourlay, with reference to the lung homogenate experiment, did you see any difference in the kinds of pneumonia in the four different groups of animals?

R.N. Gourlay

Yes, some of the pneumonias were definitely different. Some of the animals in the group of 15 calves inoculated with lung homogenate had no pneumonia at all, and some had up to 85% of the lungs affected. The animals with 85% pneumonia died, a very severe suppurative broncho-pneumonia being present. All ranges of reaction were noted.

J.M. Rutter

Did you see any differences between those calves treated with tylosin and ampicillin?

R.N. Gourlay

We saw very little in the tylosin-treated calves. I cannot really remember what sort of pneumonias there were in the ampicillin-treated calves.

J.M. Rutter

As I understand it, you were suggesting that the antibacterial substances were knocking out different components in the homogenate, and presumably this might be reflected in the lesions which you see in the lungs.

R.N. Gourlay

Of course, these were all conventional animals, so they had their own microflora, as well as the organisms which we put in, which confuses the issue.

J.B. McFerran *(UK)*

I think you demonstrated clearly the importance of mycoplasma in this condition, but did you look for virus infection? One explanation for your last slide, with the better results obtained with lung homogenate compared with pure culture, might be the presence of a latent virus.

R.N. Gourlay

We did check for viruses, both culturally and with serological studies. There seemed to be no indication that viruses were playing any part at all.

H.M. Pirie

What time after infection were the calves which were given *M. dispar* and later developed alveolitis looked at?

R.N. Gourlay

They were killed three weeks after infection, although sometimes we kill them at two weeks post infection. This may have been too early. This is an interesting point. Do you think that cuffing could develop from an alveolitis?

H.M. Pirie

Work in laboratory animals and the pig suggests that alveolitis probably comes first. When you give the calves *M. bovirhinis*, do you consider that it produces pathogenic effects in the nasal cavities and upper respiratory tract?

R.N. Gourlay

We do not know about the pathogenicity of mycoplasmas for the upper respiratory tract.

P. Pignatelli

I should like to know if you obtained the described results in your experimental challenge under normal conditions of maintenance, or did you apply some stresses to your calves?

R.N. Gourlay

Most of the work I have talked about was done in gnotobiotic calves, which are kept in large plastic isolators maintained at room temperature. Each calf is in an individual isolator. That might be called stress, but they certainly look very content in the isolators.

J.M. Rutter

You mentioned in your paper the use of the mammary gland for studying infections with mycoplasmas. Would you like to comment on the comparability of the mammary gland and the respiratory tract as far as experimental infections are concerned?

R.N. Gourlay

I think the *M. bovirhinis* work will give an indication of this. It seems to us that the mammary gland is a very good model and is probably more sensitive to infection with mycoplasmas than the respiratory tract. We obtained a definite sub-clinical mastitis with *M. bovirhinis*, which was indicated by an increased number of cells in the milk, whereas, when we inoculated it into the respiratory tract of calves, no lesions were observed. On the other hand, when we inoculate *M. dispar* and the ureaplasmas into the mammary gland, we obtain very severe clinical mastitis. I look on it as a very useful screen to test the pathogenicity of an organism, and we usually inoculate mycoplasmas into the mammary gland before going on to experiments involving the respiratory tract. That is why we never put *A. laidlawii*, which is one of the organisms which we occasionally isolate, into calf lungs; we have put it into the mammary gland and have not produced any mastitis whatsoever, from which we have inferred that it was not worth while putting it into the lungs of gnotobiotic calves.

H.J. Breukink *(Netherlands)*

You use the word "sub-clinically" even though you say that about 60% of the lungs were pneumonic. What do you mean by the word "sub-clinical"?

R.N. Gourlay

I mean that there is no clinical evidence of disease. The animal looks all right, but if it were chased around it might turn out to be a bit poorly -

H.J. Breukink

Just from a distance.

R.N. Gourlay

Yes, and most farmers would think that it was normal.

L.H. Thomas *(UK)*

We do examine these animals clinically during the course of the experiment. The rectal temperature of the animals is taken every day, and an examination is made, but you can detect no evidence of clinical pneumonia. When they are killed at the end of the experiment there is a degree of pneumonic consolidation, as Dr. Gourlay has described.

R.N. Gourlay

A great number of calves which are killed do have pneumonic lesions in their lungs, but a farmer would not know that the calves had any symptoms.

H.J. Breukink

This is true, but 40-60% consolidation is quite a large amount.

J.M. Sharp *(UK)*

I got the - possibly erroneous - impression from your earlier experiments in gnotobiotic calves involving *M. bovirhinis* and *M. bovis* that, whenever you had a bacterium there, you had a

greater percentage of pneumonia. Would it be erroneous to
suggest that the bacterium is perhaps paving the way for *M.
bovirhinis* ?

R.N. Gourlay

We do not believe that at all. I tried to point out one
case where there was 10^7 *E. coli* in one of these calves which had
no pneumonia at all.

J.M. Sharp

But it did not have *M. bovirhinis* or *M. bovis* either.

R.N. Gourlay

No, because it was a control animal. It was not inoculated.

J.M. Sharp

What I am saying is, when you have the two together, are
you then getting pneumonia?

R.N. Gourlay

No, we are not.

N.J.L. Gilmour *(UK)*

In view of the fact that pasteurellae are presumably pathogenic in the lungs, have you considered putting them in combination with mycoplasma to see if there is a synergistic effect
between the two?

R.N. Gourlay

Yes, I think we have done that, after a fashion, but I am
not too happy about the results. We are working towards it.

J.M. Rutter

After having seen all the slides of the macroscopic appear-
ances of lungs, I think it was very interesting to see what is
actually going on at the cellular level, in Dr. Allan's paper.

One point which did strike me was that in the Table which you showed there seemed to be quite a significant difference between the numbers of mycoplasmas isolated from group 1B compared with 1A, although about 50% of the pneumonic calves from both groups yielded *M. dispar* and you got lots of ureaplasmas and *A. laidlawii* from group 1B. I wondered what the differences between groups 1A and 1B were, and whether there were any differences in the histopathology.

E. Allan *(UK)*

Histopathologically there was no difference. They were examined at different times of the year.

H. Ernø *(Denmark)*

It was a beautiful paper, and we are certainly progressing. Can we safely assume that *M. dispar* is the only mycoplasma, except *M. mycoides*, which has a capsule?

E. Allan

I think you should refer to the work at Compton. They have been looking at pure cultures of mycoplasmas, and none of the other species which they have isolated have a capsule.

R.N. Gourlay

As you know, the ureaplasmas have some material outside the cell. I do not know whether this is a capsule, and I do not think anyone has described it as such, but it is certainly extra-cellular material. I do not think any of the other mycoplasmas we have looked at were capsulated.

C. Howard

None of the bovine ones we have looked at had capsules but there are other strains in other animal species which do have capsules.

R.N. Gourlay

For example, *M. meleagridis* and *M. pneumoniae*.

J.M. Rutter

Dr. Howard, in the two groups of animals which you described - the two Tables which you showed us - giving the effect of the treatment, it seemed that, in the second group of animals, the response to the intramuscular primer followed by the intra-tracheal booster was considerably less efficient than in the first one. Is that true, and if so, have you any explanation for it?

C. Howard

It certainly appeared that way. They were a different group of animals and a different batch of the mycoplasmas was used to vaccinate them. In the first experiment we did not take many pieces of lung tissue to work out the average recovery numbers but we increased sample numbers in the subsequent experiment. This led to more quantitative detail. All I can say is that there was still a significant difference in the numbers of mycoplasma in lung tissue. What is more important is that the intratracheal injection had no effects in comparison with intramuscular, followed by an intratracheal injection. It is not just a non-specific effect.

P.W. Wells (UK)

I should like to take up a point which you made about the dissimilarity between the efficacy of vaccination against myco-plasma and against PI3. You said that in your system intra-muscular followed by intratracheal was the most efficient system compared with other routes or combinations.

C. Howard

That is correct. That is doing it with the same batch of antigen and the same amounts into the two groups of calves.

P.W. Wells

You said that this was different from PI3.

C. Howard

Apparently different.

P.W. Wells

I was thinking of the work which Dr. W.D. Smith did in this Institute. He showed with PI3 in lambs that intramuscular injection with an inactivated antigen in Freunds adjuvant followed by an intranasal inoculation with inactivated antigen was more effective than the intramuscular-only route. This seems to be similar to what you have found with mycoplasm.

K. Petzoldt *(West Germany)*

Can you explain the method of killing mycoplasmas by macrophages? Is it a type of lysis?

C. Howard

I think it is a straightforward phagocytosis.

K. Petzoldt

An enhancing of phagocytosis.

C. Howard

I think so, yes. It is merely that the antibody is opsonic. Without the antibody the mycoplasmas just parasitise the surface of the cell and grow on it. You can stain infected macrophage cultures by immunofluorescence and demonstrate specific mycoplasmas growing happily on the surface of cells in quite large numbers.

K. Petzoldt

It is not, then, a direct action of the antibody.

C. Howard

No. We included controls, in which the same concentrations of specific antibody were added to mycoplasma-infected calf kidney cells. The mycoplasmas survived quite happily. We had decreases in viable counts only with the macrophage cultures, not with the calf kidney cultures.

J.M. Rutter

What about the dialysable fraction in bovine nasal secretions? Presumably that is a different system.

C. Howard

Yes, that is dealing with small molecular weights, or cations, or something like that. It is a peculiar thing which seems to be absorbed out by red cells, and it can also be absorbed out with the mycoplasmas which are not killed. It is as if it is sticking on. It sticks on to anything and then will kill perhaps some strains.

J.M. Sharp

A small practical point: how do you assess the amount of antigen incorporated into the vaccines?

C. Howard

We grow the mycoplasmas in broth, spin them down and inactivate them with formalin and then do a total protein on the final suspension, which we then divide up.

F.J. Bourne (UK)

I should like to make a point on the antibodies which you seem to have produced in the respiratory tract of these animals.

C. Howard

We seem to have a local immunity of some sort, but I am not sure whether we have shown that it is an antibody yet.

F.J. Bourne

Are you not even sure that it is humoral?

C. Howard

No, we cannot say. We have antibody in concentrated lung washes taken from vaccinated animals, but antibody is present both in intramuscularly-inoculated and intratracheally-inoculated animals.

F.J. Bourne

I think this is quite interesting. In the experience of
our work, which we have been doing principally in pigs, and
some in the calf, we find it very difficult to stimulate local
antibody in terms of an IgA response, using a non-replicating
antigen. We are not alone in this experience. It is possible
that you have here a mechanism whereby you can stimulate a local
immune system, so obviously it would be extremely useful - almost
a necessity - to determine what antibody you are playing around
with. Even to determine whether it is an antibody.

C. Howard

We have tried some preliminary fluorescence tests, by which
we certainly found that some of the antibodies seem to be IgG.

F.J. Bourne

Which one would expect to get. You quoted Pearce's work
as possibly suggesting that you could stimulate an IgA response
using a non-replicating antigen, quoting the toxin/toxoid *Vibrio*
system.

C. Howard

Yes, and we stimulated local immunity, but I do not think
that I actually related it to an antibody or to any particular
class of antibody.

F.J. Bourne

A word of caution here. What was peculiar about Pearce's
system was that, with the toxin, he could both prime and get a
secondary response, using the toxin, but he could not with the
toxoid. If he primed with the toxoid and then dosed with the
toxin, or the toxoid, there was no response. So he has a very
peculiar system and he has now changed his mind about some of
the things he said originally. He finds that he can stimulate
an antibody response using mucosal stimulation of toxin/toxoid
combinations, but he cannot determine whether this is going to
give a systemic response, a systemic and local response in terms
of intestinal juice secretion of IgA, or just intestinal juice

secretion. In other words, he can get a response at mucosal
level, which may also give a serum response, or it may give
only an intestinal juice response. He just cannot predict what
is going to happen. So, when one is talking about mucosal systems, it really is a complicated system in terms of antigen/
antibody presentation, and certainly in the response which you
are going to get.

B. Morein *(Sweden)*

The question is, are you quite sure that all the mycoplasma
are killed with formalin, because formalin does not kill in a
straight line.

C. Howard

We do check the vaccine batches to see if we can grow
anything from it, and we have been unable to grow anything.

B. Morein

It is not uncommon to find it in vaccines sometimes. You
can sometimes find living particles in vaccines.

C. Howard

It is less than 10 organisms per ml. You start off with
10^{10} organisms.

H.M. Pirie

I should like to ask you about the mycoplasmacidal factors
in the nasal secretions. Are these nasal secretions in calves?
Is there any evidence that these substances are in bronchial
secretions?

C. Howard

We have found this activity in nasal secretions taken both
from calves and from adult cows. We have also looked at bronchial
secretions and we have perceived it in this as well.

O.C. Straub *(West Germany)*

Why did you use formalin? Why did you not also try other inactivating substances? The adjuvant which you use is quite important. A question which occurs to me, working with viruses, and which should be addressed to all mycoplasmologists, is that we know that there are viruses which grow in mycoplasmas. In future experiments, could we find viruses which will kill mycoplasma, or could the reason for these different results be that some mycoplasmas are already infected with viruses?

C. Howard

There is no member of the genus *Mycoplasma* which has been demonstrated to have a virus. The known viruses all infect members of the genus *Acholeplasma*. As far as inactivation with formalin is concerned, we use it because people have had some success with injecting chickens, hamsters and mice with mycoplasmas, using formalin for inactivation of the antigen. We have compared formalin and irradiation for inactivating antigen, and the formalin was as good, perhaps even a bit better. Certainly the irradiated material was no better than the formalin inactivated material. We have tried many different ways of inactivating. We have a limited number of calves, and once we have a system which works, it is more interesting to progress on to other things rather than to work our way through lots of different inactivation procedures.

O.C. Straub

Formalin might be put on the Index. Formalin is one of those substances which we may not be able to use in future experiments.

C. Howard

We have tried two experiments with complete Freunds adjuvant. It seems to make no difference whether we use complete or incomplete Freunds. Doing different experiments you get more or less the same sort of picture. There are lots of adjuvants in the bovine field which we could try. At the present we have not tried any of the new combinations. I was talking to Dr.

Wells about adjuvants, and he seemed to think that the oily adjuvants are as good as any in terms of the ability to stimulate an antibody response.

O.C. Straub

In France they have a terrific adjuvant which they use in their foot and mouth vaccine for the ox.

G. Dannacher *(France)*

This is a foot and mouth vaccine prepared for cattle. The results with earlier vaccines were bad, and improved only when the adjuvant was changed. It may not be as effective for other species.

O.C. Straub

I feel that perhaps in the mycoplasma field, where we have trouble with inducing immunity, we should pay special attention to the use of new and possibly better adjuvants as compared with the generally known ones.

H. Ernø

I do not think that we have special difficulties in inducing immunity, at least not when we are producing antisera. We use several kinds of adjuvant - for instance aluminium hydroxide.

E. Allan

Did the vaccination prevent arthritis on challenge?

C. Howard

We did not get any arthritis in the conventionally reared calves following inoculation via the respiratory tract. We have since tried to protect against intravenous challenge, which did induce arthritis.

J.M. Rutter

Dr. Ernø has been telling me about the ways in which the International Reference Centre for Animal Mycoplasmas could be of assistance to workers in the mycoplasma field, and I am going to ask him to say a few words on this topic.

First, we would be pleased to provide limited amounts of antisera - something like 2 ml - against all the known mycoplasma species. Two ml does not sound very much, but if you use it for immunofluorescence it may be diluted perhaps 40 times, which is ample for this test.

Second, if you have strains which you cannot identify, you can send them to us for identification, preferably in a lyophilised state. These should be differentiated, as far as possible, into groups before dispatch, to save us undue work. If you have, say, 70 mycoplasma isolates which you cannot identify, try to differentiate them by biochemical tests or other methods, and then send a sample of each group to us.

Finally, we would be happy to advise newcomers to the field on which methods they should use for identification and for sero-epidemiological studies.

We would like you to follow the International Posting Code concerning the sending of mycoplasmas. We do not want to receive a crushed or broken package containing mycoplasmas - that does not make them happy back in Denmark!

SESSION 4B

BACTERIAL

Chairman:

J.M. Rutter

Co-ordinator:

G.E. Jones

PULMONARY BACTERIAL FLORA OF PNEUMONIC
AND NON-PNEUMONIC CALVES

E.M. Allan

Department of Veterinary Pathology, University of Glasgow,
Veterinary School, Bearsden Road, Bearsden, Glasgow, Scotland.

ABSTRACT

The lungs of 92 calves, ranging in age from one day to six months, were examined bacteriologically. Routine bacteriological methods were used and several sites of the lung were studied in most animals. The lungs of 62 calves were culturally positive for bacteria.

Of the 92 animals examined 63 were pneumonic macroscopically. Bacteria were isolated from 41 of these calves (65%) and 52 isolations were made. The species most commonly identified amongst the isolants were Pasteurella haemolytica (17.4%), Pasteurella multocida (11.5%), Corynebacterium pyogenes (9.6%) and Staphylococcus aureus (7.6%).

Of the remaining 29 non-pneumonic calves examined 21 (72.4%) had bacteriologically positive lungs and 29 isolations were made. The most commonly isolated species from the non-pneumonic lung tissue were P. haemolytica (10.3%), P. multocida (10.3%). Streptococcus pneumoniae (10.3%), C. pyogenes (7%) and S. aureus (7%).

Several other species of bacteria were cultured from penumonic and non-pneumonic lung tissues; no difference in the isolation frequencies between the two groups was found.

There appeared to be no association between the age of the calf and either the number of isolations made or the species isolated from pneumonic and non-pneumonic tissue.

In some animals large numbers of bacteria, usually a Pasteurella sp., were recovered and these were usually from 'typical' pasteurella lesions. ie acute exudative interstitial pneumonia. On the other hand, a few cases with similar histology were found from which no organisms could be isolated from the lung tissue.

Occasionally, profuse growth of an unusual organism, eg Corynebacterium xerosis, Actinobacillus lignieresii was made from the lung tissue of non-pneumonic calves.

The association of bacteria with bovine respiratory disease
in Great Britain has been known for many decades (Jennings
and Glover, 1952; Omar, 1966; Ide, 1970). However, the true role
played by bacteria in pulmonary disease is unclear. Potentially
'pathogenic' bacteria, for example *Pasteurella* spp., *Haemophilus
somnus, Corynebacterium pyogenes* and *Escherichia coli* have been recovered from pneumonic lung tissue of cattle. (Thorpe et al., 1942;
Carter and Rowsell, 1958, Magwood et al., 1969; Corstvet et al.,
1973; Bitsch et al., 1976), but whether these organisms are
primary pathogens is still unclear. Most have been isolated
from the tracheas and nasopharynges of healthy non-pneumonic
calves, but usually in smaller numbers than from pneumonic
animals (Hamdy and Trapp, 1967; Magwood et al., 1969; Corstvet
et al., 1973). Collier and Rossow (1964) did not isolate a
Pasteurella sp. from the lungs of 88 non-pneumonic calves.
Pasteuella spp. are considered to be important bovine respiratory
pathogens, particularly in the condition known as transit/
shipping fever or 'pasteurellosis', which is generally
recognised as an acute interstitial pneumonia (Heddleston et al.,
1962; Hetrick et al., 1963; Sørensen et al., 1964). Reisinger
et al. (1959) isolated parainfluenza-3 virus from the lung
tissue of calves with shipping fever and the combined effect of
this virus with a *Pasteurella* sp. is considered to be the pathogenic mechanism of the disease (Hetrick et al., 1963; Baldwin,
et al., 1967).

The microbial flora of the normal bovine respiratory tract
is controversial; the work below describes the bacterial
recoveries from the lungs of a series of pneumonic and non-
pneumonic calves and discusses the significance of the findings.

MATERIALS AND METHODS

The lungs of 92 calves were examined bacteriologically.
Most of these animals had been housed within the same air space
in groups of four to 20 for various periods of time. At the
time of examination the calves ranged in age from one day to
6 months. Eleven animals died and the remaining were shot and

exsanguinted. The lungs were removed into polythene bags,
avoiding contact with other surfaces, as soon after death as
possible. After macroscopic examination duplicate samples of
tissue of approximately 10mm cube were aseptically removed into
8.1 ml sterile phosphate-buffered saline (PBS, pH 7.4). The
anterior part of the right apical lobe was sampled in all cases
and tissue from the right cardiac and right diaphragmatic lobes
were sampled in many calves.

One sample of tissue was stored at -70°C, the other was
chopped lightly and incubated at 37°C for 30 - 45 minutes. A
loopful of suspension was then inoculated onto each of
MacConkey agar, 10% horse blood agar and chocolate blood agar
plates, the latter two media being inoculated in duplicate.
One horse blood agar and one chocolate blood agar plate were
incubated anaerobically at 37°C, while the other plates were
incubated aerobically at 37°C. All plates were examined 24
and 48 hours later and colonies were identified by the methods
of Cowan and Steel (1965), based on the individual biochemical
reactions of the organisms. The number of bacterial colonies
obtained from one loopful of sample was used as an indication
of the degree of infection and assessed as; +++, more than 50
colonies; ++, 20 - 50 colonies; +, 5 - 20 colonies. Tissue from
abjacent sites of the lung were fixed and processed for
histological examination.

RESULTS

The results are illustrated in Tables 1, 2 and 3.

On the basis of macroscopic and microscopic pulmonary
examination, 63 of the 92 calves were considered to have
pneumonia; four of the 11 animals which died had severe lesions
which probably caused their death. The extent of the pneumonia
in the other calves varied and several different histological
lesions were recognised. Exudative type lesions were most
characteristic of the pneumonia in the younger calves up to
about two months old, while a more proliferative reaction,

particularly of lymphocytes, was frequntly observed in the
older animals. However, several animals, some of which had
additional complications, for example, bronchiolar polyps,
bronchiectasis and abscesses, had intermediate type reactions.

TABLE 1

THE BACTERIOLOGICAL EXAMINATION OF THE LUNGS OF PNEUMONIC AND NON-PNEUMONIC
CALVES INDICATING THE NUMBER OF ISOLATIONS FROM THE CALVES POSITIVE
BACTERIOLOGICALLY.

	No. calves	No. calves positive bacteriologically	% Calves	No. Isolations
Pneumonic	63	41	65	52
Non-pneumonic	29	21	72.4	29
Total	92	62	67.4	81

Of the 63 pneumonic calves studied, 41 yielded bacteria
(65%) and 52 isolations were made (Table 1) while 29 isolations
were made from the 21 non-pneumonic calves which yielded bacteria.
Of the total 92 calves, bacteria were isolated from 67.4% and
a total of 81 isolations were made.

A total of 27 species of bacteria were isolated from the
lung tissue of the pneumonic and non-pneumonic calves (Table 2).
P. haemolytica and *P. multocida* were the most commonly isolated
species from both groups of calves. A slightly higher isolation
rate of both species was made from the pneumonic calves,
P. haemolytica and *P. multocida* being 17.4% and 11.5% of the total
isolations respectively compared with 10.3% of the total isolations for both species from non-pneumonic lungs. Five isolations
of *C. pyogenes* were made from pneumonic tissue and only two from
non-pneumonic calves. The other commonly isolated bacteria were
Staphylococcus aureus, Streptococcus pneumoniae, Strep. bovis and *Staph.
epidermidis*. There did not appear to be any differences between
pneumonic and non-pneumonic animals in the isolation frequencies
of the less commonly isolated species. Most bacteria were
isolated in small numbers from both pneumonic and non-pneumonic
tissue although profuse growth resulted from one or two

TABLE 2

THE ISOLATION FREQUENCIES OF BACTERIA FROM THE LUNG TISSUE OF 63 PNEUMONIC
AND 29 NON-PNEUMONIC CALVES.

	Pneumonic			Non-pneumonic		
	Number isolates	% Total isolates	% Total calves	Number isolates	% Total isolates	% Total calves
Pasteurella haemolytica	9	17.4	14.2	3	10.3	10.3
P. multocida	6	11.5	9.5	3	10.3	10.3
Corynebacterium pyogenes	5	9.6	7.9	2	6.9	6.9
Streptococcus pneumoniae	3	5.7	4.7	3	10.3	10.3
Staphylococcus aureus	4	7.6	6.3	2	6.9	6.9
Strep. bovis	3	5.7	4.7	1	3.4	3.4
Staph. epidermidis	3	5.7	4.7	o	o	o
Strep. mitis	1	2	1.6	2	6.9	6.9
Strep. faecalis	2	3.8	3.1	1	3.4	3.4
Aerococcus viridans	2	3.8	3.1	1	3.4	3.4
Acinetobacter sp.	3	5.7	4.7	o	o	o
Micrococcus luteus	1	2	1.6	2	6.9	6.9
Staph. sp.	1	2	1.6	1	3.4	3.4
Neisseria sp.	1	2	1.6	1	3.4	3.4
Actinobacillus lignieresii	1	2	1.6	1	3.4	3.4
Klebsiella sp.	1	2	1.6	1	3.4	3.4
C. bovis	1	2	1.6	o	o	o
C. xerosis	o	o	o	1	3.4	3.4
Strep. sp.	o	o	o	1	3.4	3.4
Aerococcus sp.	1	2	1.6	o	o	o
Haemophilus sp.	o	o	o	1	3.4	3.4
Aeromonas sp.	1	2	1.6	o	o	o
Bacillus sp.	1	2	1.6	o	o	o
Alcaligenes faecalis	1	2	1.6	o	o	o
Micrococcus roseus	o	o	o	1	3.4	3.4
Micrococcus sp.	1	2	1.6	o	o	o
Escherichia coli	o	o	o	1	3.4	3.4

animals, eg large numbers of *Actinobacillus lignieresii* were
recovered from the lung tissue of a non-pneumonic calf less
than one month of age and *C. xerosis* was abundant in the lungs
of a non-pneumonic six months old animal. Despite the high
frequency of isolation of the two *Pasteurella* spp., their
presence was associated with 'pasteurellosis' - like lesions
(ie acute exudative interstitial pneumonia) in only one case.
Pasteurella spp. were isolated from another 12 calves with
pneumonia, but none had lesions of acute interstitial
pneumonia; conversely two calves with 'pasteurellosis' - like
lesions did not yield any pasteurellae. More than one species
of bacteria was isolated from 17 calves, eight of which were
non-pneumonic.

The distribution of the isolation frequency within the
different age groups is illustrated in Table 3. These results
indicate that bacteria can be recovered with similar frequencies
from pneumonic and non-pneumonic calves, sampled at different
ages. Likewise, the 5 bacterial spp. listed show a scattered
distribution between pneumonic and non-pneumonic animals of all
ages. Although many of these calves had been housed in groups
for specific periods of time, a common bacterial flora within
the groups was not found.

DISCUSSION

In this study bacteria were isolated from the lungs of 62
and 92 calves. Sixty five per cent of the pneumonic calves
were positive bacteriologically which is comparable with the
results of Gourlay et al. (1970) who isolated bacteria from
the lungs of 42 of 65 calves. In a similar study by Bitsch
et al. (1976) 72% of pneumonic calf lungs were positive
bacteriologically.

A high proportion of the lungs of non-pneumonic calves
harboured bacteria (72%), although in general small numbers were
isolated. Collier and Rossow (1964) examined the lung tissue
of 88 healthy cattle, aged about two years, and 198 bacterial

TABLE 3

THE DISTRIBUTION OF FIVE SPECIES OF BACTERIA FROM PNEUMONIC AND NON-PNEUMONIC LUNG TISSUE OF CALVES WITHIN THE FIVE AGE GROUPS

	1 Month		1 Month		2 Months		3 Months		6 Months	
	*pn	non-pn	pn	non-pn	pn	non-pn	pn	non-pn	pn	non-pn
No. calves	4	11	11	–	7	3	17	4	24	11
No. isolates	3	12	15	–	6	3	14	4	14	10
Isolations of:										
P. haemolytica	–	1	3	–	2	–	1	–	3	2
P. multocida	1	2	2	–	–	–	–	–	3	1
C. pyogenes	–	–	–	–	–	–	3	–	2	2
Strep. pneumoniae	–	2	–	–	–	1	1	–	2	–
Staph. aureus	–	1	2	–	–	–	1	1	1	–

*pn - pneumonic: non-pn - non-pneumonic

isolations were made; 36% of the isolants were *Bacillus* spp.,
22% *Streptococcus* spp. and 18% *Streptomyces* spp. Many of these
species are soil organisms and it was suggested that the high
isolation rate may have been due to contamination from ruminal
contents. In that work *Pasteurella* spp. were not recovered and
only four isolations of *C. pyogenes* were made. This is in contrast
to the present study where 20% of the calves harboured
Pasteurella spp. in their lungs. These organisms were recovered
at a slightly higher rate from pneumonic (23.5%) than non-
pneumonic calves; this figure is lower than that of Gourlay
et al. (1970) who isolated pasteurellae from 30% of their
pneumonic calves and of Bitsch et al. (1976) who found them in
32% of pneumonic calf lungs. Most of the remaining bacterial
species isolated have been reported by other workers (Gourlay
et al., 1970; Bitsch et al., 1976) although one or two unusual
species, whose origins are unknown, were found, eg *A. lignieresii*
and *C. xerosis*.

Generally, small numbers of organisms were isolated from
the lung tissue of both pneumonic and non-pneumonic calves.
It may be important in this connection that very few of the
calves in this series actually died from pneumonia although
some had fairly extensive lesions. The number of species of
organisms isolated from a series of fatal pneumonic cases does
not appear to be available and so the importance of the numbers
of bacteria recovered is not known. More than one species of
bacteria was recovered from the lungs of 17 calves but there was
no common pattern among multiple isolations. Six of the calves
in the study of Gourlay et al. (1970) and 27 of the 50 calves
examined by Bitsch et al. (1976) harboured more than one
organism.

There appeared to be no association between the isolation
frequency of the species recovered from pneumonic and non-
pneumonic calves and the age of the animals.

Many of these organisms are considered to be pathogenic for
the bovine respiratory tract (Omar, 1966) and a profuse growth of

Pasteurella sp. was made from one calf which had typical
'pasteurellosis' lesions. However, no pasteurellae were
isolated from other animals with similar lesions.

This work has shown that potentially pathogenic bacteria
can be isolated from normal pulmonary tissue in approximately
two-thirds of animals and from a similar proportion of calves
with a non-fatal pulmonary disease. No difference in the
species isolated from pneumonic and non-pneumonic tissue was
found. Although it is likely that many bacteria play a role
in exacerbating pulmonary lesions leading to a fatal pneumonia,
as is the case with *Pasteurella* spp. in shipping fever, the
importance of the number of organisms and the species of bacteria
involved in many respiratory outbreaks is not known.

REFERENCES

Baldwin, D.E., Marshall, R.G. and Wessman, G.E. 1967. Am. J. Vet. Res. <u>28</u> p. 1773.

Bitsch, V., Friis, N.F. and Drogh, H.V. 1976. Acta vet. scand. <u>17</u>, p. 32.

Carter, G.R. and Rowsell, H.C. 1958. J. Am. vet. med. Ass. <u>132</u>, p. 187.

Collier, J.R. and Rossow, C.F. 1964. Am. J. vet. Res. <u>25</u>, p. 391.

Corstvet, R.E., Panciera, R.J., Rinker, H.B., Starks, B.L. and Howard, C. 1973. J. Am. vet. med. Ass. <u>163</u>, p. 870.

Cowan, S.T. and Steel, K.J. 1965. Manual for the Identification of Medical Bacteria, University Press, Cambridge.

Gourlay, R.N., MacKenzie, A. and Cooper, J.E. 1970. J. comp. Path. <u>80</u>, p. 575.

Hamdy, A.H. and Trapp, A.L. 1967. Am. J. vet. Res. <u>28</u>, p. 1019.

Heddleston, K.L., Reisinger, R.C. and Watko, L.P. 1962. Am. J. vet. Res. <u>23</u>, p. 548.

Hetrick, F.M., Chang, S.C., Byrne, R.J. and Hansen, P.A. 1963. Am. J. vet. Res. <u>24</u>, p. 939.

Ide, P.R. 1970. Can. vet. J. <u>11</u>, p. 194.

Jennings, A.R. and Glover, R.E. 1952. J. comp. Path. <u>62</u>, p.6.

Magwood, S.E., Barnum, D.A. and Thompson, R.G. 1969. Can. J. comp. Med. <u>33</u>, p. 237.

Omar, A.R. 1966. Vet. Bull. <u>36</u>, p. 259.

Reisinger, R.C. Heddleston, K.L. and Manthei, C.A. 1959. J. Am. vet. med. Assoc. <u>135</u>, p. 147.

Sørensen, D.K., Johnson, D.W. and Hoyt, H.H. 1964. International Meeting on Diseases of Cattle, Copenhagen, p. 5.

Thorpe, W.T.S., Shigley, J.F. and Farrell, M.A. 1942. Am. J. vet. Res. <u>3</u>, p. 342.

THE ROLE OF PASTEURELLAE IN RESPIRATORY DISEASES OF CATTLE

N.J.L. Gilmour

Animal Diseases Research Association, Moredun Institute,
408 Gilmerton Road, Edinburgh, Scotland.

ABSTRACT

Both Pasteurella multocida and Pasteurella haemolytica are the cause of pneumonia in cattle and both can be isolated from the upper respiratory tracts of clinically normal animals and from tracheal air in the case of P. haemolytica. The lungs must therefore be exposed to infection. It is postulated that the factors which interfere with clearance of those organisms from the lungs might be predisposing causes of pasteurella pneumonia. The epidemiology of some of the pneumonias in calves and of the shipping fever complex is reviewed with the aim of elucidating the role of pasteurellae in bovine pneumonias.

This paper reviews the role of *Pasteurella haemolytica* and *P. multocida* in pneumonia of cattle. Whereas a study of the epidemiology may indicate underlying contributory factors which predispose to the occurrence of pneumonic pasteurellosis, recent experimental work on the response of calves and sheep to aerosols of *P. haemolytica* has indicated possible mechanisms which alter the susceptibility of the lungs to that organism.

Two syndromes associated with pneumonia in which pasteurellae have been incriminated as causal agents are the so-called 'enzootic pneumonia' of calves and the 'shipping fever' complex. Pasteurellae are also responsible for acute, sporadically-occurring pneumonia in individual animals. The term enzootic pneumonia has been used to describe outbreaks of pneumonia which occur in housed calves, generally in the first six months of life. A variable proportion of such calves develop acute respiratory disease with pyrexia and tachypnoea, hyperpnoea or dyspnoea, followed in some cases by death. Other calves in the group usually have evidence of a milder respiratory disease manifested by mucopurulent nasal and ocular discharges.

The term shipping fever arose because of the association between the disease and recent transportation, especially following the long journeys involved in feed-lot cattle operations in USA and Canada. However, a syndrome similar to shipping fever can occur in older animals when stress due to transportation is not a factor. Both enzootic pneumonia of calves and shipping fever are complex diseases insofar as a range of micro-organisms has been isolated from affected animals. Thus parainfluenza 3 (PI3) virus, adenovirus, infectious bovine rhinotracheitis (IBR) virus, rhinovirus, reovirus, enterovirus, respiratory syncytial virus, mucosal disease virus, influenza virus, chlamydiae and mycoplasmas have all been isolated from cases of enzootic pneumonia by various researches. PI3 or IBR virus infections have been reported frequently in investigations into shipping fever. The bacterial species isolated are almost invariably *P. haemolytica* or *P. multocida* and there is little doubt now that the crucial tissue damage is done by these pasteurellae.

Collier (1968) noted that the lung lesions which result from either *P. haemolytica* or *P. multocida* are identical and postulated that the lesions of fibrinous pneumonia were due to endotoxin. Subsequently, therefore, both syndromes will be treated as a single entity for which the term pneumonic pasteurellosis will be used.

P. haemolytica and *p. multocida* are commonly isolated from the upper respiratory tract and tonsils of healthy cattle but not from healthy lung tissues (Collier, 1968). Thomson et al. (1969) recovered pasteurella spp. from nasopharyngeal swabs from 6 to 10 month old healthy calves maintained under conditions where shipping fever might be expected. The carrier rate for both organisms was similar and was in the region of 75%. Magwood et al. (1969) examined calves fom herds affected with pneumonic pasteurellosis and from healthy herds and found the overall isolation rate for *P. haemolytica* was 23% and for *P. multocida* 61.3%. Carrier rates were unaffected by the presence of disease in the individual calves nor did they predict future disease. There was some evidence of a cycle in the nasopharyngeal carriage of *P. haemolytica* but not of *P. multocida*.

Pass and Thomson (1971) found that *P. haemolytica* was widely distributed over 15 sites on the nasal mucosa of healthy animals examined at post-mortem and that the organism was present in cases where nasal swabs taken in vivo had been negative. This suggests that carrier rates based on single swabs will be underestimates. They also found that *P. haemolytica* was present on the surface but never between or within epithelial cells.

The types of *P. haemolytica* most commonly recovered from both nasopharyngeal swabs from healthy carriers and from pneumonic lungs are biotype A, serotypes 1 and 2. These comprised 80% of strains isolated from post-mortem material and 87% of strains from nasal swabs in a survey by Wray and Thompson (1971). In North America the predominant serotype associated with bovine respiratory disease is Al (Lillie, 1974).

The *P. multocida* serotype associated with bovine pneumonias is principally type A, whereas types B and E are implicated in haemorrhagic septicaemia(Carter, 1967).

The question now to be considered is what converts an animal which is a carrier of *P. haemolytica*, for example, but which is apparently healthy, into a case of pneumonia. From the work of Grey and Thomson (1971) who found *P. haemolytica* in tracheal air, it is postulated that the lung is repeatedly exposed to small numbers of organisms from droplets formed in the nasal passages. The defence mechanisms are normally competent enough to remove the bacteria which have penetrated the bronchioles and alveoli in this manner.

Epidemiological studies of pasteurellosis have, on circumstantial evidence, identified both physical and infectious agents which are thought to predispose to pneumonic pasteurellosis. Hoerlein (1973) considered that both types of 'stressor' might be necessary under some conditions, and postulated that the shipping fever complex was due to a combination of stress, non-bacterial (listed above) and bacterial infections. The physical factors listed include heat, cold, dust, damp, trauma, fatigue, dehydration, hunger, anxiety, fear and surgery. In practice it is most likely that combinations of these factors will operate; for example, outbreaks of pneumonia among housed calves tend to occur where such factors as overcrowding and ventilation can be incriminated.

To determine how these physical factors might affect the host's resistance to pneumonic pasteurellosis we must consider how organisms enter the lungs from the upper respiratory tract where they occur in healthy animals. They may be carried either in aerosols of droplet nuclei (Wilson and Thomson, 1968) or in infected exudates generated in the upper respiratory tract (Wright, 1961). Interference with the mucociliary tracheal elevator, due to dehydration for instance, might allow pasteurella-laden exudate from the upper respiratory tract to descend to the lungs and overwhelm the local defence mechansims. Concurrent

PI3 virus infection may also be implicated in increasing the
susceptibility of the lung to pasteurella infection, since it
has been shown experimentally in mice that clearance of bacteria
from lungs can be reduced especially at the period around 7
days after virus infection (Green, 1965).

Gilka et al. (1973) investigated the clearance of *P.
haemolytica* administered in an aerosol from the lungs of calves
pretreated with the oedema-inducing agents - histamine, endotoxin
and croton oil, and found that clearance was impaired in each
instance and also when a dose of hydrocortisone which induced
oedema, was used.

Prior infection of calves with PI3 virus has been found to
interfere with pulmonary clearance of *P. haemolytica* at 7 and 11
but not 3 days after the virus administration (Lopez et al.,
1976). Bacterial retention did not correlate with the development of pulmonary changes due to the virus, but appeared to be
due to actual malfunction of alveolar macrophages. Despite
these findings, experimental infections of calves with PI3 virus
and either *P. haemolytica* or *P. multocida* with the aim of reproducing pneumonic pasteurellosis have not been uniformly successful.

Jericho et al. (1976) produced pneumonia with an aerosol of
P. haemolytica given 4 days after inoculation with IBR virus.
Pneumonia induced in this way was prevented by prior vaccination
with commercial IBR vaccine. This suggests that IBR was a
contributory factor in the production of the pneumonia.

A reliable method of reproducing pneumonic pasteurellosis
in a high proportion of calves is of prime importance in
investigating factors which predispose to the disease. Failures
encountered in the past might be attributable to the use of
calves which could have had antibodies acquired from colostrum
and from prior experience of pasteurellae. Our findings in
sheep suggest that the use of specific pathogen free,
colostrum-deprived experimental calves might be prerequisite
for further studies into predisposing factors.

At this Institute we have used both conventional and specific pathogen free (SPF) lambs to study the effect of aerosols of *P. haemolytica:* acute pneumonic pasteurellosis was produced only when SPF lambs were used. Pretreatment with PI3 virus was found to increase the susceptibility of lambs to aerosols of *P. haemolytica* given 4 to 7 days after the virus, and pneumonia occurred in 90% of lambs treated in this way. The experimental disease produced was identical with the natural disease. This model has been used to investigate the efficacy of possible vaccines against pneumonic pasteurellosis, and has proved to be highly reproducible. The use of SPF calves might allow similar progress in investigation of pneumonic pasteurellosis in that animal.

REFERENCES

Carter, G.R. 1967. Ad. Vet. Sci. 11, p. 321.

Collier, J.R. 1968. J. Am. vet. med. Ass. 153, p. 1645.

Gilka, F., Thomson, R.G. and Savan, M. 1974. Can. J. comp. Med. 38, p. 251.

Green, G.M. 1965. Antimicrobial Agents and Chemotherapy, Ed. C.L. Hobby, American Society for Microbiology Ann. Arbor. USA. p. 26.

Grey, C.L. and Thomson, R.G. 1971. Can. J. comp. Med. 35, p. 121.

Hoerlein, A.B. 1973. J. Am. vet. med. Ass. 163, p. 825.

Jericho, K.W.F., Magwood, S.E. and Stockdale, P.H.G. 1976. Can. vet. J. 17, p. 194.

Lillie, L.E. 1974. Can. vet. J. 15, p. 233.

Lopez, A., Thomson, R.G. and Savan, M. 1971. Can. J. comp. Med. 40, p. 385.

Magwood, S.E., Barnum, D.A. and Thomson, R.G. 1969. Can. J. comp. Med. 33, p. 237.

Pass, D.A. and Thomson, R.G. 1971. Can. J. comp. Med. 35, p. 181.

Thomson, R.G., Benson, M.L. and Savan, M. 1969. Can. J. comp. Med. 33, p. 194.

Wilson, M.R. and Thomson, R.G. 1968. Res. vet. Sci. 9, p. 467.

Wray, C. and Thompson, D.A. 1971. Br. vet. J. 127, p. lxvi.

Wright, C.W. 1961. Bact. Rev. 25, p. 219.

DISCUSSION

<u>J.M. Rutter</u> *(UK)*

You mentioned, Dr. Allan, that there was an increase in the numbers of bacteria in the diseased animals compared with the normal animals. Have you any evidence of the location of the bacteria in the diseased animals?

<u>E. Allan</u> *(UK)*

Samples in pneumonic cases were taken from pneumonic lesions, which were generally found in the anterior lobes, and also from the middle and diaphragmatic lobes, which were generally non-pneumonic. Most of the isolations were from the anterior lobes.

<u>J.M. Rutter</u>

Do you have any histopathological evidence showing how the bacteria might be distributed within the pneumonic lesions on a microscopic basis?

<u>E. Allan</u>

No.

<u>N.J.L. Gilmour</u> *(UK)*

Did you classify pneumonia on gross or on microscopical examination, and did you find any difference in the number of organisms between pneumonic and non-pneumonic areas in the same animal?

<u>E. Allan</u>

We classified them as pneumonic on both macroscopic and microscopic examination. The answer to your second question is no.

<u>J.M. Rutter</u>

The results which you have presented seem to be rather different from those of Collier and Rosser, who did not isolate pasteurella from lungs. Have you any idea what the explanation for this might be?

364

E. Allan

No.

J.M. Rutter

Yesterday we were talking about adult pneumonias. The Glasgow workers were referring to chronic suppurative pneumonia in adults. We did not hear very much about the possible aetiology of that. Have there been any comparative studies between the kinds of cases which you have been seeing in young animals and the chronic cases in adults which we were hearing about yesterday?

H.M. Pirie *(UK)*

We do not have detailed microbiological results on adult cattle.

C. Holzhauer *(Netherlands)*

We have examined a lot of lungs from young calves. When animals die after being ill for only a few days, we find pasteurella in about 85 or 90% of the animals examined. We always find fibrinous pleurisy and pneumonia in these animals, but in calves which have been sick for a period of 2-3 weeks we see other things such as catarrhal pneumonia. In these cases we isolate pasteurella only in about 10-20% of animals. We also find *Staphylococcus* and *Haemophilus*.

J.M. Rutter

Professor Straub was telling us this morning about mixtures of bacteria, mycoplasmas and viruses in the cases which he was looking at. Were the animals which you describe in the bacterial study the same as the ones which you described earlier in the mycoplasma study, and was there any correlation between isolations of mycoplasmas and bacteria from them?

E. Allan

There was no common bacterium isolated with any specific mycoplasma. In answer to your second question, the animals were the same.

P. Pignatelli *(Italy)*

I should like to know if there is some specific test to ascertain the pathogenicity of the strains of pasteurella isolated from calves with and without pneumonia. You have isolated many strains of pasteurella in animals with and without pneumonia. I would like to know whether the various strains are of the same pathogenicity or not.

E. Allan

There are specific tests but I did not do them.

L.H. Thomas *(UK)*

I should like to make two observations. I think the results which Dr. Allan has given us very closely resemble the bacterial isolations which have been made from pneumonic lungs at Compton. Dr. Gourlay did a survey which was published some years ago which gave much the same results.

The second observation is a rather subjective one, and that is the observation of the effectiveness of antibiotic therapy. I was in general practice for a short while and found it to be effective, and it seemed to me probably indicative that bacteria were playing a part in this disease.

A. Andrews *(UK)*

I think that antibiotics help in many cases, but not in every case. Supportive therapy is quite useful and general nursing is particularly helpful, including the use of such drugs as aspirin. In many cases we must not always assume that you can just administer antibiotics. This did come up whilst discussing Dr. Allan's paper. Had any of these calves ever had any sort of antibiotic?

E. Allan

No.

N.J.L. Gilmour

Could I ask Dr. Allan what tests she would use to differentiate the pathogenicity of strains of P. haemolytica. She said
there were tests - I wondered which ones she would actually do.

E. Allan

I believe that they can be typed antigenically.

N.J.L. Gilmour

But that does not tell you the pathogenicity. You only
differentiate the serotypes.

E. Allan

You could then group them from pneumonic and non-pneumonic
calves.

W.B. Martin (UK)

In defence of Dr. Allan, may I say that there are certain
serotypes which Dr. Gilmour associates with pneumonia, certainly
in sheep, and therefore one might consider that certain serotypes
are more liable to be pathogenic than others in certain circumstances. What is important, Dr. Allan, would be to know the
numbers of bacteria which are present. I think this would be
very significant, because there must obviously be vast differences between pneumonic lesions in so-called pneumonic animals,
and normal lung tissue in what we are calling normal animals.
I cannot believe, when you talked about Corynebacterium pyogenes
being present in a normal lung, that if it were present in
significant numbers one would really be talking about a normal,
non-pneumonic animal.

E. Allan

That is why I feel that this subject should be studied in
much more detail, taking the different areas of the lung and
quantifying the number of bacteria present. You can isolate
P. haemolytica and put it down as the cause of pneumonia, but if
you do not know the numbers which are present, it does not
really mean very much.

N.J.L. Gilmour

Could I just add one thing, in case I was misunderstood.
I think that within an arbitrary serotype of *P. haemolytica* there
is no experimental way at the moment of determining whether it
is pathogenic or not, apart from the administration of the
organisms to mice in conjunction with mucin. We have some
evidence that some serotypes have different LD50's for mice,
and at the moment that is the only way that you can test them.

J.M. Rutter

With reference to the mixed infection work with PI3 and
pasteurella, I think that Professor McKercher referred to the
successful production of lesions in America using the PI3/
pasteurella combination. Is that correct?

D.G. McKercher *(USA)*

The only thing I can recall is the fact that in the study
which was carried out on those 400 000 cattle, pasteurellae
were recovered from 50% of the lungs which were cultured.

J. Harkness *(UK)*

Speaking as a virologist, I wonder if there is anyone here
who would care to comment on the significance or pathogenicity
of the organism known as *Haemophilus somnus*. This was first
isolated in America, and has recently been isolated in this
country, I think from Dumfries. Workers in Weybridge have
inoculated this organism into calves and obtained rather dramatic
results including fibrinous bronchopneumonia and deaths. I
wondered if anyone had encountered it and would care to comment.

W.B. Martin

I have been involved in the investigation of one outbreak
in cattle in which acute death and some form of encephalitis
occurred. We failed to find any virus, although we were looking
for the possibility of IBR. Large numbers of gram-negative
organisms were visible in the brains of affected animals but I
have a feeling that they were not cultured, or not cultured very
well.

J.M. Rutter

Could I stimulate the Glasgow and the Compton workers to comment on the lesions that Dr. Gilmour has described in the calf which was inoculated with PI3 and *P. haemolytica* ?

H.M. Pirie

The one thing which struck me was that there did not seem to be much fibrinous pleurisy.

N.J.L. Gilmour

No, there was no pleurisy. The calf died 5 to 6 days after the aerosol administration of *P. haemolytica* . We have only infected three calves, so I cannot claim to be an expert on the bovine situation, but the response of this one calf was different from the response we generally obtain from sheep. When we administer an aerosol of *P. haemolytica* to sheep we get acute deaths in 30-40% of treated animals. In our experiments we have normally been killing 7 to 10 days after challenge with *P. haemolytica*. Lesions of pneumonia are seen in those animals which have not died, although these sheep are clinically sick. This was not the case in this particular calf, as it did not become acutely ill shortly after aerosolisation but rather 6 days later. It was a colostrum-deprived but not SPF calf, which had been born on a farm, and it may therefore have had some other infection.

H.M. Pirie

You may have said this - did you recover the organism in large numbers from this calf?

N.J.L. Gilmour

In moderate numbers: the lesions present are consistent with its being a pneumonic bacillosis.

L.H. Thomas

At Compton, we have inoculated four gnotobiotic calves with *P. haemolytica*: extensive lesions of bronchopneumonia were present in two calves and nothing in the other two. We recovered *P.*

haemolytica from the two affected animals. Inoculation was by the intratracheal route and the dose approximately 10^8 organisms. A variable result is our conclusion.

J.B. McFerran *(UK)*

May I suggest that an important and interesting step might now be to combine pretreatment with virus at the appropriate time and then subsequently with the infection. We have worked with IBR virus and, though this does not imply that IBR is necessarily the predisposing cause of pneumonic bacillosis in all cases, it is probably important in the field. Furthermore we at least have an agent which makes animals susceptible to pasteurella, and I think this is important, if only as an experimental tool, even if it does not elucidate what actually happens on the farm.

C. Howard

I thought the general conclusion from the earlier papers and discussions was that PI3 was of no importance in calves, and that pasteurellas occur in so few animals that they are probably not important in a large number of cases anyway.

J.M. Rutter

I think Dr. Stott was suggesting that PI3 was not very important in calves.

E.J. Stott *(UK)*

That is the conclusion of our work in a field situation.

B. Morein *(Sweden)*

The PI3 virus causes a "decreased escalating" effect of the mucus escalator at 7 days post infection. If the pasteurella infection is superimposed on this, pneumonic symptoms occur, but by this time it might be 14 days after the initial infection with PI3. Any serological reaction to PI3 will therefore have occurred before you take the first serum sample, and then you do not appear to get a significant rise.

E.J. Stott

We were taking the samples continuously, every three weeks.

B. Morein

If you do that it would be all right, but then the antibody rise does not appear to be connected with the disease: it comes 14 days before.

E.J. Stott

That would still correlate with the incidence of disease in the way we analysed our results.

A. Andrews

This is rather a naive question: in your sheep work, what happens if you put the organisms in the reverse order?

N.J.L. Gilmour

We have not put them in the other way round because SPF lambs are very scarce and expensive. Having obtained a system which works, we did not think it necessary to examine fully all the permutations which are possible. We wanted to exploit the system which worked.

J.B. McFerran

As I remember, Dr. Stott showed a correlation between respiratory syncytial and disease and, to a lesser extent, some correlation between PI3 and disease, but he also emphasised the fact that large numbers of animals showed antibody rises to PI3 without the correlation. Am I right in saying that?

E.J. Stott

That is correct.

J.B. McFerran

Are you sure that every strain of PI3 has the same pathogenicity? Could it not have been that some of these strains were pathogenic, causing respiratory illness, and others were non-pathogenic strains. This occurs in other organisms - why should it not occur in PI3?

E.J. Stott

The evidence from the survey work was that there was a correlation between PI3 infection and disease. That is positive data _for_ PI3. The evidence _against_ PI3 was the vaccine trial on the farm, in which we reduced the incidence of PI3 infection significantly, and did not reduce the incidence of disease. It seems to me that that data speaks against the importance of PI3 in the disease which we were seeing on that farm.

J.B. McFerran

If I remember rightly, there was a 50% reduction in the isolation of PI3 in the first year. There could still be some strains of PI3 which were not being protected against by your vaccine. In other words, the vaccine was giving a sufficiently good immunity to protect against the non-pathogenic strains of the virus but not against the invasive strains of PI3.

E.J. Stott

Can you give me any data for PI3 virus in which people have compared different strains under identical conditions and have shown that there is a significant difference in their virulence and in their ability to resist vaccine-produced antibody?

J.B. McFerran

What I am suggesting is only a possibility. This work has not been done, though I think it should be.

B. Morein

I am not saying that this implies pathogenicity, but we know that some strains differ in their neuraminidase activity. For example, I know that I cannot infect a calf under 6 weeks old with a neuraminidase-weak strain, but if I take, for example, the Tübingen E6 or SLP strains, these can infect any calf under 6 weeks of age, regardless of whether they have maternal antibodies or not. Furthermore, in the lymphoblast transformation test, if we take lymphocytes from animals which are immunised against a neuraminidase-strong strain but use a neuraminidase-weak strain in the test, we do not get any blast transformation; blast transformation will only occur with a neuraminidase-strong strain. A similar finding is obtained if another test for cell mediated immunity, the leukocyte migration inhibition test, is used. There are certainly differences among strains of PI3 which cannot be detected by antibody tests.

E.J. Stott

I am sure that there are in vitro differences between strains. As soon as you isolate and begin manipulating viruses in vitro you will induce enormous differences. I think the crucial question is, are these differences related to variations in the severity of field outbreaks with PI3 infection. I don't think that we know.

B. Morein

That has been shown by Bilkie. He was unable to infect calves under the age of 6 weeks, whereas we have successfully accomplished this using a different strain of virus.

H.M. Pirie

Coming back to bacteria and to Dr. Allan's paper, I think the point is that we all believe that bacteria are important in calf respiratory conditions. Where is the evidence for this, either from our own laboratory, or in the literature? I would accept that pasteurellae are important, and Dr. Allan did say that in one of the cases which had this type of pneumonia there were vast numbers of pasteurella. The point is that there is very little information about the numbers of organisms recoverable from pneumonic lungs, nor as to whether bacteria are the cause of death in pneumonic cases.

N.J.L. Gilmour

This comes back to what Mr. Thomas said on the first day - that we must have a system whereby we can put back these agents into the animals to see what they do. This applies to viruses, mycoplasma and bacteria.

H.M. Pirie

I think that someone should first recover the bacteria from pneumonic lungs in significant numbers.

J.M. Rutter

This is the point which Dr. Allan was making, that in acute bacterial pneumonia there has not been a study made of the bacteria which one can isolate.

Summary by Dr. Sherwin Hall (UK) of papers presented on Day 2

I think that initially it might be of some help if I attempted to define some sort of structures, some sort of skeleton on which we might hang some flesh at this stage in the discussion.

The point I wish to make is this: we are concerned with disease, specifically respiratory disease. There would be few who would argue that there are three major components of respiratory disease. First of all, you have to have the host; you have to have an agent of some kind, not necessarily infectious; and, I think most people would agree, you have to consider the environment in which the two elements find themselves.

First of all, I am going to say something about the host, in the hope that it will give some classification to the ideas. Yesterday, Dr. Eyre from Canada made the point that he was concerned with the molecular level of investigation. At the other extreme we can consider the populations of animals. In between those two we can consider an intact animal, or we might consider the cellular level within organs. In other words, you have a hierarchy, if you like. Within that hierarchy you have 'ologies'. Thus, the 'ology' associated with population studies - that is, numerous calves and watching what happens when you get groups of them together, we call 'epidemiology'. When we are concerned with the single, alive, intact animal, we are really concerned with the clinical science of it, the clinical aspects, and then

when we are concerned with changes and structures in organs at
cellular levels we are concerned with the gross and micro
'pathology'. The micropathology itself can be sub-classified
into what you can see with a light microscope and what you can
see with an electron microscope. At molecular level we have
what Dr. Eyre mentioned - the biochemistry, and I put it to you
that this includes serological changes, which involve simply
antibody molecules.

Today we have been concerned with living agents, mycoplasmas
and bacteria, as distinct from non-infectious agents such as
are associated with, say, fog fever or milk allergy. I was
delighted to hear Dr. Gourlay from Compton mention Koch's
Postulates. My usual challenge is that Koch's Postulates are
largely of historical interest. That is what I think Dr. Gourlay
implied. He made the point that Koch's Postulates were really
of importance only when you consider organisms that simply require inoculation into the host in order to produce disease.
At the other extreme, you have organisms in the host which do
not produce disease. Your dilemma is to ascertain if it is
there in any causal relationship whatever.

I think we might consider a scale of probability from 'O'
probability to 'l' probability, where the simple presence of an
organism in a host is equivalent to disease. You might like to
put any particular organism which you are concerned with some-
where along that scale of probability and it may well be that,
of the organisms which we have heard about today, IBR might be
somewhat higher up the scale of probability in terms of a simple
infection causing disease than possibly PI3 and all the other
organisms.

It seems to me that the crucial problem has been that we
are talking about organisms which are at the lower end of the
scale of probabilities. As soon as you get into that end of the
scale you are in trouble in terms of your experimental systems,
because you can no longer apply what you might call determinative
pathology - determinative in the sense that all you have to do

is to take your host and your single factor and experiment in
single factor situations. You now have to consider what you
might call a stochastic pathology - the pathology of probabilities. As soon as you start getting into that field, you are in
trouble, because it gets expensive. You have to think in terms
not only of single animals, but of populations. But if you are
going to understand disease, and be able to explain it, we should
be able to go right through the whole series of the hierarchy
and explain the disease in terms of how it behaves in populations, in single animals, in organs, at cellular levels and
indeed right down to the molecular level. If you can understand
it that way, then you begin to really know something about disease.

If I may be provocative, I suggest that one of the general-
isations which comes out of this is that there has been far too
much emphasis on the serology without attempting to relate it
higher up the scale. Professor Straub made a plea this morning
that more attention should be given to serological standardisation. Dr. McFerran was not too happy about this, and my bet
is that every laboratory thinks that its methods are right.
You would have a difficult time getting that kind of standardisation, desirable though it may be.

I think that there is an even more important priority. I
think that, whatever serological tests are used, they should
bear much closer correlation with what is going on up the scale.
If we are concerned with stochastic pathology, you are at the
lower end of the scale and you have to take into account far
more about the interactions between the environment and the agent,
and the environment and the host. You have to think about the
age of the host, and about the interaction between host and
agent. A lot of emphasis has been given today to the interaction between agents and the host in terms of the serum response
and this kind of thing. Dr. Gourlay put in another plea for
caution. He went so far as to say that you cannot even assume
that because you have seroconversion there is necessarily a
causal assocation. You cannot assume that, simply because you

can isolate an organism from a diseased tissue, it is necessarily causal. That is an extreme caution which I applaud.

I would like now very briefly to look back over today's papers and pick out some points.

This morning, Dr. Bitsch from Denmark made a serological approach. Indeed, his was a serological approach in animals which were quite old - 2 to 2½ years old. I think it is quite important to relate the serological results to the status of the disease. This did not come through too clearly to me. He did make a point on technique, which he was very firm about. It was challenged, but it seems to me that here is fruitful ground for some co-operation.

We heard from Dr. Holzhauer of the Netherlands about 'pinkengriep', and the suggestion, again largely on serological evidence, that this is associated with bovine syncytial virus.

Dr. le Jan from France - again from serological studies but with a difference - was looking particularly at local anti-bodies. He was able to demonstrate that local antibodies develop quite quickly, and that there was a very good correlation between the local antibodies and subsequent seroconversion. But he con-cluded that it is difficult to say which agent is actually causing the disease. That was a note of caution.

Dr. Stott from Compton, interestingly, approached this in the first place as a hypothesis he had established, and then he looked at it from the different levels of organisation. He looked at it from epidemiological level, and then took this epidemiological evidence as a basis on which to design experi-ments in the laboratory. I think this is surely the primary role of epidemiological work, to try to put up markers which need to be further investigated in laboratory conditions. Hav-ing done that, he made certain conclusions which clearly have been challenged here, including the view that we should question whether or not PI3 vaccine should be used.

This morning also developed into something of a debate between live and inactivated virus vaccines. As the Chairman pointed out, we could argue this one until long after the bar has opened!

Professor Straub took an interesting line. Quite apart from the question of any serological evidence, he made an interesting approach to protection, in using IPV virus which has been highly passaged, to stimulate the production of interferon. He also mentioned that 'mucosal disease' was a better name for the disease than 'bovine viral diarrhoea'. I agree with him, because I think I am right in saying that mucosal disease interferes with the reticulo-endothelial system, and that it can interfere with the basic response of the animal to any other challenge. Nonetheless, Professor Straub did make the plea that the environmental aspects of respiratory disease are important.

From Brussels, Dr. van Opdenbosch presented some interesting slides showing fluorescent antibody work with the respiratory syncytial virus which quite clearly stimulated a lot of interest. Dr. van Opdenbosch also made the point that he thought that bovine viral diarrhoea virus was indeed an important pathogen in respiratory disease.

This afternoon we had sessions on mycoplasmosis, and the role of bacteria. My impression was that the mycoplasmologists were far more cautious than the virologists. They were putting up all kinds of reasons, and attempting to adduce what I would regard as firmer evidence for their conclusions that mycoplasma were playing an active role in disease than some of the virologists. I applaud that.

Dr. Ernø made a plea that we require an up-to-date catalogue of what is actually going on within the EEC countries, and he made the point that the evidence for pathogenicity of some mycoplasmas is weak. The Compton workers provided some evidence that there were some mycoplasmal agents which are of importance, if only in starting off some reaction in the lungs which can then prepare a seedbed for other seeds to get in and do some damage.

I thought the bacteriologists also showed a worthy caution. They pointed out this question of interactions. It seems to me that, if we are dealing with organisms which are down the end of the scale of probability of actually producing disease, then we have to consider interactions, in particular environmental interactions, far more because it seems to me that if we do not, somebody else will. We have had a lot of emphasis in this conference on living agents. In the last century, in the great sanitary awakening, when Sir Edwin Chadwick had a lot of executive power, he believed that disease was caused by smell. On that basis he was able to execute a policy which went a long way towards removing the burden of infectious disease. I put it to you also that when John Snow took the handle off the Broad Street pump and stopped the cholera outbreak he did not know what strain it was, what it did or anything about it. But he stopped disease. It may well be that we are putting a bit too much emphasis on organisms and the strains of this and that, and are not paying sufficient attention to these environmental aspects. It may well be that knowledge of these can solve, or go a long way towards reducing, the overall burden of respiratory disease.

SESSION 5A

PATHOLOGY

Chairman:

H. Frerking

Co-ordinator:

N.J.L. Gilmour

THE PATHOLOGY OF CALFHOOD PNEUMONIAS

L.H. Thomas

ARC Institute for Research on Animal Diseases, Compton,
Nr. Newbury, Berkshire, England.

ABSTRACT

The predominant histopathological finding in a series of 65 autopsies carried out on housed calves dying of respiratory disease on a large beef rearing farm was an acute to chronic exudative bronchopneumonia. No evidence of the inclusion body pneumonia reported by Jarrett (1954) or by Omar (1965) was found and the degree of peribronchiolar lymphoid hyperplasia (cuffing) was minimal.

A similar picture of exudative bronchopneumonia was found in pneumonic lung material obtained from all but one outbreak of enzootic calf pneumonia investigated over the last 7 years on 18 different farms. In the one outbreak the findings were of acute pulmonary oedema and haemorrhage.

In another survey of pneumonic lung material, this time at slaughter of 935 animals from the same large beef rearing farm above, the predominant lesion was a proliferative 'cuffing' pneumonia. An additional macroscopic lesion also observed at slaughter was a variable degree of fibrinous pleurisy (11% of animals). The cuffing pneumonia may be a longstanding lesion related to earlier respiratory disease. A correlation was found between the incidence during life of enzootic calf pneumonia and cuffing pneumonia at routine slaughter in these animals (p< 0.01).

Parasitic bronchitis of calves has been encountered only infrequently by this author. This histopathological findings have included an acute foreign body reaction to the presence of lung worm larvae in the bronchioles and closely resemble those described more fully by Jarrett et al. (1960).

INTRODUCTION

The four respiratory disease syndromes described in this paper represent the personal experience of the author during 8 years research. For a more comprehensive description of the calfhood pneumonias the reader is referred to the paper by Jarrett (1956).

Enzootic Pneumonia

A series of 65 autopsies were carried out over 4 years on housed calves dying of enzootic pneumonia on a large beef rearing farm. Macroscopic findings included 60% or more consolidation of the anterior lung tissue, frequently with interstitial emphysema and emphysematous bullae in the remaining posterior parts of the diaphragmatic lobes. The consolidated areas varied from red to red/grey hepatisation often with variable degrees of abscessation and bronchiectasis in the cranial lobes, especially the right apical lobe. Fibrinous or fibrotic adhesions were often present on the serosal surface of the lung and thorax. Mild to severe inflammation of trachea and bronchi was seen, with accumulation of frothy fluid.

The microscopic findings from 46 of the 65 deaths ranged from acute bronchopneumonia to a chronic suppurative broncho-pneumonia. Cellular changes included catarrhal bronchiolitis and alveolitis with accumulation in the air-spaces of alveolar macrophages, polymorphonuclear leucocytes and round cells. Interstitial alveolitis with oedema and cellular infiltration was also seen. More chronic changes included abscessation, fibrosis and bronchiectasis. Peribronchiolar round cell infiltration was not marked in any of the lungs examined and no evidence of lympho-reticular hyperplasia (cuffing) was seen. These changes represent what may be described as the typical or classicial picture of exudative, purulent bronchopneumonia. But in nine of the 65 autopsies the exudative changes were less marked and comprised focal or diffuse interstitial alveolitis.

A disturbing inability was experienced by this author
to recognise certain atypical proliferative changes reported by
several authors (Jarrett, 1954; Omar, 1966 and Stevenson, 1967)
to be commonly present in pneumonic calf lungs. Such changes
include alveolar epithelialisation and the presence of
eosinophilic or phloxinophilic inclusion bodies. Technical
difficulties might explain the lack of inclusion bodies but
failure to find proliferative lesions such as alveolar
epithelialisation suggests a rather more fundamental difference
between the material from this one farm and that examined by
the other workers. However a similar picture, essentially of
exudative bronchopneumonia, was also found by this author
in natural outbreaks of enzootic pneumonia investigated over
the last 7 years on 18 different local farms (Thomas, 1973 and
unpublished observations).

Acute Respiratory Distress

One outbreak of respiratory disease investigated in a
group of 40 yarded, single suckled, beef calves differed from
the pattern of exudative bronchopneumonia described above. Here
the clinical and pathological findings more closely resembled
the acute respiratory distress syndrome (ARDS) defined by
Breeze et al. (1976). The gross pulmonary lesion was a
substantial increase in lung weight due to fluid accumulation
and microscopic changes recognised were interstitial emphysema
with marked congestion, intra-alveolar haemorrhage, hyaline
membrane formation but not apparent alveolar epithlialisation.

Cuffing pneumonia and Pleurisy

The other type of atypical proliferative reaction described
by Jarrett (1954) as extensive peribronchiolar lymphoid hyperplasia or 'cuffing', although not present in the 65 animals
dying of enzootic pneumonia, was however frequently recognised
in material taken at routine slaughter of adult cattle from the
same farm. Eleven per cent of 935 animals slaughtered had 5%
or more of the lung space consolidated. Macroscopically the
lesion was grey/red and indurated. The cut surface consistently

revealed a mottled appearance due to accumulation of pale grey coloured peribronchiolar tissue. Microscopic examination of these areas revealed marked peribronchiolar lymphoreticular hyperplasia (cuffing). (39% of these lungs were examined microscopically).

The cuffing lesion, although recognised only at slaughter when the cattle were adult, may be a longstanding lesion related to earlier respiratory disease. A correlation was found between the incidence during life of enzootic pneumonia and the cuffing pneumonia seen at routine slaughter of the same animals ($p < 0.01$). Gourlay et al. (1970) lend support to the hypothesis that the lesion develops earlier in life. They observed extensive peribronchiolar lymphoid hyperplasia in 45 clinically healthy veal calves routinely slaughtered around 3 months of age. (These workers also failed to recognise phloxinophilic inclusion bodies in either the healthy veal calves or in 20 other calves that died with lesions of exudative purulent bronchopneumonia).

A macroscopic lesion frequently recognised in association with the pneumonic consolidation of the 935 adult cattle surveyed above was a variable degree of fibrinous pleurisy. There was a significant correlation between the incidence of the two lesions ($p < 0.01$). When present, the pleurisy was located at the caudal borders of the diaphragmatic lobes and in severe cases extended cranially involving over 50% of the visceral and parietal serosa. Interlobular fibrotic adhesions were often present in these severe cases. No clinical signs of ill health were recognised in these animals immediately prior to slaughter, although the presence of both lesions is associated with reduced growth performance (Thomas et al., 1977). Marginal pleurisy has been noted before by Michel and Mackenzie (1965) as an undefined condition of fairly common occurrence in cattle.

Parasitic Bronchitis

Parasitic bronchitis of calves has been encountered on
only 3 occasions by this author. The histopathological findings
included an acute foreign body reaction to the presence of lung
worm larvae and closely resembled those described more fully
by Jarrett et al. (1960).

DISCUSSION

Four respiratory disease syndromes have been described
in this paper. The close correlation between enzootic
pneumonia, cuffing pneumonia and pleurisy would suggest common
factors in their aetiology and indeed the same mycoplasmas and
bacteria may be found in association with both enzootic and
cuffing pneumonia (Gourlay et al., 1970). Research into these
conditions should clearly continue to follow convergent paths.
The other two syndromes are apparently distinct and past
research into both has reflected this.

In addition to the essential function of defining
respiratory disease syndromes, pathology and more particularly
histopathology may give an indication of the possible aetiology
of a disease.

The presence of inclusion bodies in a substantial proportion of enzootic pneumonias and their similarity to those
seen in virus pneumonias of other species has led Jarrett (1954)
to suggest a virus aetiology for the inclusion body pneumonia
of calves. Similar inclusion bodies have been reported in the
experimental pneumonitis of calves produced by parainfluenza
type 3 (PI-3) infection (Dawson et al., 1965). However apart
from unpublished serological surveys referred to by Darbyshire
and Roberts (1968) which have shown PI-3 and other viruses to
be common in the cattle population, the evidence for 'virus
pneumonia' being an important respiratory disease of calves
in the field still remains essentially a histopathological
observation and one that cannot be confirmed by this author.
More recent virological and serological evidence collected in

parallel with the autopsy material described in this paper will
be presented in session 3 of this seminar (Stott and Thomas et
al., vide supra).

The peracute exudative reaction of bovine lung described
by Jubb and Kennedy (1970) as a 'Pasteurellosis' was recognised
in a small proportion of the 46 cases of exudative bronchopneumonia described in this paper. However some doubt may be
cast on the value of separating these reactions into two syndromes
and stronger reservations may be levelled at the term
'Pasteurellosis'. Microbiologists would maintain, with some
justification, that the term should be reserved for conditions
from which species of Pasteurellae may be isolated. Because
these organisms may be isolated in association with a number
of different respiratory syndromes including enzootic pneumonia
and cuffing pneumonia (Gourlay et al., 1970) and the ARDS
described above (Thomas, unpublished observations) the term
would appear to have a limited descriptive value.

Jarrett (1954) draws attention to the marked similarity
between cuffing pneumonia of calves and similar reactions in
mice and pigs, now known to be the result of a mycoplasmosis.
Although Gourlay et al. (1970) were not able to correlate mycoplasma infections with the presence or absence of cuffing lesions
in calf lungs, it seems probable that mycoplasmas play an
important part in the cuffing pneumonia of calves (Gourlay
et al., vide supra and Pirie and Allan 1975).

The acute respiratory distress syndrome is generally
considered to be an anaphylactic reaction. Another allergic
reaction of bovine lung, seen in more adult cattle and
described by Pirie et al. (1971) as closely resembling Farmer's
Lung is extrinsic allergic alveolitis. It is considered to be
an Arthus type reaction. Both allergic conditions are quite
distinct histologically and neither reaction may be recognised
in the histopathology of enzootic pneumonia. There would
appear to be no evidence therefore that allergic reactions are
involved in the pathogenesis of enzootic pneumonia.

The aetiology of parasitic bronchitis and the involvement of the nematode worm, *Dictyocaulaus viviparus* is well established. However the marked cuffing reaction that also occurs in this disease sounds a suitable cautionary note with which to close. There are dangers in ascribing one pathological response to a single cause.

CONCLUSION

The clinical and pathological description of any disease syndrome is a prerequisite for polarising research on that disease. Essentially this paper has attempted no more than to remind readers of descriptions well made, in the past, by other workers. But in addition I have sought to query some descriptive boundaries and observations, to lend emphasis to the more important and frequently seen pathological changes and to add a few new observations.

ACKNOWLEDGEMENT

I am grateful to Mr. Stephen Shaw of this Institute for the statistical calculations.

REFERENCES

Breeze, R.G., Pirie, H.M., Selman, I.E. and Wiseman, A. 1976. Vet. Rec.
98, p. 138.

Darbyshire, J.H. and Roberts, D.H. 1968. J. clin. Path. 21, suppl. No. 2.
p. 61.

Dawson, P.S., Darbyshire, J.H. and Lamont, P.H. 1965. Res. Vet. Sci. 6,
p. 108.

Gourlay, R.N., Mackenzie, A. and Cooper, J.E. 1970. J. Comp. Path. 80, p. 575.

Jarrett, W.F.H. 1954. J. Path. Bact. 67, p. 441.

Jarrett, W.F.H. 1956. Br. Vet. J. 112, p. 431.

Jarrett, W.F.H., Jennings, F.W., McIntyre, W.I.M., Mulligan, W., Sharp,
N.C.C. and Urquhart, G.M. 1960. Vet. Rec. 72, p. 1066.

Jubb, K.V.F. and Kennedy, P.C. 1970. Pathology of Domestic Animals, 1, p. 221.

Michel, J.F. and Mackenzie, A. 1965. Res. Vet. Sci, 6, p. 344.

Omar, A.R. 1966. Vet. Bull, 36, p. 259.

Pirie, H.M., Dawson, C.O., Breeze, R.G., Wiseman, A. and Hamilton, J. 1971.
Vet. Rec. 88, p. 346.

Pirie, H.M. and Allan, E.M. 1975. Vet. Rec. 97, p. 345.

Stevenson, R.G. 1967. J. comp. Path. 77, p. 263.

Thomas, L.H. 1973. Vet. Rec. 93, p. 384.

Thomas, L.H., Wood, P.D.P. and Longland, J.M. 1977. Br. Vet. J. (In press).

SOME PULMONARY LESIONS OF CALVES AND THEIR SIGNIFICANCE

H.M. Pirie
Department of Veterinary Pathology, University of Glasgow
Veterinary School, Bearsden Road, Bearsden, Glasgow, Scotland.

ABSTRACT

Although the traditional systems for classifying pulmonary lesions in calves have been useful, they should be reviewed taking into consideration new information about the cell populations that exist in the lungs and current concepts of inflammation.

Amidst the profusion of changes that can be seen in the lungs of calves with pulmonary disease, some can be recognised as landmarks. These may be helpful in assessing the disease process and may be used for classification purposes. The following identifiable lesions are described and their usefulness reviewed

1) cuffing pneumonia

2) viral pneumonia associated with inclusion bodies

3) exudative interstitial or fibrinous pneumonia

4) exudative pneumonia with or without suppuration

5) atypical interstitial pneumonia or the respiratory distress syndrome

6) fungal granulomas

7) plasma cell bronchitis and bronchiolitis

8) bronchiolitis obliterans

9) bronchiectasis

10) interstitial eymphysema and

11) pulmonary oedema.

INTRODUCTION

In this paper some of the pulmonary lesions found in bovine animals, up to approximately six months of age, will be discussed. Although most of the material to be described refers to pneumonia occurring in calves indoors the abnormalities have been found in calves outside, particularly single-suckled calves. In this connection it should be remembered that pulmonary lesions in calves outside must always be differentiated from those caused by *Dictyocaulus viviparus;* these have been described earlier.

The pathological changes in calf pneumonia are diverse making this one of the most difficult groups of diseases to classify satisfactorily and usefully on a histopathological basis. Current classification and nomenclature are controversial and it is easy to find fault with them. Indeed it might be asked whether or not any classification will serve a useful purpose. However most clinically significant problems are associated with definite vascular, exudative and cellular changes in the lungs and by studying these we should be able ultimately to understand more about these reactions even if a universally acceptable classification based on them is not immediately obvious. Other criteria for classifying calf pulmonary diseases are no better. The aetiological agents that initiate these changes are not known in many cases nor are the mechanisms which mediate inflammatory and immunological reactions in the bovine lung as well understood as those in some other species.

In spite of the difficulties, several distinct lesions can be recognised which can be used as guidelines when trying to unravel the complexities of the problem and it is these which will be considered here. It should be remembered that in any given case of pulmonary disease more than one of these lesions can be seen, for example, bronchiolitis obliterans may exist with cuffing pneumonia and the lesions characteristic of the respiratory distress syndrome may be found with exudative

pneumonias. One fundamental aspect of the calf pneumonia
problem is to resolve whether or not, in these cases, we are
dealing with independent or interrelated processes.

Cuffing pneumonia

Cuffing pneumonia is a lesion that, in its fully developed
form, is usually seen in calves three months of age or older.
The changes occur in the anterior parts of the lungs and,
although clinically significant, are not usually extensive
enough to be responsible for death. Peribronchiolar lesions
that almost certainly represent an earlier phase of cuffing
pneumonia are seen in calves from two months of age.

The reaction was initially described by Jarrett et al.
(1953) and further details were given later (Jarrett 1954, 1956).
Essentially the term applies to a lesion recognised by the
large number of lymphocytes which have accumulated in and
around bronchioles forming a cuff. At its maximum development
the lesion encloses the affected bronchiole in a sheath of
lymphocytes which narrows its lumen and compresses surrounding
alveoli. The cuff eventually becomes follicular with germinal
centre-like areas. Plasma cells can be seen in the lamina
propria of the bronchi and bronchioles along with the lymphocytes.
In affected lobules the alveoli are either collapsed or there
is an alveolitis. The alveolitis results in collections of
neutrophils and macrophages in the alveolar air spaces sometimes accompanied by oedema fluid; multinucleate macrophage
giant cells are found in some animals. Complicating lesions
may also be found but they do not affect the basic diagnosis.

Cuffing pneumonia is considered to be strongly suggestive
of mycoplasma infection. Peribronchiolar lymphoid hyperplasia
was found in 75% of a series of 45 three month old calves from
which mycoplasmas including *Mycoplasma dispar* and *Ureaplasma spp.*
were isolated (Gourlay et al., 1970). A significant association
between fully developed cuffing lesions and infection with
M. dispar and *Ureaplasma spp.* was shown in a group of calves by

Pirie and Allan (1975). *Mycoplasma dispar* has also been shown to be present in other groups of calves with naturally occurring cuffing pneumonia from two months of age upwards and mycoplasmas have been demonstrated on the surface of affected bronchial epithelium in these animals by electron microscopy (Allan and Pirie 1977, Allan et al., 1976).

Small peribronchiolar accumulations of lymphocytes can be found in non-pneumonic calves (Pirie and Allan 1975) and even in pneumonic animals a major problem when identifying this lesion is deciding when the accumulations are large enough and numerous enough to warrant the diagnosis cuffing pneumonia. Nevertheless at one end of the spectrum this is a readily recognised change in calf lungs. It has been suggested that agents other than mycoplasma will produce marked peribronchiolar lymphocytic accumulations but there is as yet no good evidence that all the features implied by the term cuffing pneumonia can be found in lesions produced by other organisms. Conversely severe pneumonic reactions not characterised by peribronchiolar lymphocytic accumulations can be produced in mice by infection with a high dose of *Mycoplasma pulmonis* (Lindsey and Cassell 1973) who demonstrated that the severity, duration and pathological character of the pulmonary disease was dependent on the dose of infecting organisms.

Virus Pneumonia with Inclusion Bodies

Although pulmonary changes suggestive of virus infection can be found in calf lungs one cannot be sure that they are associated with virus infection when using microscopy, unless inclusion bodies are seen or viral antigen can be detected by immunofluorescence. Another consideration is the fact that, in our experience, viruses such as parainfluenza (PI3) virus can be isolated from calf lungs when inclusion bodies can not be detected and specific lesions are absent.

Lesions of virus pneumonia may be found in calves one week old which contrasts with the age of animals in which cuffing

lesions are seen. Usually in natural or experimental infections with viral agents the lesions produced are comparatively
localised and extensive pulmonary consolidation, when it
occurs, is attributed to secondary bacterial infection initiating
a widespread inflammatory response. Therefore in animals
dying with extensive pneumonic lesions it is often considered
that the original viral lesion might be difficult to find.
Nevertheless in one investigation (Omar 1966) 16% and 17.6%
of 125 outbreaks of pneumonia in calves in East Anglia were
thought to be associated with PI3 virus and adenovirus
respectively on the basis of finding typical lesions in lungs
from the farms studied.

Lesions which are useful diagnostic markers are found in
infections with PI3 virus, bovine adenovirus, infectious
bovine rhinotracheitis (IBR) virus and bovine respiratory
syncytial virus (BRS).

Experimental infection of calves with PI3 virus (Betts
et al., 1964, Dawson et al., 1965, Omar et al., 1966) results
in a reaction that is mainly proliferative and involves the
bronchiolar and the alveolar epithelium. Hyperplasia of the
alveolar epithelium (epithelialisation) is a well recognised
feature of this infection and epithelial syncytial giant cells
can be found. Eosinophilic intracytoplasmic inclusion bodies
are also seen; they are found mainly at five days post infection
and persist for only two days. Giant cells have also been
reported in bronchial lymph glands (Omar 1966). During our
own investigations calves infected with PI3 virus were found
to have a bronchiolitis characterised by focal degeneration
of the epithelial cells and infiltration by neutrophils; along
with this there was either alveolar collapse or a neutrophilic
alveolitis. In these animals, although intracytoplasmic
inclusion bodies were found in the bronchial and bronchiolar
epithelium, there was no alveolar epithelial hyperplasia or
giant cell formation.

The pneumonic lesion characteristic of adenovirus infection

in calves (Darbyshire et al., 1966, 1969) is a bronchiolitis
with necrosis of bronchial epithelium, occlusion of bronchioles
and alveolar collapse; eosinophilic or basophilic intranuclear
inclusion bodies are seen in the bronchial epithelial cells
and cells of the alveolar walls. The inclusions are most
numerous seven days after infection. Cells containing intranuclear
inclusion bodies may also be seen in the bronchial lymphnodes.

The virus of infectious bovine rhinotracheitis (IBR) will
also produce intranuclear inclusion bodies in the epithelial cells
of the respiratory tract particularly those of the trachea
and bronchi (Crandell et al., 1959). This disease is usually
associated with marked changes in the upper respiratory tract
and pneumonia in the absence of these is uncommon.

Another virus induced pulmonary lesion of calves is that
of BRS virus. Microscopically it is characterised by large
multinucleated giant cells, syncytial cells, which are larger
and have many more nuclei than those usually seen in PI3 virus
infections. These have been described in the lungs of
experimentally infected calves (Mohanty et al., 1975) although
eosinophilic cytoplasmic inclusion bodies, which occur in
tissue culture cells infected with this virus, were not seen.
The syncytia were found 14 and 21 days after infection.

Jolly and Ditchfield (1965) and Wellemans (1976)
demonstrated PI3 virus infection and BRS virus infection in
field cases using fluorescent antibody methods.

Interstitial emphysema has been found in animals with
viral pneumonias; this is referred to later.

Exudative Interstitial Pneumonia or Fibrinous Pneumonia

Exudative interstitial pneumonia was the term used by
Jarrett (1956) to describe a pneumonia of calves which is
also referred to as fibrinous pneumonia (Omar 1966, Jubb and
Kennedy 1970). This is an easily recognised lesion characterised by an acute inflammatory reaction in the lung with marked

exudation of fluid, in which fibrin formation is a prominent
feature into the alveolar air spaces and the interstitial
tissue of the interlobular septa and pleura; the latter is
seen as fibrinous pleurisy. Additionally there is severe
pulmonary congestion, thrombosis of small blood vessels,
necrosis of alveolar walls and bands of inflammatory cells
outlining connective tissue structure such as bronchiolar
walls, blood vessels and interlobular septa. The overall effect
leads to the lung having a marbled appearance as has been
mentioned earlier when the pneumonias of adult cattle were
discussed.

In most instances in Britain this lesion is considered
to be due to *Pasteurella multocida* or *Pasteurella haemolytica*
infection and in our experience these organisms can be
isolated in large numbers from lungs with exudative interstitial pneumonia. However cases do occur when the *Pasteurella*
spp. are not found. *Pasteurella spp* are often found in lungs
which do not have the changes described above but in these
instances they are usually present in small numbers.

Fibrinous pneumonia can be fatal and has been seen in
calves indoors and calves outdoors (Wiseman et al., 1976).
There may or may not be a history of recent movement and it is
not always possible to show that PI3 virus has been involved
in the development of the lesion.

Exudative Pneumonia with or without Suppuration

Exudative pneumonias are those in which the foundation of
the lesion is the acute inflammatory response without marked
proliferative changes in the cell populations of either the
lung tissue itself or the immune-inflammatory infiltrate.
Traditionally these are considered to be caused by bacterial
colonisation of the lung and mostly have been called bronchopneumonias. Depending on the character and distribution of
the reaction it is sometimes possible to classify them further
into interstitial or suppurative or necrotising. This in turn

may be related to the nature of the infecting organism. This momenclature can be used for pneumonias with a wide variety of exudative or cellular reactions and the variation is usually ascribed to the fact that the inflammatory process is seen at different stages. In some animals neutrophils are the main cell types present, in others the cells of the mononuclear phagocytic system predominate. Often the cellular infiltrate appears to be more significant than the fluid exudation. In all cases there is fluid or cells or both within the alveolar and bronchiolar air spaces.

Exudative pneumonias can spread to involve as much as 75% of an animal's lung tissue. When this degree of damage is produced they can be fatal without the development of complicating lesions such as those associated with the acute respiratory distress syndrome (ARDS). Although exudative pneumonias are generally attributed to primary or secondary bacterial infection in fact the aetiology is not often identified nor is their development adequately explained.

Atypical Interstitial Pneumonia or the Acute Respiratory Distress Syndrome

Some calves indoors develop respiratory distress and die due to any combination of the following pulmonary lesions

1) congestion and oedema

2) hyaline membranes

3) alveolar epithelial hyperplasia

4) interstitial emphysema.

This group of lesions is characteristic of the bovine acute respiratory distress syndrome (ARDS) (Breeze et al., 1976). Earlier descriptions of this type of pulmonary change in indoor calves in Britain used the term atypical interstitial pneumonia (AIP) (Omar and Kinch 1966) and one type of atypical pneumonia described by Jarrett (1954) was also in this category.

This syndrome has not been investigated in Britain in any detail and only a few cases have been reported although the condition may not be uncommon. Most animals with ARDS are between four and five months old although younger animals can be affected and it has been found in single-suckled calves in a straw yard (Omar and Kinch 1966) or an open court (Wiseman et al., 1975). What could be termed a standard death rate from calf pneumonia was assessed, on one farm with a problem, as 4% of the animals at risk (Thomas and Swann 1973). When AIP is involved it has been stated that mortality can be as high as 38% within a group (Omar and Kinch 1966); the total number of calves at risk in the latter investigation was not given. The pulmonary changes characteristic of this condition can occur on their own but there may be areas in the lung with other acute or chronic bronchopulmonary damage such as cuffing pneumonia (Omar and Kinch 1966) or exudative interstitial pneumonia (Wiseman et al., 1976). Many lungs with ARDS are bacteriologically sterile although some have been found to contain *P. haemolytica* or *M. dispar* or *Ureaplasma spp.* The aetiology of this reaction in calves is not known and any association between it and the other pulmonary lesions of calves is unproven. The term ARDS is preferable to AIP since the latter has been used for other pathologically distinct conditions such as bovine farmer's lung and diffuse fibrosing alveolitis.

Fungal Granulomas

Granulomas containing fungi, usually similar to *Aspergillus spp.*, are seen in calf lungs. In our experience the animals have not been less than two months old but Jarrett (1956) described one case one month old. Usually the granulomas are few and when they are the only lesion present they are probably of no consequence. Their significance when they are accompanied by other lesions is not known. It is commonly supposed that acute respiratory damage may develop in calves as a result of hypersensitivity to fungal or actinomycetal organisms in mouldy hay or mouldy bedding but there are no unequivocally confirmed cases in the literature.

Plasma Cell Bronchitis and Bronchiolitis

A lesion affecting the anterior parts of the lungs and recognised by marked accumulations of plasma cells in peri-bronchiolar tissues and the lamina propria of bronchioles and bronchi has been found in calves three to four months of age. The calves with this lesion have been in groups whose other members have had cuffing pneumonia. The distribution of cells is similar to that seen in cuffing pneumonia but plasma cells are by far the most numerous cell type present; the peri-bronchiolar lesions are diffuse in nature and not follicular.

Bronchiolitis Obliterans

Bronchiolitis obliterans can be a major component of pneumonic reactions in calves two months of age and older. The lesion is seen in animals with cuffing pneumonia but also occurs in exudative pneumonias. It is not an uncommon abnormal-ity and apart from its intrinsic effect in disturbing lung functions it may be important in delaying resolution of any accompanying alveolar reaction. Why it should develop in some animals is not clear but it is interesting that some of the microbiological agents that infect calves can damage bronchiolar epithelium for example *M. dispar*, PI3 virus, bovine adenovirus and RSV. Bronchiolitis obliterans is seen in adult cattle with farmer's lung and in young animals in the later stages of parasitic bronchitis.

Bronchiectasis

Although bronchiectasis is usually found in older cattle it has been seen in calves only four months old. In calves the dilated bronchi may be full of viscid clear or grey mucus instead of purulent exudate. The lesions are usually in the anterior part of the lungs. This type of abnormality produces permanent lung damage and if bronchiectasis is extensive the animal will not thrive.

Interstitial Emphysema

Interstitial emphysema is found in calves in the following circumstances

1) as part of the bovine ARDS

2) with severe pneumonias and

3) less frequently as the only abnormality.

When it is severe it will cause considerable interference with normal ventilation and afflicted animals usually have marked clinical signs. Although interstitial emphysema can affect a localised area of lung and in some incidents has been described as predominantly affecting the anterior lobes only (Omar and Kinch 1966) it is more frequently found in the diaphragmatic lobes and is usually most severe in this situation. Interstitial emphysema is probably produced following mechanical damage to the respiratory acini as a result of increased resistance in the conducting airways, particularly on expiration, brought about by either contraction of smooth muscles of the bronchi and bronchioles or exudate in the lumen of these structures or thickening of their lamina propria by inflammation. The possible role of uninhibited proteolytic enzymes in weakening the respiratory acini is not known.

Severe interstitial emphysema has been recorded in calves naturally infected with PI3 virus (Jolly and Ditchfield) and with BRS virus (Wellemans 1976). The latter cases were usually seen in autumn.

Pulmonary Oedema

Massive pulmonary oedema is included in this discussion since it may be found as the only lesion to explain sudden death in calves which may or may not have had clinical signs of respiratory embarrassment. In some instances the pulmonary oedema is obviously secondary to a cardiac lesion such as a ventricular septal defect. However morphologically detectable cardiac lesions are not always present and it is then very difficult to ascertain whether the pulmonary oedema is secondary to acute left heart failure or just a primary change in the haemodynamics of the pulmonary circulation such as that brought about during bovine anaphylaxis. These calves do not have the combination of lesions of the bovine ARDS.

REFERENCES

Allan, E.M. and Pirie, H.M. 1977. J. med. Microbiol. 10, p. 469.

Allan, E.M., Pirie, H.M. and Selman, I.E. 1976. Proceedings 9th International Congress on Diseases of Cattle: Paris. p. 381.

Betts, A.O., Jennings, A.R., Omar, A.R., Page, Z.E., Spence, J.B. and Walker, R.G. 1964. Vet. Rec. 76, p. 382.

Breeze, R.G., Pirie, H.M., Selman, I.E. and Wiseman, A. 1976. Vet. Rec. 98, p. 138.

Crandell, R.A., Cheatham, W.J. and Maurer, F.D. 1959. Am. J. Vet. Res. 20, p. 505.

Darbyshire, J.H., Jennings, A.R., Dawson, P.S., Lamont, P.H. and Omar, A.R. 1966. Res. Vet. Sci. 7, p, 81.

Darbyshire, J.H., Kinch, D.A. and Jennings, A.R. 1969. Res. Vet. Sci, 10, p. 39.

Dawson, P.S., Derbyshire, J.H. and Lamont, P.H. 1965. Res. Vet. Sci. 6, p. 108.

Gourlay, R.N., Mackenzie, A. and Cooper, J.E. 1970. J. Comp. Path. 80, p. 575.

Jarrett, W.F.H. 1954. J. Path. Bact. 67, p. 441.

Jarrett, W.F.H. 1956. Brit. Vet. J. 112, p. 431.

Jarrett, W.F.H., McIntyre, W.I.M. and Urquhart, G.M. 1953. Vet. Rec. 65, p. 153.

Jolly, R.D. and Ditchfield, J. 1965. Can. Vet. J. 6, p. 295.

Jubb, K.V.F. and Kennedy, P.C. 1970. Pathology of Domestic Animals; 2nd Edition Academic Press, New York and London, p. 270.

Lindsey, J.R. and Cassell, G.H. 1973. Am. J. Path. 72, p. 63.

Mohanty, S.B., Ingling, A.L. and Lillie, M.G. 1975. Am. J. Vet. Res. 36, p. 417.

Omar, A.R. 1966. Vet. Bull. 36, p. 259.

Omar, A.R., Jennings, A.R. and Betts, A.O. 1966. Res. Vet. Sci. 7, p. 379.

Omar, A.R. and Kinch, D.A. 1966. Vet. Rec. 78, p. 766.

Pirie, H.M. and Allan, E.M. 1975. Vet. Rec. 97, p. 345.

Thomas, L.H. and Swann, R.G. 1973. Vet. Rec. 92, p, 454.

Wellemans, G. 1976. Proceedings 9th International Congress on Diseases of Cattle: Paris, p. 373.

Wiseman, A., Selman, I.E., Pirie, H.M. and Harvey, I.M. 1976. Vet. Rec. 98, p. 192.

A. van Nieuwstadt *(Netherlands)*

I would like to put a question to Dr. Thomas. In those
cases of typical interstitial pneumonia which you mentioned,
have you carried out any serological survey in the same herd
for the possible aetiological role of an RS virus infection in
those cases?

L.H. Thomas *(UK)*

Are you referring to the one outbreak which I described as
the acute respiratory distress syndrome?

A. van Nieuwstadt

As an instance, yes, but possibly you have seen other cases
of acute respiratory distress.

L.H. Thomas

That is the only one I have seen.

A. van Nieuwstadt

Was there a serological survey during this work?

L.H. Thomas

I can say that that particular outbreak was something of
a microbiological feast, in that we had evidence of infection
with respiratory syncytial virus, with parainfluenza 3 virus,
with at least 3 species of mycoplasm, and *Pasteurella haemolytica*
was isolated also. It is the usual complex story. As to the
other rather larger series which I described, those were in
fact taken from the same farm which Dr. Stott was describing
yesterday.

J.M. Sharp *(UK)*

This is a question for Dr. Thomas and for Dr. Pirie. I
have not formed an opinion from the talk of the relative importance which they attach to different types of pneumonia.
Which do they think are the predominant types we are dealing with?

From the pathology, which agents do they think are causing this type of pneumonia? Is it viruses and mycoplasmas, which we heard a lot about yesterday, or is it the bacteria, which no one in this gathering is really prepared to speak about?

H.M. Pirie *(UK)*

From the material which we have looked at we think that the cuffing pneumonia is the most important one. The term 'cuffing pneumonia' really refers to a morphological lesion which could be an end-stage lesion. This does not exclude the possibility that it goes through an earlier phase at which these cuffs are not as big, only we cannot identify this at the moment on a histological basis. Dr. Thomas has mentioned the fact that we find these lesions in cows. If you take the pig situation which is better worked out, we know that sows have cuffing lesions just in the same way as do pigs at 6 months of age. Our view is that this is the important background pneumonia which is not necessarily always lethal.

L.H. Thomas

I think it rather depends what criteria one uses for assessing importance. As Dr. Pirie said, the cuffing lesions do not tend to kill calves. The acute exudative bronchopneumonia does. Nevertheless, the cuffing lesion is a frequent one, and it is undoubtedly associated with a reduction in performance of the animals. I think it is an unfair question to ask what the microorganisms might be, from the histological appearance. You do not see many microorganisms when you actually look down the microscope. You can infer from other observations what might be going on. I think you can perhaps infer that the cuffing lesion may have as its basis a mycoplasma infection, for instance, on the basis of other work which has been done to show that, if you experimentally infect animals with mycoplasmas you get a cuffing lesion as a result. I do not think we have the same sort of information to put with the lesion of acute exudative bronchopneumonia.

J.B. McFerran *(UK)*

Could I ask Dr. Thomas to elaborate a little on the aetiology of pneumonia on the beef farm. You mentioned that these calves come on to it at 16 to 18 days of age. You suggested that this would give you a sample of the virus infections within a 200 mile radius. Do you infer by this that the calves are bringing the organisms in with them, or do you think that your organisms are endemic on this farm, and these calves are infected once they arrive there?

L.H. Thomas

I do not think I can answer the question. All I can say is that that is the set-up. These animals are collected from a wide area and I would expect that they bring in various infections and also acquire various infections when they come on to the farm. I cannot be more precise than that.

J.M. Sharp *(UK)*

I would like some further evidence on the undoubted import-ance of cuffing pneumonia. I do not dispute that it is preval-ent, and that it is the most common lesion which you see. Could you expand a little further on its undoubted importance, in terms of a reduction of performance.

H.M. Pirie

One of the papers which I quoted was Dr. Gourlay's. Seventy five percent of the animals had cuffing lesions.

L.H. Thomas

I can only repeat that in the sample of just under 1 000 animals we have found that, in animals with the cuffing lesion, the performance is reduced by up to 7.6%. This is a reduction in liveweight gain. If you compare the animal with a pneumonic lesion with an animal without a lesion, it will not put on weight as quickly as the healthy animal. This was during a controlled trial which we have carried out on this farm. Eleven percent of the 1 000 had a pneumonic lesion at slaughter. By pneumonic lesion I mean 5% or more of the lung tissue was consolidated.

A. Andrews *(UK)*

How many of those animals were clinically ill during their life, and how many were treated, out of the 11%?

L.H. Thomas

There was a significant correlation at the 1% level, between treatment of enzootic pneumonia during life.

A. Andrews

Yes, but that is not quite the same thing. How many were actually treated, or virus ever seen? Was this out of the whole 1 000?

L.H. Thomas

I cannot remember the exact figure of how many it was, but if you do a statistical calculation on the 1 000 animals, there was a significant correlation at the 1% level betwen treatment for enzootic pneumonia and the appearance of the pneumonic lesion at slaughter.

SESSION 5B

THERAPY

Chairman:

H. Frerking

Co-ordinator:

N.J.L. Gilmour

PHARMACOLOGICAL CONSIDERATIONS
OF CURRENT METHODS OF THERAPY

P. Eyre
Ontario Veterinary College, University of Guelph,
Ontario, Canada.

ABSTRACT

The two classes to true anti-inflammatory drugs are (1) glucocorticoster-oids and (2) non-steroid (salicylate-like) anti-inflammatory agents. Other classes of drugs which are used as anti-allergics are the sympathomimetics or adrenaline-like compounds and the cromones.

Corticosteroids stabilise cellular and lysosomal membranes and there-by inhibit release of the chemical mediators of inflammation and proteolytic enzymes. Other glucocorticoid effects include inhibition of antibody synthesis; suppression of activity of fibroblasts; elevation of circulating neutrophil count and reduction in eosinophil count. Steroids also increase microvascular tone and decrease permeability thus reducing exudation and oedema formation.

Non-steroid anti-inflammatory drugs (NSAID) act principally to inhibit the biosynthesis of prostaglandins. The salicylate-like compounds also inhibit kallikrein activity and kinin formation and at the same time pharmacologically antagonise the tissue effects of kinins, prostaglandins and slow-reacting substance of anaphylaxis (SRS-A). NSAID are, with some exceptions, analgesic and antipyretic: effects not shown by corticosteroids.

The glucocorticoids have been utilised extensively in acute and chronic inflammation, particularly in afflictions of the skin, musculo-skeletal system and lung. These drugs are of no value in acute anaphylaxis or histamine stock. Salicylate-like drugs are used mainly for musculo-skeletal disorders. NSAID have been shown to be effective in controlling respiratory hypersensitivity in cattle and horses and are worthy of greater prominence in this respect. Adrenaline and related drugs are most often employed in situations involving allergic respiratory and cardiovascular impairment. Cromones, which prevent release of histamine, have not been employed in clinical veterinary medicine.

410

INTRODUCTION

Anti-inflammatory and anti-allergic drugs possess widely
differing mechanisms of action which in part determine their
clinical usefulness. 'Classical' anti-inflammatory steroids
have been used most frequently in controlling inflammation of
the respiratory tract, as well as in many other organ-systems.
Salicylate-like drugs have recently been shown to possess
useful pulmonary anti-inflammatory properties while sympathomimetic agents are reserved for the acute allergic reaction.

ADRENOCORTICOSTEROIDS

Commonly used corticoids include: Cortisone, Hydrocortisone,
Prednisone, Prednisolone, Betamethasone, Dexamethasone and
Triamicinolone. All are of similar chemical structure and
mechanism of action. The biological effects of glucocorti-
costeroids are numerous and complex and it will not be possible
to review them comprehensively within the scope of this brief
presentation.

Anti-inflammatory actions are probably the most widely
recognised properties of the glucocorticoids. They suppress
inflammation at all levels including early phenomena (vasodilation,
oedema formation, leukocyte migration); later events (collagen
deposition, fibroblast and capillary proliferation) and finally
cicatrisation. Furthermore, corticosteroids inhibit inflammation
irrespective of the cause (physical, chemical or immunological
trauma).

It is widely accepted that glucocorticoids perform their
anti-inflammatory action by stabilising cellular and lysosomal
membranes (Weissman and Thomas, 1964), thus preventing the
release of the chemical mediators of inflammation (histamine,
5-hydroxytryptamine, slow-reacting substance of anaphylaxis,
kallikreins, prostaglandins) from target cells (mast cells and
basophil leukocytes) and of proteolytic enzymes from lysosomes
(in polymorphonuclear neutrophil leukocytes, for example).

This unitary hypothesis, however, does not adequately explain
all the actions of corticosteroids. For example the steroids
are immunosuppressant and have a pronounced inhibitory action
on fibroblasts. Another striking glucocorticoid effect is on
cell-mediated immunity; principally to cause 'lysis' of lymphoid
tissue and to interfere with the function of macrophages.
(When activated by antigen, sensitised lymphocytes produce a
lymphokine; macrophage migration inhibition factor (MIF) which
causes macrophage accumulation by inhibiting their mobility).
Glucocorticoids block the action of MIF on macrophages whose
migration is no longer inhibited. Macrophages therefore do
not accumulate (Barlow and Rosenthal, 1973). Glucocorticoid
drugs increase the numbers of circulating neutrophil (PMN)
leukocytes, while at the sime time reducing the numbers
of basophils, eosinophils and mononuclear leukocytes. A very
important and often overlooked property of the corticosteroids
is their ability directly to increase the tone and decrease the
permeability of the microvasculature, thus reducing exudation
and oedema formation.

Therapeutic uses.

    The principal clinical use of corticosteroid drugs in
veterinary medicine is in the treatment of lameness and
musculo-skeletal diseases in general. Acute and chronic
diseases of the eye, skin and lung, and acute mastitis and
metritis are also indications for corticosteroid therapy.
Numerous other conditions cannot be covered in the scope of
this discussion. It is important to make the often-repeated
statement that corticosteroid therapy is palliative not curative
and therefore largely empirical. Special caution is required
with infectious conditions owing to suppression of the immune
system and the risk of dissemination of micro-organisms. In
addition, abrupt cessation of prolonged steroid therapy
carries a significant risk of adrenal insufficiency which may
be life-threatening.

NON-STEROID (SALICYLATE-LIKE) ANTI-INFLAMMATORY DRUGS (NSAID)

Compounds under consideration include: - Phenylbutazone
(butazolidin), Acetylsalicyclic acid (Asa, Aspirin), Indomethacin
(Indocin), Mefenamic acid and Ibuprofen. All these compounds
have in common the ability to block prostaglandin biosynthesis.
Fundamental in the mediation and modulation of inflammation
are the prostaglandins; a series of biologically potent
endogenous lipids. Prostaglandins (PG) produce vasodilation
and whealing, increase vascular permeability, sensitise pain
receptors, release histamine and increase chemotaxis. PGE
is synthesised by macrophages in response to stimulation by
lymphocyte-derived MIF. This macrophage PG is responsible for
negative feedback (inhibition) of lymphocyte MIF production.

Prostaglandins are synthesised by a variety of cell types
which includes leukocytes, mast cells, epithelial and
endothelial cells. The disruption of cell membrane integrity
caused by vasoactive amines, kinins complement and lysosomal
enzymes liberates phospholipases and lipid substrates which
together produce arachidonic acid. Arachidonate, the principal
substrate (precursor) for PG synthesis, is converted by cyclo-
oxygenase to cyclic prostaglandin endoperoxides (PGG or H):
compounds with very short biological lives. PGG or H are further
converted to three possible products: (i) prostacyclin (PGX)
another short-lived lipid which is thought to have a protective
effect on vascular endothelium and to prevent platelet aggregation, (ii) prostaglandins which are largely pro-inflammatory
in nature and (iii) thromboxanes (TX-synthesised from endoperoxide mainly in platelets) which are potent aggregating factors
(Bunting et al., 1976;Gryglewski et al., 1976; Moncada et al.,
1976; Kuehl et al., 1977). Non-steroid anti-inflammatory drugs
inhibit the enzyme cyclo-oxygenase, thus inhibiting the biosynthesis of endoperoxide and blocking the major inflammatory
pathways (Vane, 1971; Ferriera and Vane, 1974).

In addition to their blocking PG synthesis, NSAID also
inhibit kinin formation and may also antagonise pharmacologically

the actions of histamine, kinins and SRS-A on smooth muscle and vascular endothelium (Burka and Eyre, 1977). Many NSAID (especially salicylates) are both antipyretic and analgesic; properties which are not shared by corticosteroids.

Therapeutic uses

NSAID have been confined in veterinary medicine almost exclusively to the treatment of lameness and musculo-skeletal disorders in general. Recent studies however have shown that NSAID effectively block cardiorespiratory manifestations of anaphylaxis in cattle and horses (Eyre, 1971; Eyre et al., 1973; Eyre, 1976) and control the clinical and pathological signs of helminth-induced interstitial pneumonia in cattle (Eyre et al., 1975). This is logical in view of the known importance of lipids and kinins in bovine hypersensitivity (Eyre et al., 1973). NSAID should be given more consideration in the control of acute respiratory disease in cattle (see review: Chand and Eyre, 1977). Being both analgesic and antipyretic, the salicylate-like drugs offer considerable symptomatic relief in addition to their anti-inflammatory properties.

SYMPATHOMIMETICS (ADRENALINE-LIKE COMPOUNDS)

The so-called direct-acting sympathomimetics include Adrenaline, isoprenaline and salbutamol among others. Indirect acting sympathomimetics include Methylxanthines (eg theophylline) and Amphetamines.

Adrenaline, isoprenaline and salbutamol stimulate cell membrane adenylate cyclase and thus elevate the concentrations of cellular cyclic adenosine, 3', 5' monophosphate (cyclic AMP). These drugs thus mimic the body's sympathoadrenal response to stress. However, although adrenaline and isoprenaline are both powerful cardiostimulants and bronchodilators, salbutamol is a specific bronchodilator only. Xanthines and amphetamines possess essentially similar properties to adrenaline. Their mode of action is to inhibit the enzymatic degradation of cyclic AMP.

Therapeutic uses

Adrenaline has been widely employed and is highly effective
in the treatment of acute anaphylactic shock and of acute
allergic pulmonary oedema. Adrenaline reverses the fall in
blood pressure and cardiac insufficiency and also causes
constriction and decreased permeability of micro-blood vessels,
thus reducing oedema formation. Bronchoconstriction associated
with acute histamine release is also reversed by adrenaline,
isoprenaline and salbutamol. Salbutamol is a true anti-
asthmatic, causing specifically bronchodilation without
significant cardiovascular actions. Xanthines and amphetamines
may be employed in similar circumstances as adrenaline.

CROMONES

The only cromone in current clinical use is Disodium
cromoglycate(Intal, Lumodal, cromolyn). This drug interferes
with the immunological release of histamine and SRS-A.
Cromoglycate is inhaled by human asthmatic subjects and
provides long term relief from chronic bronchospasm and pulmonary
vascular lesions. So far, the drug has not proved useful in
experimental pulmonary hypersensitivity in cattle but may be
more promising in the horse and dog.

REFERENCES

Barlow, J.E. and Rosenthal,A.S. 1973. Glucocorticoid suppression of macro-
    phage migration inhibitory factor. Journal of Experimental Medicine,
    137, 1031-1039.

Bunting, S., Gryglewski, R., Moncada, S. and Vane, J.R. 1976. Arterial walls
    generate from prostaglandin endoperoxides a substance (prostaglandin
    X) which relaxes strip of mesenteric and coeliac arteries and
    inhibits platelet aggregation. Prostaglandins, 12, 897-913.

Burka, J.F. and Eyre, P. 1977. Effects of bovine SRS-A (SRS-A[bov]) on
    bovine respiratory tract and lung vasculature in vitro. European
    Journal of Pharmacology, 44, 169-177.

Chand, N. and Eyre, P. 1977. Non-steroidal anti-inflammatory drugs; A
    review. New applications in hypersensitivity reactions of cattle and
    horses. Canadian Journal of Comparative Medicine, 41, 233-240.

Eyre, P. 1977. Pharmacology of bovine, pulmonary vein anaphylaxis in vitro.
    British Journal of Pharmacology, 43, 302-311.

Eyre, P. 1976. Preliminary studies on the antagonism of anaphylactic
    hypersensitivity in the horse. Canadian Journal of Comparative
    Medicine, 40, 149-152.

Eyre, P., Lewis, A.J. and Wells, P.W. 1973. Acute systemic anaphylaxis in
    the calf. British Journal of Pharmacology, 47, 504-516.

Eyre, P., Nymeyer, D.H., McCraw, B.M. and Delin, T.R. 1976. Protection by
    acetylsalicylic acid (Aspirin) and other agents in experimental acute
    interstitial pneumonia of calves. Veterinary Record, 98, 64-66.

Ferriera, S.H. and Vane, J.R. 1974. New aspects of the mode of action of
    non-steroid anti-inflammatory drugs. Annual Review of Pharmacology,
    14, 57-73.

Gryglewski,R.J., Bunting, S., Moncada, S., Flower, R.J. and Vane, J.R. 1976.
    Arterial walls are protected against deposition of platelet thrombi
    by a substance (prostaglandin X) which they make from prostaglandin
    endoperoxides. Prostaglandins, 12, 685-713.

Kuehl, F.A., Humes, J.L., Egan, R.W., Ham, E.A., Beveridge, G.C., and
    Van Arman, C.G. 1977. Role of prostaglandin endoperoxide PGG_2 in
    inflammatory process. Nature (London), 265, 170-172.

Moncada, S., Needleman, P., Bunting, S. and Vane, J.R. 1976. Prostaglandin
    endoperoxide and thromboxane-generating systems and their selective
    inhibition. Prostaglandins, 12, 323-335.

Vane, J.R. 1971. Inhibition of prostaglandin synthesis as a mechanism of action of aspirin-like drugs. Nature (London), <u>231</u>, 232-235.

TREATMENT OF INFECTIOUS RESPIRATORY DISEASE OF CALVES

B. Martin

21 Hill Street, Kilmarnock, Scotland.

ABSTRACT

The term 'Infectious Respiratory Disease' is used to refer to the complex of upper and lower respiratory infections generally recognised as being associated with a range of viral and bacterial agents and occurring, classically, in the indoor calf.

For the clinician, the aetiological and pathological complexities of the syndrome may present problems to his therapeutic approach which cannot always be guided either by clinical assessment or laboratory investigation. Some aspects of causation and pathology are discussed within the context of treatment.

Treatment is aimed at the infectious agents likely to be involved and also at their penumonic effects, while environmental features contributing to the occurrence and persistence of clinical disease cannot be disregarded.

INTRODUCTION

The disease is thought to be the most commonly occurring
entity in bovine clinical practice in this country, and in
one survey of 4 426 cases of disease in dairy cattle, 750
cases (16.9%) of infectious respiratory disease were recorded.
In the same series, when the incidence of diseases affecting
dairy cattle under one year was studied, the condition
accounted for 41% of 1 819 cases of all diseases recorded in
that age group. (Martin, 1973).

The complex offers a unique example of bovine disease
which may affect virtually every animal under one roof at
one time, so that the need for treatment often involves large
numbers to be treated as a group or separately as individuals,
according to the clinical severity.

Clinical Aspects

The common clinical picture is one of a group of calves
all or most of which, in the early stages, have a relatively
mild upper respiratory syndrome characterised by frequent
coughing and by the absence of clinical evidence of pneumonia.
As the disease progresses, a varying number of animals become
frankly pneumonic, showing tachypnoea and dyspnoea with
evidence of lung involvement on auscultation.

These upper and lower respiratory manifestations of the
syndromes are quite distinct in individual animals, and while
both forms are likely to co-exist in an established outbreak
of disease, their identification may influence the clinician's
approach to treatment without offering specific guidance as
to the pathogens likely to be involved.

Treatment

Whatever the complexities of the multifactorial causation
of the infectious respiratory syndrome may be, the antimicrobial aspect of treatment is directed at the causal agents,

and while it may seem that any consideration of the multiplicity of agents which have been reported as being involved, might serve to confuse the clinician in his selection of an appropriate antimicrobial, in effect the selection is immediately simplified by the absence of effective antivirals, and the therapeutic approach, in this respect, is singularly antibacterial.

Where a group of calves is presented with the early coughing syndrome in the absence of clinical evidence of pneumonia, and while the calves are still eating, group-therapy is simplified by the administration of oxytetracycline or chlortetracycline in the feed, in milk or water at a dose rate of 800 mg per 50 kg.

Treatment for a period of 5 to 10 days seldom abolishes coughing but, normally, progression of the disease to its subsequent pneumonic stages can be expected to be controlled effectively.

The frequent failure of antibacterial therapy to abolish the coughing associated with the upper respiratory form of the disease may suggest that non-bacterial agents play the major role in infection at this stage, and that the essential usefulness of antibacterial treatment lies in its control of secondary bacterial invasion of upper and lower respiratory structures already under viral assault.

Where some members of an affected group are observed to be pneumonic, they are likely to be inappetant so that their intake of medicated feed is sub-therapeutic, and in any case, the route and dose rate of oral antibiotic is unlikely to be adequate for the treatment of active pneumonia. Consequently, the administration of antibiotic by systemic routes to selected individuals is indicated.

Oxytetracycline, administered intravenously at a dose rate of 1.0 to 1.5 g per 50 kg, and maintained by daily injections

as required, results in the rapid recovery of the great
majority of cases. Largely, the response of cases of
pneumonia to oxytetracycline and other broad-spectrum antibiotics is highly satisfactory, so that doubts about the
part which non-bacterial pathogens play in the ultimate onset
of clinical pneumonia, seem fully justified. While there is
little dispute that non-bacterial agents do play a part at
some stage in the pathogenetic events leading to clinical
pneumonia, the overall response to antibacterial preparations
is such as to offer evidence that it is bacteria which play
the final major role. This observation is consistent with
the findings reported by Thomas in 1973.

Notwithstanding the overall success of administering
broad-spectrum antibiotics to pneumonic calves, individual
cases are encountered which fail to respond adequately unless
corticosteroid is given along with the selected antibiotic.
Doses of 20 to 40 mg of dexamethasone given intravenously
per 50 kg may be necessary to obtain a satisfactory response
in those animals failing to respond to antibiotic alone. The
failure of severe cases of pneumonia to respond to antibiotic
alone is not uncommon in the odd individual animal in an
affected group and seems likely to be due in some part to the
obstructive effects of oedema and cellular proliferation which
are features of the pathology of the pneumonias of young
cattle. Certainly, corticosteroid enhances the action of antibiotics in these cases, presumably by its anti-inflammatory
action on cellular proliferation, although it may be also,
that the physiological effects of unidentified aspects of
stress which has been implicated as a contributory aetiological
factor, are also controlled.

Following the treatment so far described, a satisfactory
clinical response may be expected over a period of 24 to 72 h,
although a small percentage of cases will fail to show any
worthwhile response. These do not often die but simply fail
to improve and the subsequent use of tylosin at a dose rate of

500 mg   per 50 kg frequently results in an almost spectacular
improvement in a significant number of these cases.

A further small percentage of affected calves fails to
respond adequately to any treatment whatsoever and these
continue to survive as chronic cases, mildly tachypnoeic and
dyspnoeic, with an infrequent cough but permanently unthrifty
and commercially useless.

Mortality is not a feature of infectious respiratory
disease where appropriate antibiotic treatment is carried
out. When the administration of oxytetracycline is followed
by absence of response and deaths in the 48 h period after the
first administration, the diagnosis should be revised with
consideration of Salmonellosis. This latter infection is
presented frequently as an acute pneumonic syndrome which is
clinically similar to infectious respiratory disease, but its
high mortality rate is a distinguishing feature.

Treatment directed at bacterial pathogens and their
pneumonic effects is an obvious and necessary approach to the
respiratory disease problem, and while the immediate response
is largely satisfactory, failure to identify and minimise
environmental faults is likely to be followed by repeated
exacerbations of disease and an ultimate increase in the
number of chronic refractory cases within an affected group.

In practical terms there is little doubt that environmental
factors contributing to the conditions which favour the
occurrence and extension of infectious respiratory disease
include inadequate cubic space and ventilation as these
relate to stocking density. Also, inadequate comfort,
inadequate feeding space, and the exposure of young animals
to older age groups under the same roof, would seem to be
significant contributory factors.

Consequently, as an adjunct to chemotherapy, it is

422

necessary as far as is possible, to correct shortcomings in
these areas of management so that clinical improvement brought
about by appropriate treatment might be maintained.

CONCLUSIONS

At this time the continuing problem of infectious
respiratory disease is a complex of many causal factors, infectious
and environmental, interrelated in such a way that we still
seem far from understanding its epidemiological features to
the point of establishing a formula for prevention.

Fortunately, mortality is not a problem if appropriate
treatment is applied, but the continuing morbidity and loss
of productivity have remained unaltered over the past 25 years.
It is to be hoped that renewed and co-ordinated research effort
within the Common Agricultural Policy will be stimulated and
guided by this European gathering of veterinary interests.

REFERENCES

Martin, B. 1973. Vet. Rec. 92, p. 164.
Thomas, L.H. 1973. Vet. Rec. 93, p. 384.

DISCUSSION

P. Pignatelli *(Italy)*

Mr. Martin: in Italy, 10 mg per kg of bodyweight of tylosine are not enough to obtain a good result. Normally we use 25, or sometimes 50 mg per kg bodyweight. Would you care to comment?

B. Martin *(UK)*

I feel that you, Dr. Pignattelli, have a much wider experience of the use of mycoplasmacides than I have. I have no direct evidence that mycoplasmas are seriously involved in the kind of respiratory diseases which I see, and only in the odd case which fails to respond to antibacterials do I then come in with the macrolide which, hopefully, is a mycoplasmacide, and this sometimes works. It may very well be working as a bactericidal agent in my case, I have no way of telling. I fully accept your opinion about the necessity for a higher dose rate.

S. Hall *(UK)*

In any equivalent human disease there would be some sort of oxygen therapy given. Generally speaking, it is regarded as being impracticable, but I would like to suggest that we should give closer consideration to oxygen therapy, even in young animals, and certainly in large ones which can be quite valuable. I suggest it can be administered quite easily. About fifteen years ago I developed some apparatus for doing this, and I believe it was very effective and quite practical.

B. Martin

Perhaps Dr. Eyre might wish to say something about the usefulness of oxygen.

P. Eyre *(Canada)*

There is no question that, by raising the tension in the inspired air, you are likely to get a better oxygen exchange, although you are still not necessarily improving carbon dioxide efflux. It is certainly useful, and it is employed all the time in human medicine, as Dr. Hall has said. Personally, I do not know about the practicality of carrying oxygen tanks around in the field.

S. Hall

This is the difficult part. The method I developed did not use a mask. You must do away with the mask. The other advantage it does have is that you can actually inject into the inspired oxygen any drug, bronchodilator, or antibiotic, as an aerosol, and get at the infection from the other side, as well as through the blood.

O.C. Straub (West Germany)

When we try to treat those animals from the other side we are sometimes puzzled by the influences which the corticosteroids have. We tried some of them to determine their influence on the blood picture. If we use Prednisolone, for example, we get a general lowering of all the blood elements, lymphocytes as well as neutrophils. We then found out that, if we gave Dexamethasone in the same group, we maintained the very high level of the granulocytes and only got a lowering of the lymphocytes. If we use Prednisolone we have to use more antibiotics because then we have the trouble of secondary infections. If we use Dexamethasone we did not have to give additional antibiotics. Obviously, only the lymphocytes were affected. Do you have an explanation for that?

P. Eyre

No, I do not have a specific explanation for that, but my comment would be that wherever possible you should not use high levels of corticosteroids without antibiotic cover.

O.C. Straub

If we use Prednisolone we do use antibiotics, but if we use Dexamethasone we can forget about administering antibiotics, in the experiments which we performed.

P. Eyre
   I did not know about this difference. That is interesting.

O.C. Straub
   If you treat a horse which has been chronically infected
with equine anaemia for a number of days, with either Prednisolone
or Dexamethasone you get febrile attacks, and you can recover the
virus. But at the same time with the Prednisolone you get a
drop in all the blood elements and the serum elements, but with
Dexamethasone you only get a lowering of the lymphocytes. I
thought it might help you in a practical way.

B. Martin
   What kind of frequency of dosing are you talking about,
using Prednisolone?

O.C. Straub
   With the Prednisolone we went as high as 250 mg per day for
5 days. We really wanted to double the maximum dose, because we
wanted to see if we had the virus present, or if it had gone.
In horses, we used a whole vial of Dexamethasol - 20 cc - per
day, and we have used it for as long as 15 days consecutively,
without using antibiotic. After the fourth or fifth day I
always have to add something with the Prednisolone.

B. Martin
   I think it is worth making the point, Mr. Chairman, that in
clinical practice one would not be thinking in terms of giving
this kind of dose rate of any steroid for a period of 5 days.
It would be given once or perhaps twice in a critical period of
48 hours early on in the disease.

O.C. Straub
   We used the extremes on purpose because under experimental
conditions we can use the extremes in order to find out where
the borderline is.

P. Eyre

I think it is important to emphasise what Mr. Martin said when he was talking about one or two shots of a high level of corticosteroid, over a very brief period of time. Frankly, there are not likely to be very severe blood changes, immuno-suppression or adrenocortical suppression in the regime which he described. When you have a week or so of treatment then you will begin to get these dramatic changes, in electrolytes in the blood, cellular changes, immune responses and so on. But I do not think you will get the changes at the level he is talking about.

O.C. Straub

When using Prednisolone you see the drop in the leukocytes on the second day. It is drastic with the Prednisolone, but is not so drastic with the Dexamethasone.

H.M. Pirie *(UK)*

I think both speakers have stressed the usefulness of using anti-inflammatory agents in these lesions as a general rule. Both speakers have put forward evidence that this can be a good thing to do. Even in some instances where the microbiological agents may be lost, certainly it is possible for inflammation to get out of control, and this may be responsible for some of these extreme lesions we get without organisms.

You mentioned using aspirin. I wonder if you have any experience of using this in the field. Also I know that you have done some experiments in which aspirin diminished the signs of experimental infections of lungworms, but have you also any experience of where the clinical disease has been made worse with aspirin - because this can happen in some cases of asthma.

P. Eyre

I think we are talking about something quite different when we talk of asthma. Asthma is essentially a bronchial smooth muscle problem. You have quite a different kind of syndrome in acute pneumonia. Admittedly you can get acute exacerbations of asthma, with oedema and excessive mucus and so on. We have to be rather careful here. The exacerbations of asthma may be caused by changing the ratio of different kinds of prostaglandins which have been synthesised by the smooth muscle. A lot of work has been done on this. We simply do not know whether this occurs in acute bovine pneumonias. It is a very good point. We have never seen it experimentally, and the limited amount of clinical trials which I have persuaded some of my colleagues to do does not bear out any idea that aspirin will induce this untoward reaction in the acute pneumonias, but I agree it may do in the asthmatic. The nearest animal model to an asthmatic human is the horse with broken wind - I know they are not identical but they are pretty close. I do not think that you should necessarily extrapolate from one species into another.

SESSION 5C

IMMUNITY

Chairman:

F.J. Bourne

Co-ordinator:

N.J.L. Gilmour

PARAINFLUENZA-3 VIRUS NEURAMINIDASE AND ANTINEURAMINIDASE IN INFECTION AND PROTECTION OF THE BOVINE RESPIRATORY TRACT

B. Morein

Institute of Virology, Royal College and National Veterinary
Institute, Stockholm, Sweden.

ABSTRACT

The respiratory tract is covered by a mucus layer. It consists of a superficial gel phase and a liquid phase beneath. The gel phase contains inhibitors to parainfluenza-3 virus (PIV-3). The majority of these are sensitive to neuraminidase. The PIV-3 particle has to pass through (penetrate) the mucus layer to infect the respiratory epithelium. It has been suggested that PIV-3 penetrates the gel phase by aid of its neuraminidase which releases the virion from the inhibitors.

Evidence that neuraminidase-sensitive inhibitors can prevent infection was found in an experiment where calves under the age of 4 weeks could not be infected with a neuraminidase weak (NAW) strain of PIV-3 but with either of two neuraminidase strong (NAS) strains. The criteria for infection were virus excretion, antibody mediated and cell mediated immune responses. Nasal secretion (NS) from these calves had comparatively high HI-titres of non-immune globulin nature, which decreased considerably after neuraminidase treatment.

Calves above the age of 6 weeks could be infected with both NAW and NAS strains, they have also a low content of neuraminidase sensitive inhibitors in NS.

A neuraminidase inhibition assay for PIV-3 was developed using the gel phase of NS from calves as substrate. In a kinetic study a rapid release of N'acetyl neuraminic acid (NANA) occurred from the gel of NS from non-immune calves when exposed to PIV-3, but the release of NANA was slow from the gel phase of immune animals.

The respiratory tract is a portal of entry of infection
for parainfluenza-3 (PI-3) virus and some other viruses. In
order to infect the epithelial cells of the respiratory tract
the virion must pass through the mucus layer. This layer
consists of a superficial gel phase with a liquid phase beneath.
In the liquid phase, cilia of epithelial cells perform beating
movements which transport the gel phase and foreign bodies
entrapped in it towards the pharynx where they can be
swallowed.

A particle situated in the remotest part of the respiratory
tract of a human is transported and cleared out within 20 - 240
minutes (for review see Rylander, 1970). Figure 1.

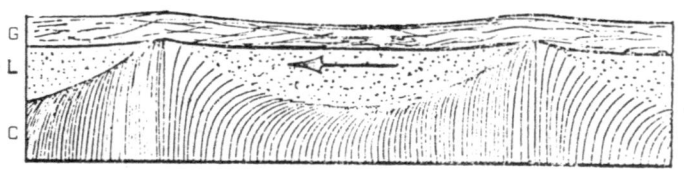

Fig. 1. An illustration of the transport mechanism of the mucociliary
         system as conceived by Hilding, 1957. The arrow indicates the
         transport direction. G=gel phase; L=liquid phase; C=cilia.

It is obvious that a virion landing in the respiratory
tract is likely to come into contact and interact with the
mucus. Furthermore it is known that both the liquid and the
gel phases of mucus contain components which participate in
the defence system. Some of these might belong to the immune
system and some are non-specific inhibitors. (For review see
Morein, 1975).

The interactions between PI-3 virus and mucus were studied
in the following ways:

1) The ability of PI-3 virus (a neuraminidase strong

strain) to release N'acetyl neuraminic acid (NANA) from
the gel and liquid phases.

2) The effect of PI-3 virus on the rheological properties
of the liquid and gel phases, ie the effect on the
viscosity.

3) The effect of PI-3 virus on the electrophoretic mobility
of the gel phase.

4) Scanning electron microscopy (SEM) of untreated gel
phases and phases treated with PI-3 virus.

It was found that:

1) NANA could be released from the gel phase of adult
animals, but not from the liquid phase (Morein and
Bergman, 1972).

2) PI-3 virus neuraminidase caused increased viscosity
of the gel phase but not of the liquid phase (Friberg
et al., 1973).

3) Following treatment with PI-3 virus there was a
decreased mobility of the gel phase towards the anode in
free electrophoresis (Höglund and Morein, 1974).

4) Using SEM, the smooth appearance of the network
structure was changed to a rough appearance. (Höglund and
Morein, 1974), (Figure 3).

The effects of PI-3 virus mentioned above can all be
explained by the reactions which are catalysed by the PI-3
virus neuraminidase. It is, however, difficult to estimate
what importance these effects have for the pathogenicity
following an infection with PI-3 virus or a secondary infection.

How is the immune response interacting with PI-3 virus in
the very early stage of infection ie in the gel phase and
liquid phases of mucus?

It is known that the liquid phase from naturally infected

animals will inhibit agglutination of PI-3 virus, a reaction
which also can be due to non-immunoglobulin inhibitors (Morein
1972, Smith et al., 1975, 1976). The neutralisation of PI-3
virus is a more specific immunological activity of the liquid
phase than the haemagglutination inhibition (HI) activity
(Frank and Marshall, 1971, Marshall and Frank, 1971). It was
also shown that purified IgA from the liquid phase of PI-3
virus-immunised cattle aggregated the virions at certain
concentrations, and at higher concentrations of IgA the
virions might be saturated with IgA molecules and therefore not
found in aggregates (Morein et al., 1973). (Figure 2).

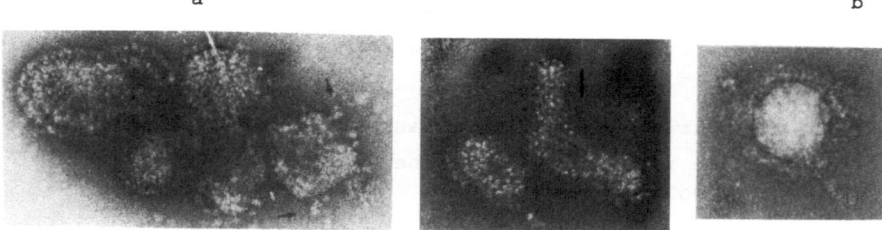

a   b

Fig. 2.   PIV-3 particle
        a)   partial inhibition with IgA
        b)   total inhibition.

        Arrows indicate that at a partial inhibition only a minority of
        peoplomers are covered with IgA molecules.

In immunological tests directed against PI-3 virus
neuraminidase it was found that the anti-neuraminidase activity
of the liquid phase is more sensitive and specific than the
HI test.

Generally it is difficult to measure an immune response
in the gel phase, but by developing an anti-neuraminidase test
using the gel phase as a substrate for the enzyme this was
possible. (Morein et al., 1973). It was found that the gel

phase from an animal which was non-immune to PI-3 virus released
NANA fast during the first two hours following incubation with
PI-3 virus. Hardly any NANA was, however, released from the
gel phase obtained from cattle immunised against PI-3 virus by
natural infection.

a   b

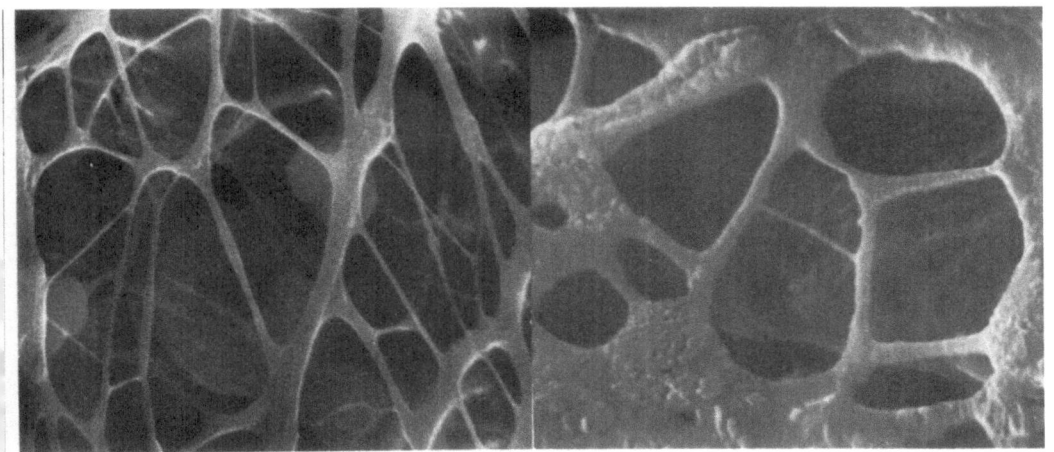

Fig. 3.   Effect of neuraminidase on the morphology of the gel phase of
          nasal secretion studied by SEM. Samples were incubated for 2 hrs
          at 37°C with a) 0.15 M NaCl (x 7 500), b) PIV-3 (x 7 500).

It appears that the PI-3 virus neuraminidase aids the
virus particle to penetrate the mucus by releasing the virion
from inhibitors in the gel phase. It seems then logical that
the anti-neuraminidase activity might aid in the protection of
PI-3 virus in the early stages by indirectly binding the virion
to the inhibitors in the gel phase.

The liquid phase of bovine nasal secretion (NS) contains
inhibitors. These are generally sensitive to neuraminidase.
In NS of adult cattle these inhibitors are not so abundant, but

in NS of newborn animals they might cause high HI titres
(Table 1). It was found that this non-immunoglobulin HI
activity was highest during the first days of life and decreased
to a low level at the age of 15 to 20 days. By analysis in
polyacrylamide electrophoresis at least three proteins were
shown in NS from new-born calves, which appears to be absent,
or present at much lower concentrations, in NS from adult
cattle. One of these proteins has been characterised and found
to be fetuin and a second has the same mobility in polyacrylamide
gel electrophoresis as α_1- fetoprotein. Although fetuin could
be a potential inhibitor that seems not to be the case with PI-3
virus. The inhibitor appears to be a high molecular weight
protein, probably analogous to that found by Smith et al. (1975,
1976) in ovine nasal secretions.

TABLE 1

THE EFFECT OF *Vibrio cholera* NEURAMINIDASE ON THE NON-IMMUNOGLOBULIN HI
ACTIVITY OF BOVINE NS FROM NEWBORN AND OLDER ANIMALS

Cattle	HI[1] relation to treatment by NA	
Age	Before	After
O days	32	2
O days	16	4
1 day	16	2
4 days	256	4
2½ years	128	64
2½ years	128	64
3 years	64	64
4 years	128	128

1) Reciprocal of dilution.

These inhibitors appear to have a function. It has been
reported (Bürki et al., 1975) that calves under the age of six
weeks can not be infected with PI-3 virus. However, others

have been able to infect calves as young as one week with PI-3
virus (Moreno et al., 1976). This discrepancy is certainly
due to the fact that different strains of PI-3 were used. It
is known that PI-3 virus strains differ in their neuraminidase
activity, some having strong enzyme activity and others having
weak activity (Drzeniek et al., 1967, Morein and Bergman 1972).
To investigate these phenomena an experiment was designed in
which young calves were immunised with either a NA-weak (U23)
or NA-strong (SLP or Tüb E6) strain. It was then found that
calves under the age of four weeks could not be infected with
the NA-weak strain but could be infected with the NA-strong
strains, regardless of whether the calf had maternal immunity
against PI-3 virus or not. Calves over the age of six weeks
could be infected with either of the strains (Manus, in
preparation). The criteria of infection were virus recovery
antibody-mediated immune response and cell-mediated immune
response (Table 2).

TABLE 2A

CAPACITY OF NA-WEAK PI-3 VIRUS TO INFECT YOUNG CALVES

Group	Calves No	Age	PI-3 strain	Virus recovery	Titre increase	Fed colostrum
A	4	3-4 w	Um-23	No	No	No
B	4	3-4 w	Um-23	No	No	Yes
C	3	1½-4 m	Um-23	Yes[a]	Yes[b]	Yes
D	1	3-4 w	No	No	No	Yes

a) Haemadsorbing activity was detected from days 3 to 6 after infection.
   The virus isolated was identified as PI-3 virus by HI test with a
   rabbit antiserum.

b) Increased titres were observed in all calves.

TABLE 2B

CAPACITY OF NA-STRONG PI-3 VIRUS TO INFECT YOUNG CALVES

Calves			PI-3	Virus	Titre	Fed
Group	No	Age	strain	recovery	increase	colostrum
E	4	3-4 w	SLP	Yes[a]	Yes[b]	Yes
F	3	3-4 w	Tüb-E6	Yes[a]	Yes[b]	No
G	4	3-4 w	Tüb-E6	Yes[a]	Yes[b]	Yes
H	2	3-4 w	No	No	No	No

a) Haemadsorbing activity was detected within days 2 to 7 after infection. The virus isolated was identified as PI-3 virus by HI test with a rabbit antiserum.

b) Increased titres were observed in all calves.

I conclude that during the first step of infection, PI-3 virus utilises neuraminidase for penetration of mucus, and consequently the antibody activity against neuraminidase is a first, but not the only, step in immunity to reinfection with PI-3 virus.

REFERENCES

Bernhardt, D., and Bengelsdorff, H.J. 1973. Zentbl. Vet. Med. Reihe. B, 20, p. 102.

Bürki, F.I., Backman, W., Miklav and Sibalin, M. Wien. Tierärztl. Mschr. 62, Heft 2, p. 41.

Drzeniek, R., Bögel, K., and Rott, R. 1967. Virology 31, p. 725.

Frank, G.H. and Marshall, R.G. 1971. Am. J. Vet. Res. 32, p. 1707.

Friberg, S., Morein, B. and Rydhag, L. 1973. Am. Rev. resp. Dis. 108, p. 1010.

Hilding, A.C. 1957. Am. J. Physiol. 191, p. 404.

Höglund, S. and Morein, B. 1974. Infect. Immun. 10, p. 877.

Marshall, R.G. and Frank, G.H. 1971. Am. J. Vet. Res. 32, p. 1699.

Morein, B. 1975. Folia vet. Lat. 5, p. 133.

Morein, B. and Bergman, R. 1972. Infect. Immun. 6, p. 174.

Morein, B., Höglund, S. and Bergman, R. 1973. Inf. Imm. 8, p. 650.

Moreno-Lopez, J.W., Törnqvist, M., Möllerberg, B. and Morein, B. 1976. Zentbl. Vet Med. Reihe B, 23, p. 801.

Rylander, R. 1970. Archs. Int. Med. 126, p. 496.

Smith, W.D., Wells, P.W., Burrells, C. and Dawson, A.M. 1975. Archs. Virol. 49, p. 329.

Smith, W.D., Wells, P.W., Burrells, C. and Dawson, A.M. 1976. Clin. exp. Immunol. 23, p. 544.

THE RESPIRATORY TRACT IMMUNE SYSTEM

K.L. Morgan and F.J. Bourne

Department of Animal Husbandry, University of Bristol,
Langford House, Langford, Bristol, England.

ABSTRACT

The immunoperoxidase technique was used to study the development of the local immune system of the bovine respiratory tract from one week of age to maturity. The predominant immunoglobulin type within cells was IgG_1, although IgA and IgM containing cells were also present in high proportions. This distribution differed from the relative concentrations of immunoglobulins in tracheobronchial secretions collected from five calves, in which IgA clearly predominated. The possible reasons for this are discussed and the roles of IgA and IgG_1 in local and systemic immunity considered.

Studies on attempts to stimulate local production of antibody will be described and mucosal protection in the ruminant will be compared with other species.

INTRODUCTION

In spite of the continuing problems of respiratory disease
in the calf and considerable interest in, and work on, the
formulation and efficacy of vaccines, little basic work has
been carried out on the nature and development of the local
immune system of the bovine respiratory tract.

IgG_1 is recognised as the predominant immunoglobulin of
bovine colostrum and milk (Pierce and Feinstein, 1965) and
although IgA plasma cells are present in the lamina propria of
the intestinal tract, IgG_1 is the quantitatively more
significant immunoglobulin class both in the lamina propria and
in intestinal juice (Newby and Bourne, 1976).

However, IgA has been shown to be the predominant immunoglobulin class in the secretion of the upper respiratory tract
of the ox (Mach and Pahud, 1969; Duncan et al., 1972). Antibodies of this class have been demonstrated in nasal secretions
following either natural infection or intranasal administration
of attenuated parainfluenza 3 virus (Morein, 1970). Similar
results have been found with the virus of bovine virus diarrhoea
(Goedemans, 1970). The response to vaccination by parenteral
and intranasal routes has been reviewed by Todd (1973).

The purpose of the present study was to follow the
development of the immune system of the respiratory tract using
immunohistochemical and immunoquantitative techniques.

MATERIALS AND METHODS

Tissue samples
      Channel Island bull calves were purchased at 4 - 7 days
of age and penned either singly or in pairs until slaughter.
Tissues were taken immediately after death from four sites;
the nasal mucosa (middle concha of the turbinate bones), trachea,
primary bronchus and lung parenchyma. These samples were

fixed in pre-cooled methanol and processed according to the
method of Sainte-Marie (1962).

Nasal and Tracheal Washings

Nasal and tracheal washings were collected weekly from 7
calves under basal narcosis.

Endotracheal intubation was carried out, using a McGill
cuffed endotracheal tube, in order to separate and facilitate
collection from the two sites. 10 ml of PBS pH 7.4 was
sprayed onto the mucosa of the left and right distal nares via
a plastic catheter. The head was held so as to enable the
collection of nasal secretions under gravity.

Similarly a catheter, previously calibrated by fibre optic
bronchoscopy so as to reach the carina, was introduced via the
endotracheal tube into the trachea. The animal was held
vertically with its head down and 20 ml of PBS pH 7.4 introduced
and the washings collected.

Immediately after collection the washings were centrifuged
at 500 g for 5 min to remove cellular material and debris. The
latter was smeared onto glass microscope slides and examined
using Leishmann's stain. The supernatant was sonicated for
20 sec at 4° in order to homogenise the mucous secretion.
Following this the samples were concentrated 20 - 50 times
using ultrafiltration (Minicon Amicon) and stored at -20°
until use.

Immunoglobulin levels were measured by rocket immuno-
electrophoresis (Laurell, 1972). Samples were treated with
formaldehyde before quantitation of IgG_1 and IgM in order to
ensure cathodal migration (Slater, 1973).

Isolation of immunoglobulins and preparation of antisera

IgG_1 and IgG_2 were isolated by the method of Mach and
Pahud (1971) and IgA and IgM by an immunosorbent method
(Newby et al., 1974). Antisera to the purified proteins were

raised in rabbits and rendered specific by cross-absorption.

Immunoperoxidase technique

Specific antisera were conjugated with horseradish peroxidase enzyme (HPO) (Sigma, London, Type VI) using glutaraldehyde (Avrameas, 1969).

Tissue sections were pre-treated to inhibit endogenous peroxidase activity prior to incubation with the HPO-antiserum conjugates, with a methanol/sodium nitroferricyanide mixture (Straus, 1971). Following incubation, peroxidase activity was revealed using diaminobenzidine reagent (DAB) which gives a dense brown reaction product (Avrameas, 1969). Suitable controls were carried out on each batch of conjugate to determine the specificity of the reaction and the degree of non-specific background staining.

Quantitation

All labelled cells were identified and counted in 30 randomly selected high power fields (x 25 objective) except in the lung parenchyma where, due to the low numbers of immunoglobulin-containing cells, 300 high power fields were counted. Serial sections were used wherever possible to allow a more direct comparison to be made between classes.

RESULTS

As seen in Table 1, immunoglobulin-containing cells were present in all sites by one week of age, although IgG_2 cells were not detected in the tracheal mucosa until two weeks of age. IgG_1, IgA and IgM containing cells were present in roughly equal numbers until six weeks of age, with very few IgG_2 containing cells. Background staining was very noticeable for IgG_1 and IgM, the former staining the whole of the lamina propria with the exception of the glandular acini. Background staining for IgG_2 and IgA was weak. Occasional surface staining of IgG_1 was seen in tracheal sections.

TABLE 1

BOVINE RESPIRATORY TRACT TISSUE

Mean numbers and ratios of cells stained for IgG_1, IgA and IgM in bovine respiratory tract					
Birth - 6 weeks, 11 animals			Ratios		
A	G	M	G_1:A	A:M	P
Nasal mucous $\quad$ 42.5$\pm$2.0	36.4$\pm$4.5	34.5$\pm$14.2	0.9	1.2	> 0.1
Trachea $\quad$ 18.1$\pm$1.0	36.7$\pm$32.8	24.4$\pm$18.0	2.0	0.7	> 0.1
Lung $\quad$ 33.8$\pm$34.0	57.5$\pm$53.0	37.4$\pm$34.0	1.8	0.9	> 0.1
Adult. 4 animals - 2 years					
Nasal mucous $\quad$ 6.8$\pm$2.5	14.0$\pm$9.0	6.8$\pm$5.0	2.1	1.0	> 0.1
Trachea $\quad$ 6.5$\pm$2.0	2.8$\pm$19.0	7.0$\pm$8.0	4.3	1.0	> 0.1
Lung $\quad$ 24.0$\pm$7.0	87.0$\pm$44.0	23.0$\pm$9.0	3.6	1.0	> 0.05

Staining for IgA was detected in serous acinar and ductule cells of the nasal and tracheobronchial glands but no detectable staining of glandular elements could be seen for either IgM or IgG. The cytoplasm of members of the plasma cell series showed dense staining for all classes; most of these cells showed the typical morphology of the mature plasma cells and were round to oval in shape with a round, eccentric nucleus and abundant cytoplasm.

The majority of these cells were located in the lamina propria immediately beneath the epithelium, although some, especially those staining for IgA, were situated close to the glandular acini. In the deeper regions of the tract, plasma cells were relatively scarce, and were rarely found in the alveolar walls themselves.

In mature animals the relative proportions of G_1, A and M containing plasma cells are similar to those found in the young animal with the possibility of a trend to G_1 predominance.

Owing to the method of collection of nasal and tracheal washings absolute immunoglobulin concentrations could not be determined. Thus the results are described as ratios of IgG_1 : IgA and IgA : IgM (Table 2).

TABLE 2

NASAL WASHINGS						
Ratio IgG_1 : IgA						
	Week 1	Week 2	Week 3	Week 4	Week 5	Week 6
155N	-	8.8	2.8	blood contaminated	1.9	1.3
156N	-	23.5	11.7	11.6	8.8	6.1
157N	-	12.6	9.5	6.6	8.8	5.8
175N	4.1	23.1	15.4	8.2	6.0	N.D.
982N	23.8	11.0	11.6	9.3	+	+
896N	29.0	15.0	11.2	+	+	+
897N	10.1	15.8	9.1	6.3	4.2	N.D.
Mean	$25.0^{+}_{-}12.6$	$15.7^{+}_{-}5.7$	$10.2^{+}_{-}3.8$	$8.6^{+}_{-}2.2$	$6.1^{+}_{-}2.7$	$4.4^{+}_{-}2.7$
Ratio IgA : IgM						
155N	-	0.6	1.6	1.2	1.5	1.4
156N	-	0.3	1.9	1.0	2.3	2.3
157N	-	0.4	1.0	1.0	1.5	1.9
175N	0.6	1.2	1.3	1.5	2.1	N.D.
892N	0.7	0.3	1.0	1.9	+	+
896N	0.2	0.9	1.2	+	+	+
897N	0.4	1.5	1.4	1.6	1.9	N.D.
Mean	$0.5^{+}_{-}0.2$	$0.7^{+}_{-}0.5$	$1.3^{+}_{-}0.3$	$1.4^{+}_{-}0.4$	$1.9^{+}_{-}0.3$	$1.5^{+}_{-}0.4$
TRACHEAL WASHINGS						
Ratio IgG_1 : IgA						
155T	-	12.3	7.5	3.2	1.2	1.1
156T	-	57.5	10.0	7.5	2.2	2.2
157T	-	19.1	12.2	10.1	4.5	3.6
175T	21.1	15.8	13.9	12.6	8.2	N.D.
892T	29.4	23.9	17.2	18.1	+	+

TABLE 2 (continued)

TRACHEAL WASHINGS						
	Week 1	Week 2	Week 3	Week 4	Week 5	Week 6
Ratio IgG_1 : IgA (cont)						
896 T	18.9	12.3	10.9	+	+	+
897 T	25.3	18.8	12.6	8.4	5.9	N.D.
Mean	$23.7{\pm}4.7$	$22.9{\pm}15.7$	$12.0{\pm}3.1$	$9.9{\pm}5$	$4.4{\pm}2.8$	$2.3{\pm}1.3$
Ratio IgA : IgM						
155T	−	0.5	2.7	2.2	2.0	2.1
156T	−	0.5	3.6	2.0	1.8	2.0
157T	−	0.7	1.0	2.1	3.4	3.1
175T	0.9	1.8	2.0	2.4	2.1	N.D.
892T	1.0	3.3	2.3	2.9	+	+
896T	0.3	0.3	0.7	+	+	+
897T	0.2	0.5	1.6	3.0	3.0	N.D.
Mean	$0.6{\pm}0.4$	$1.1{\pm}1$	$1.9{\pm}0.9$	$2.4{\pm}0.4$	$2.5{\pm}0.7$	$2.4{\pm}0.6$

During the whole period of collection, IgG_1 was the predominant immunoglobulin class in nasal and tracheal washings, although the relative concentration of IgG_1 decreased markedly during the six week period. At one week of age IgM was present in greater concentration than IgA, although this position was reversed by 2 - 3 weeks of age.

DISCUSSION

A feature of this work is the predominance of IgG_1 in respiratory secretions during the first 6 weeks of life, although towards the end of this period IgA was assuming quantitative significance and observations after this period and up to 2 years of age show IgA as the major immunoglobulin in secretions (unpublished data). This would support the published observations of Duncan (1972) and Mach and Pahud (1971).

The presence of immunoglobulin cells in respiratory tissues at the end of the first week of life indicates an ability by the calf to form these immunoglobulins; however, plasma cell numbers do not correlate with immunoglobulin levels in nasal and tracheal secretions. IgG_1, IgA and IgM containing plasma cells are present in approximately equal numbers up to 6 weeks of age at a time when IgG_1 is by far the predominant immunoglobulin class and when IgM levels predominate over IgA.

Two factors will influence this. It is likely that IgG_1 and IgM are colostrum derived; this is indicated in the present study by the intensity of the background staining to both of these immunoglobulins and by the similarity of the IgG_1 : IgM ratio in secretions compared to serum (Porter, 1972). The observation of Smith (1976) that colostrum deprived lambs have no immunoglobulin in nasal secretions until 3 weeks of age, after which IgA emerges as the predominant class, would confirm this view.

The second factor is that plasma cells in the lamina propria are not necessarily secreting at the same rate.

It has been known for some time that passive immunity may protect the young calf against Infectious Bovine Rhinotracheitis (Kahrs, 1966) parainfluenza virus (Bogel and Liebelt, 1963; Dawson, 1966) and adenovirus (Burkl, 1971) for up to 4 months and against bovine viral diarrhoea for 6 - 10 months (Kahrs, 1966; Malmquist, 1968; Phillip, 1973). Furthermore, this protection is correlated to serum antibody levels (Dawson, 1966; Sinha, 1962; Malmquist, 1968; House and Manley, 1973; Casselberry, 1968).

The persistence of IgG_1 as the predominating immunoglobulin is in accord with the above observations and the recorded serum half life of colostrum derived IgG_1 in the calf of 21 days (Logan et al., 1973), 18 days (Mcdougall and Mulligan, 1969) or 11.5 days (Sasaki et al., 1976) is not inconsistent with the thesis that colostral IgG_1 affords protection to the respiratory tract of the young calf.

From this, one might postulate the existence of an
effective local defence mechanism based on colostrum derived
IgG_1 and IgM which persist at the mucosal surface for some
time. That IgG_1 can protect against infection at the mucous
surface is suggested by the protective effect of intracheal
administered hyperimmune serum to parainfluenza and adenovirus
(Haralambiev et al., 1972). Both IgG_1 and IgM fix complement
and are opsonising agents; could it be significant that a
large percentage of cells from the respiratory tract of the
young calf are polymorphs, probably engaged in phagocytic
defence (unpublished data)?

The persistence of maternal antibody has frustrated
vaccination attempts using attenuated viral vaccine (Phillip,
1975). Would it be possible to vaccinate effectively a calf
immediately it is born, and before it has suckled, by nasal or
intratracheal presentation of attenuated viral antigen?
Experiments conducted in the piglet have shown that human
colostral IgA appears in the serum 2 h after feeding and after
another 2 h appears in bronchial secretions (unpublished data).
Before this time it might be possible to initiate infection
and cell priming; hours later antibody appears on the surface
of the respiratory tract to prevent the swamping of the immune
system by antigen and the development of overt disease.

In the older animals IgG_1 containing cells predominate
over IgA and IgM containing cells. However, an IgA : IgG_1
ratio of 13 : 1 has been recorded in nasal secretions. A
similar discrepancy between submucosal immunoglobulin synthesising cells and immunoglobulin in secretions has been reported
in the pig (Bradley et al., 1976) and rabbit (Hand and Contey,
1974). This discrepancy may be accounted for by differences
in rate of synthesis, transudation and degradation in secretions
of the different classes.

The large number of IgG_1 containing cells raises the

question once again of the importance of IgG_1 in local immune systems. Two possible roles of IgG_1 in the local site can be considered. The distribution of plasma cells containing IgG_1 immediately beneath the respiratory epithelium suggests the possibility that it may form a 'second line' of mucosal defence behind the surface protection offered by IgA, which is apparently transported into secretions via the serous cells of the mucosal glands, according to the evidence of this survey. It has been suggested (Brandtzaeg, 1973) that a similar role exists for human IgG in the nasal mucosa. In addition locally produced IgG_1 may represent an important contribution to the systemic immunoglobulin pool. It has been shown that locally produced IgA contributes to serum levels in a number of species which have IgA-dominated local immune systems, including the dog (Vaerman and Heremans, 1970), man (Bull et al., 1971) and the rat and guinea pig (Vaerman et al., 1973) and it is conceivable that a similar situation exists with bovine IgG_1. This would not eliminate the possibility that IgG_1 has a secretory role in the respiratory tract in the same way that it appears to have in the gut. The biological advantage of systemic immunity arising from a local system is plain, especially as they are associated with sites of major antigenic challenge. It is also becoming increasingly clear that it is an over-simplification to consider local immune systems as entirely separate from systemic immunity, a concept which is likely to be important in the development of efficacious mucosal vaccines.

450

REFERENCES

Avrameas, S. 1969. Immunochemistry. 6, p. 43.

Bogel, K. and Liebelt, J. 1963. Zbl. Bakt. I Abst. Orig. 191, p. 133.

Bradley, P.A., Bourne, F.J. and Brown, P.J. 1976. Vet. Pathol. 13, p. 90.

Brandtzaeg, P.1973. Ann. Immunol. (Inst. Pub). 124C, p. 417.

Bull, D.M., Bienenstock, J. and Tomasi, T.B. 1971. Gastroenterology. 60,
    p. 370.

Burkl, F. 1971. Wien. Tierärtzl. Mschr. 58, p. 122.

Casselberry, N.H. 1968. J. Am. Vet. Med. Ass. 152, p. 853.

Dawson, P.S. 1966. J. Comp. Path. 76, p. 373.

Duncan, J.R., Wilkie, B.N., Hiestand, F. and Winter, N. 1972. J. Immunol.
    108, p. 965.

Goedemans, W.T. 1970. Zbl. Vet. Med. 17B, p. 508.

Haralambiev, H., Draganov, M. and Zwetkov, P. 1972. Alch. Exp. Vet. Med.
    26, p. 273.

Hand, W.L. and Conley, J.R. 1974. J. Clin. Invest., 53, p. 334.

House, J.A. and Manley, M. 1973. J. Am. Vet. Med. Ass. 163, p. 819.

Kahrsk, R.F. 1966. Cornell Vet. 56, p. 288.

Laurell, C.B. 1972. Scand. J. clin. Lab. Invest., 29, p. 21.

Logan, E.T., Penhale, W.J. and Jones, R.A. 1973. Res. Vet. Sci. 14, p. 394.

Mach, J.P. and Pahud, J.J. 1971. J. Immunol., 106, p. 552.

Malmquist, W.A. 1968. J. Am. Vet. Med. Assoc. 152, p. 763.

McDougal, D.F. and Mulligan, W. 1969. J. Physiol. 201, p. 770.

Morein, B. 1970. Int. Arch. Allerg., 39, p. 403.

Newby, T.J., Bourne, F.J., Chidlow, J. and Steel, M.J. 1974. Res. Vet. Sci.
    17, p. 39.

Newby, T.J. and Bourne, F.J. 1976. Immunology, 31, p. 475.

Phillip, J.I.H. 1973. Ph.D. Thesis, London.

Phillip, J.I.H. 1975. Devel. Biol. Stand., 28, p. 501.

Pierce, A.E. and Feinstein, A. 1965. Immunology, 8, p. 106.

Porter, P. 1972. Immunology, 23, p. 275.

Sainte-Marie, G. 1962. J. Histochem, Cytochem. 10, p. 250.

Sinha, S.K. 1962. Adv. Vet. Sci., 7, p. 225.

Sasaki, M., Davis, C.L. and Larson, B.L. 1976. J. Dairy Sci., 60, p. 623.

Slater, L. 1975. Archs. Clin. Biochem., 12, p. 19.

Smith, W.D. 1976. Res. Vet. Sci., 21, p. 341.

Straus, W. 1971. J. Histochem. Cytochem. 19, p. 682.

Todd, J.D. 1973. J. Am. Vet. Med. Ass, 163, p. 807.

Vaerman, J.P., Andre, C., Bazin, H. and Heremans, J.F. 1973. Eur. J. Immun. 3, p. 580.

Vaerman, J.P. and Heremans, J.F. 1970. Immunology, 18, p. 27.

ANAPHYLACTIC ANTIBODIES IN CATTLE - THEIR COLOSTRAL TRANSMISSION TO CALVES AND POSSIBLE LOCALISATION IN THE RESPIRATORY TRACT

K. Petzoldt and C. von Benten

Institut für Mikrobiologie and Tierseuchen der Tierärztlichen
Hochschule Hannover, 3000 Hannover 1, Germany.

ABSTRACT

There are many reports on the acquirement of maternal antibodies by the newborn calf, but little is known about the transfer of anaphylactic antibodies of the class IgE. Hammer and coworkers (1971) and Eyre (1973) have presented evidence for a bovine IgE-class. After the detection of such an IgE-activity in bovine colostrum (Hammer et al., 1971) we have performed some experiments concerning the colostral transfer of anaphylactic activity from mother to young. Using an antigen extracted from liver fluke (Fasciola hepatica) it could be demonstrated that newborn calves - and possibly lambs too - were passively sensitised against this naturally occurring antigen due to the oral intake of maternal anaphylactic antibodies. Besides the natural transfer of skin reactivity against liver fluke antigen, experimental transfer of this anaphylactic reactivity was shown by intracutaneous injections. Three-day old calves gave a positive reaction in the Prausnitz-Küstner-Test (PK) and Passive Cutaneous Anaphylaxis (PCA). The technical conditions for the detection of anaphylactic activity in the skin of the newborn calf by PK and PCA were investigated.

After application of a bacterial autogenous vaccine in 60 calves with respiratory disease, 6 cases of anaphylactic shock occurred. It was possible to demonstrate anaphylactic antibody activity in two of these calves by the direct skin test as well as in colostrum-deprived calves by passive sensitisation. Preliminary experiments were performed to demonstrate the presence of antibacterial anaphylactic antibodies in the respiratory tract. Neither by direct provocation with the vaccine nor by aerogenic passive sensitisation of lambs with aerosols of this vaccine was it possible to reproduce respiratory anaphylaxis. Antibody detection in vitro was not successful.

INTRODUCTION

Anaphylactic antibodies may belong to the immunoglobulin class G or E (Watanabe and Ovary, 1977). Our knowledge concerning allergies in domestic animals, especially antibody-mediated anaphylaxis in cattle, is limited. The main cause of anaphylaxis in cattle might be IgE as reported by Wells and Eyre (1970 and 1972), Hammer et al. (1971) and Eyre (1973). Even though you will find a lot of references about colostral immunoglobulins there are few reports of the role of IgE in bovine colostrum. Only Mossmann and his co-workers in Freiburg, Germany (1974) have given the results of some work on the colostral transfer of an experimentally-induced bovine IgE from cow to calf. On the other hand, we have performed experiments in the bovine species concerning the colostral transfer of naturally occurring anaphylactic activity from mother to young because up to this time there has been no information given about maternal anaphylactic antibodies in the newborn calf (Stanworth, 1973). Preliminary experimental data have been discussed (Petzoldt et al., 1975) but not yet published in detail.

Only *in vivo* methods are available for the detection of bovine anaphylactic antibodies. This limits experimental work. Referring to allergic reactions *in vivo*, recently, Watanabe and Ovary (1973) claimed: 'The only reaction still used for detection of antigens and antibodies *in vivo* is passive cutaneous anaphylaxis or the PCA reaction'. This is true for the bovine species too. At the beginning of our experiments we tested the PCA- and Prausnitz-Küstner methods for detecting anaphylactic antibodies using 27 newborn colostrum-deprived calves and 14 lambs. An aqueous extract of liver fluke (*Fasciola hepatica* = Fh) was used as antigen. In 3 day old calves intracutaneous injections of their mother's serum containing Fh-anaphylactic antibodies resulted in positive PCA reactions. The technical conditions of this method have been reported elsewhere (von Benten et al., 1976).

We investigated two aspects of anaphylaxis in cattle:

1) Does a passive sensitisation against natural antigens in calves occur due to colostral intake?

2) Are there any anaphylactic antibodies involved in reactions of the respiratory tract of calves vaccinated against bacterial pneumonia?

The transfer of anaphylactic antibodies from mother to young under natural conditions.

The antigen used in our tests was a complex one as we could show by means of polyacrylamide gel electrophoresis. For detection of anaphylactic antibodies serum samples of blood or colostrum were diluted up to 1 : 640 and tested by the PCA reaction in newborn calves according to the usual technique (Stanworth, 1973). Using the Fh-antigen for direct skin tests we identified pregnant cows and sheep which were naturally infected with Fh. From positive mothers this skin reactivity was transmitted to their offspring due to the oral intake of colostrum (Table 1). In experiments with two cows and their calves it could be demonstrated repeatedly that the serum of calves which were PCA - negative before colostrum intake, afterwards contained the antibody activity from the colostrum of the dam (Table 2). This sensitising antibody activity in the colostral whey of cows and in the serum of their suckling calves was heat labile (56°C for 30 min.) and persisted in the skin of colostrum-deprived calves for a period of 3 to 5 weeks at least (Table 3). Hence these antibodies fulfil two of four requirements for IgE-antibodies (Watanabe and Ovary, 1977). Reduction of alkylation trials or molecular weight estimation were not tried. But one can say that in calves, and also in lambs, under natural conditions a passive anaphylaxis can occur. The significance of colostrum-derived anaphylactic antibodies in calves directed against naturally occurring antigens like bacteria is still questionable. With regard to aerosol vaccination and other vaccination procedures in calf-production units the risk of anaphylactic reactions mediated by maternal antibodies must be taken into account.

TABLE 1

SKIN REACTIVITY AGAINST *Fasciola hepatica* ANTIGEN AFTER ORAL INTAKE OF COLOSTRUM

Animal	Colostrum Intake	After Colostrum Intake Positive skin reaction up to antigen dilution	Time interval till provocation
Calf 1	3160 ml	1 : 10 000	12 hours
Calf 2	3120 ml	1 : 10 000	22 "
Calf 3	2740 ml	1 : 10 000	26 "
Lamb 1	Ad libitum	1 : 10 000	28 "
Lamb 2	185 ml	1 : 500	29 "

TABLE 2

DETECTION OF ANAPHYLACTIC ANTIBODIES IN SERA OF CALVES AFTER INTAKE OF COLOSTRUM FROM SKIN TEST POSITIVE COWS

Cow	PCA Experiment	Cow Colostrum	Positive PCA Reactions with Calf. Blood serum before intake	Calf blood serum after intake
1	1	≥ 1 : 300	No	1 : 30
	2	1 : 30	No	1 : 30
2	1	Undiluted	No	Undiluted
	2	1 : 10	No	Undiluted

TABLE 3

PERSISTENCE OF ANAPHYLACTIC ANTIBODIES IN THE SKIN OF CALVES (PCA SKIN REACTIONS REPRESENTING THE MEAN VALUE OBTAINED FROM TWO MEASUREMENTS)

Time after injection (days)	Antibodies derived from	Dilution Undiluted	1:4	1:40	1:160	1:640
		Diameter of skin reactions (mm)				
21	Colostral whey	33	29	15	14	9
21	Serum	9	17	10	N.D.	N.D.
35	Colostral whey	43	39	18	Neg.	Neg.
35	Serum	27	12	Neg.	N.D.	N.D.

Possible involvement of anaphylactic antibodies in reactions of the respiratory tract against bacterial antigens

In a calf-raising unit vaccinations against chronic pneumonia with an autogeneous vaccine were performed. The vaccine contained inactivated *Staphylococci* and *Proteus*. After revaccination of 60 three month old calves 6 calves showed shock symptoms, eg expiratory dyspnoea. Three calves died. Two of the calves which survived were examined for the presence of anaphylaxis.

In the direct skin test with intradermal injection of the vaccine (after centrifugation to exclude particulate matter) in dilutions up to 1 : 1 000, both animals showed a local positive immediate type allergy. Positive reactions (edema with a mean diameter of 8 mm) were observed half an hour after challenge in calf 1 (antigen dilution 1 : 10) and in calf 2 (antigen dilution 1 : 100). Positive delayed-type reactions were not detectable.

The application of the vaccine by aerosol failed to induce anaphylactic symptoms of the respiratory tract in these 2 calves. In the tracheal secretions sampled according to the technique of Schatzmann and co-workers (1972) anaphylactic antibody activity was detectable neither before nor after the respiratory challenge. The presence of anaphylactic antibodies in sera of both vaccinated calves could be demonstrated by PK-reactions using three month old colostrum deprived calves as recipients. Sera of calf 1 induced positive PK-reactions up to a titre of 1 : 10; serum of calf 2 was positive up to a titre of 1 : 500. In a repeated PK-test with another calf which was challenged 24 h after the intradermal injection of anaphylactic sera, it showed a systemic anaphylaxis reaction instead of a local one. Only immediate treatment with 5.0 ml Fluomethason, 5.0 ml antihistamine and 50.0 ml Calcium gluconate (24%) saved the calf.

These observations made us look for the possibility of passive sensitisation by the aerosol route with the serum of

calf 2. Two colostrum-deprived four day old lambs were
exposed to an aerosol of about 13.5 g calf serum and were
challenged three days later with 4.9 g antigen (autogeneous
vaccine diluted 1 : 10 with phosphate buffered saline). Apart
from a transitory rise in the respiratory rate to 104/min no
abnormalities could be observed. On the other hand another
colostrum-deprived lamb used for PCA-reactions with the
anaphylactic calf sera showed a systemic anaphylactic reaction
when it was challenged with the autogeneous vaccine by the
intravenous route. Therefore it is not possible to say whether
or not anaphylactic antibodies were responsible for the
incidents following vaccination with autogeneous vaccine in the
calves mentioned above. Results of the experiments for demonstrating anaphylactic antibodies in these calves are summarised
in Table 4.

TABLE 4

ANAPHYLACTIC REACTIVITY OF TWO CALVES AFTER REVACCINATION WITH AN AUTO-
GENEOUS ANTIBACTERIAL VACCINE

Calf	Test		
	Direct skin test (positive reaction up to antigen dilution)	Pk-reaction (positive re-action up to serum dilution)	Passive sensitisation of lambs by aerosol
1	1 : 10	1 : 10	Negative
2	1 : 100	1 : 500	Negative

REFERENCES

Benten, Ch. von, Floer, W. and Petzoldt, K. 1976. Aentbl. Vet Med. Reihe, B, $\underline{23}$, p. 200.

Butler, J.E. 1973. J. Am. Vet. Med. Ass. $\underline{163}$, p. 795.

Eyre, P., Lewis, A.J. and Wells, P.W. 1973. Br. J. Pharmac. $\underline{47}$, p. 504.

Hammer, D.K., Kickhöfen, and Schmid, T. 1971. Eur. J. Immunol. $\underline{1}$, p. 249.

Mossmann, H., Meyer-Delius, M., Vortisch, U., Kicköfen, B. and Hammer, D.K. 1974. J. Exp. Med. $\underline{140}$, p. 1468.

Petzoldt, K., Floer, W. and Von Benten, C. 1965. Übersichten zur Tierernah-rung, $\underline{3}$, p. 293.

Schatzmann, U., Straub, R. and Gerber, H. 1972. Schweizer. Arch. Tierheilk. $\underline{114}$, p. 395.

Stanworth, D.R. 1973. Front. Biol. $\underline{28}$.

Watanabe, N. and Ovary, Z. 1977. J. Immunol. Meth. $\underline{14}$, p. 381.

Wells, P.W. and Eyre, P. 1970. Vet. Rec. $\underline{87}$, p. 173.

Wells, P.W. and Eyre, P. 1972. Immunochemistry $\underline{9}$, p. 88.

IMMUNOLOGY IN CALF RESPIRATORY DISEASE

C. Le Jan and J.M. Asso

INRA Station de Recherches de Virologie et d'Immunologie,
Route de Thiverval, 78850 - Thiverval-Grignon, France.

ABSTRACT

The experimental inoculation by the nasal route of infectious bovine rhinotracheitis (IBR) virus in 8 days old calves provokes immunological response at systemic and local level. These calves were selected for their absence of serum antibodies against IBR virus.

By the serum neutralisation test we were able to evaluate the onset of neutralising activity in nasal secretion and in serum. We considered the activity in nasal secretion to be the local response and the activity in the serum to be the systemic response.

There is no correlation between the local and systemic response. With the virus we used, about 90% of calves showed local antibodies between the eighth and fourteenth day after inoculation and the neutralising activity vanished after the fourteenth day.

At the general level we observed antibodies after the fourteenth day which persisted for 3 or 4 weeks but not in all the animals and not always in the calves which have shown a local response.

The independence of local from systemic response is also found when we give a local booster inoculation of the same virus after one month. We measured regularly an increase in the level of neutralising activity in the nasal secretion between the fifth and the fifteenth day and in some animals an increase of neutralising activity in the serum. When the calves were inoculated 3 or 4 times by the nasal route, the neutralising activity in the mucus persists for a long time (one month). Many of these animals have no reaction at the systemic level.

In the same calves we have studied the peripheral blood lymphocytes (PBL). These cells are able to protect a layer of cells infected with IBR *if given at the moment of the release of the virus from cells (6h). These cells must not come from an infected or immunised calf : the PBL of a new-born calf (2h) have the same activity. The in vitro incubation of IBR virus with PBL showed a decrease in the titre of infectivity of the virus.*

The PBL were cultivated in the presence of killed virus. After 4 days' culture, these cells, when in contact with sheep red blood cells, form thermostable rosettes. This phenomenon appears only in calves inoculated with IBRV for 8 or 14 days.

There is no correlation with the blastogenesis stimulation measured by thymidine incorporation.

There is no correlation with the antibody response at the general or local level.

We tried to look for these thermostable rosettes with cells obtained at the slaughter house from lymph node spleen and lung washings.

The growth of viruses which are the causes of respiratory
disorders like rhinitis, tracheitis, bronchitis, pneumonitis,
is usually restricted to the respiratory system.

It is believed that the characters determining the phenomenon of protection are related to the local distribution of
the infection.

We compared the kinetics of the local and systemic responses
at the level of immunoglobulin production and at the level of
changes in the properties of lymphocytes following primary and
repeated inoculations of the virus.

Such respiratory infections are known to be commonly
prevalent among calves, and have been much talked about in
recent times. On the basis of the above we studied an experimental
infection in eight day old calves with a laboratory strain of
Infectious Bovine Rhinotracheitis (IBR) virus.

MATERIALS AND METHODS

1. Animals

Twenty-six calves, Holstein Friesian breeds of eight days
of age, reared under industrial scale conditions, were screened.
All of them had IBR-specific antibodies of colostral origin.

2. Virus

The virus strain used was propagated in the MDBK cell line.
We obtained 5.10^5 PFU/ml in 24 h, at 37°C. We have thus far
observed no evidence of clinical manifestations following
inoculation of this virus into calves under test.

3. Experimental infection

5.0 ml of the undiluted virus suspension was given intranasally to each calf at each inoculation, at intervals of one
month.

4. Collection of samples

Serum and nasal swabs were collected at regular intervals, immediately frozen and inactivated at $56^{\circ}C$ before the tests.

5. Neutralisation tests

Infection reduction tests were carried out with 100 $TCID_{50}$ of IBR virus, after 18 h incubation at $37^{\circ}C$.

6. Isolation and culture of lymphocytes

Lymphocytes were isolated, purified and cultured from peripheral blood, bronchial washings, thymus, spleen and lymph nodes.

Peripheral blood leucocytes were obtained by the Ficoll-triosil (density : 1.076) technique; for lymphocytes of other origin, Ficoll-triosil was used at a density of 1.09.

Cells were suspended at a concentration of 1×10^6 /ml in Eagle's medium supplemented with 10% calf serum and 1% L-glutamine, and incubated in a humidified atmosphere of CO_2. In our test system we used the Falcon micro tissue culture plate No. 3040, with 0.2 ml of the sample per well, employing 12 wells per sample and in Costar plates (Tissue culture, cluster 24) using 1 ml of sample per well, employing at least three wells per sample.

We studied the cell viability by Trypan blue exclusion and E-rosette formation. Using the glass adherence or carbonyl-iron ingestion technique, we eliminated the macrophages in some cases. The cells were maintained in culture medium for three days with mitogenic agents like Phytohemagglutinin M, Concanavaline A or UV inactivated IBR virus.

7. In vitro properties of cultivated lymphoid cells

a) Lymphoblastogenesis

One microcurie of tritiated thymidine for 0.2 ml of cell suspension was added, and incorporation of DNA precursor was evaluated by the usual techniques. Stimulation index is expressed by the ratio ; CPM in 6 wells with stimulation/ CPM in the 6 wells without stimulation.

Thermostable rosettes : cells were suspended in foetal calf serum (2 x 10^6 cells/ml) and mixed with a same volume of 1% sheep erythrocytes (SRBC) in Earle's medium with lactalbumin 10% FCS, 10% T70 Dextran. The mixture was incubated for 1 h at + 4^OC and 15 m at 37^OC; rosette-forming lymphocytes were counted with a haemocytometer. These thermostable rosettes were different from the E rosettes, which were destroyed at 37^OC.

b) Virus inactivation

The lymphocytic cell suspension was mixed with different dilutions of IBR virus and incubated for different times at 37^OC. The residual virus was tested on MDBK cells.

The cell suspension was put onto a MDBK monolayer infected at different time intervals with IBR virus (10 lymphocytes for one infected cell). The plaque counts and size were evaluated after 24 and 48 h incubation at 37^OC.

RESULTS

Humoral Responses

1. Systemic antibodies. Almost all the animals we used showed the presence of specific antibodies in their serum before intranasal inoculation of the IBR virus.

The level of anti-IBR antibodies was the result of decrease of colostral antibodies and active synthesis of specific immunoglobulins (Figure 1).

Two animals which did not have serum antibodies showed a response three weeks after virus administration.

Most of them exhibited a constant level or a slight decrease of serum antibodies even after multiple virus inoculations.

In four calves, we were able to observe a phase of decline
of the anti-virus activity between 30 and 45 days after the
first inoculation, followed by an increase of the level of
anti-IBR antibodies in the serum.

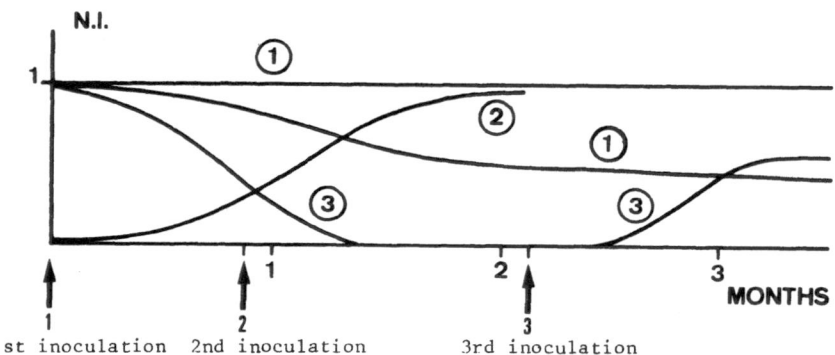

Fig. 1. Kinetics of serum antibody levels.

1) in 20 calves, serum antibodies stayed at the same level, or
decreased slightly.

2) in two calves, serum antibodies were absent at the beginning : they
begin appearing three weeks after the first local inoculation.

3) in 4 calves, serum antibodies disappeared at days 30 - 45 ; the phase
of decline followed by a new increase.

NI neutralising index

intranasal inoculations of IBR virus.

2. Local antibodies in nasal mucus. We evaluated the anti-
virus activity of nasal mucus at different times after intranasal virus inoculation.

We have obtained very reproducible results. The mucus
showed some activity on the tenth day following inoculation.
This activity persisted for one to two weeks. The level was
maximum from the beginning (1/5 dilution of mucus reduced ten
fold the infectivity of the 100 TCID 50 dose used).

TABLE 1

KINETIC OF LOCAL RESPONSE

	First inoculation	Second inoculation	Third inoculation
Delay before appearance or increase of antibodies	6 - 12 days (mean : 10 days)	6 - 12 days (mean : 10 days)	6 - 12 days (mean : 10 days)
Persistence of antibodies at a high level	8 - 15 days (mean : 11 days)	15 - 30 days (mean : 22 days)	>45 days

TABLE 2

DISTRIBUTION OF LOCAL AND SYSTEMIC RESPONSES

		Serum antibody kinetics (according to Fig. 1.).		
		1	2	3
Local antibodies (according to Fig. 2)	A	12 calves	2 calves	1 calf
	B	8 calves	0 calf	3 calves

After the second and third intranasal inoculations we observed the same kind of local response with certain anamnestic characters: rise of antibodies after 10 days with maximum level from the beginning, but each time with an activity more and more persistent. (Figures 2 and 3).

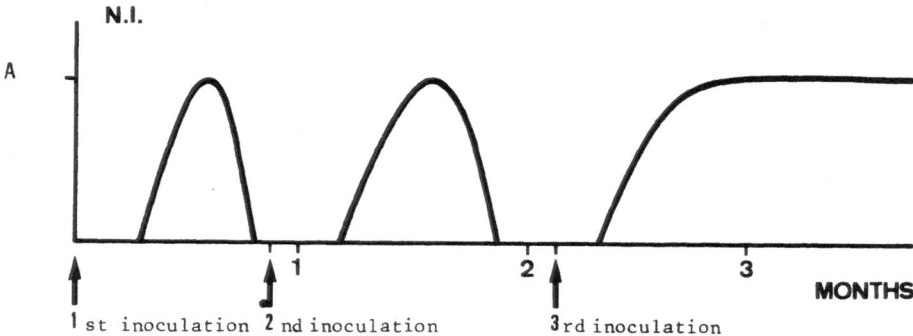

Fig. 2. Kinetics of local antibodies in 15 calves.

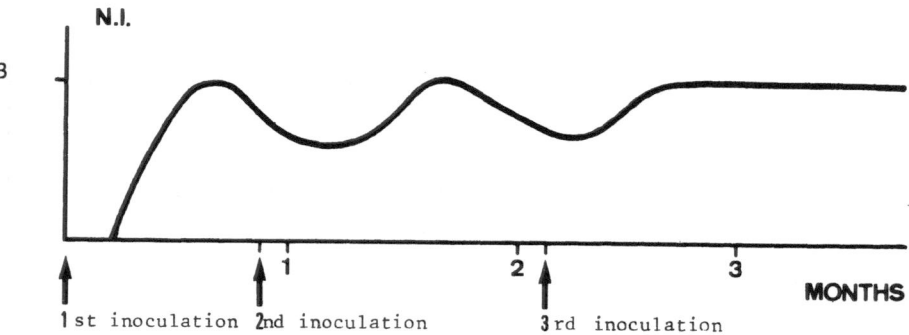

Fig. 3. Kinetics of local antibodies in 11 calves.

3. Discussion. We find that there is no correlation between local and systemic humoral response after the inoculation of the IBR virus intranasally in calves.

The local stimulation is apparently independent of the serum antibody level. The animals with maternal or active antibody react locally just like animals devoid of IBR specific immunoglobulins.

Comparison of kinetics show the same independence: after the first inoculation the local antibodies disappear before the increase of systemic antibody levels. After several inoculations the level of local antibody remains high and serum antibody level falls to the initial status. Each virus administration stimulates a local response even in the presence of residual antibodies, but has no effect on the systemic response.

The results are in accord with the general consensus about the independence of the local immunological system from the systemic one. The antibodies producing cells are not the same, they have not the same course of development nor the same synthetic activity.

The local barrier inhibits the spread of virus or of antigens and could prevent contact with systemic cells.

Lymphocyte responses to viral infection

Each virus inoculation stimulates the same cellular reaction. We did not find any difference in the stimulation at the primary and booster inoculations.

We used two *in vitro* tests with IBR virus:

1) The inactivation of IBR virus by lymphocytes. This is a non-specific reaction. This reaction takes place even if there was no previous specific stimulation.

2) The lymphocytes in contact with killed IBR virus undergo blastogenesis if the donor has been previously in contact with the infectious virus. In that case the virus evokes a response similar to non-specific mitogens like PHA or Con A.

1. The non-specific activity of lymphocytes on IBR virus

PBL and lymphocytes from bronchial washings destroy the infectivity of IBR virus: this is shown by direct incubation of various dilutions of virus with the suspended cells, or by putting lymphocytes on a layer of IBR infected cells. These lymphoid cells are active when taken from the animal or after three days of culture with or without antigenic stimulation. The lymphocytes are active without macrophages which stick to glass and without serum.

The activity on infected cell layers is limited to the phase of the viral cycle at which the virus is freed from cells, that means between the sixth and eighth hour after the beginning of infection.

We obtained the same result with MDBK infected cells and with autologous testicular cells: there was no histocompatibility effect.

These properties are not linked with previous immunisation of the donor: we obtained the same results with lymphocytes of a colostrum-deprived 2 h old calf.

2. Specific reactivity of lymphocyte against IBR virus
Peripheral blood leucocytes. We have observed a time-linked lymphocyte reactivity after virus inoculation: the *in vitro* properties of the PBL depend on the time of the sampling.

Thymidine incorporation. The incorporation of thymidine corresponds to the DNA synthesis in the lymphocyte during blastic transformation. The PBL in presence of inactivated IBR virus incorporate tritiated thymidine at a higher degree than the controls. This reaction takes place between the seventh and the fourteenth day after intranasal virus inoculation. From 14 animals, 9 reacted on the seventh day, 7 on the four-teenth day.

Thermostable rosettes. Culture of PBL with inactivated virus evokes thermostable rosette forming cells between the seventh and the fourteenth day after intranasal inoculation. These rosette forming cells do not exist in control unstimulated

TABLE 3

THYMIDINE INCORPORATION AND THERMOSTABLE ROSETTES FORMATION: RESULTS AFTER
PRIMARY INOCULATION

Calf number	J - 1, + 2, + 5 R	I	J + 7 R	I	J + 14 R	I	J + 17 R	I
81	O	1	O	2	5	1	O	1
82	O	1	14	1	7	1	O	1.5
83	O	1	O	1	9	2	O	1.4
84	O	1	11	5.3	11	6	O	1
85	O	1	ND	4.5	7	2	O	1
86	O	1	3	6	10	2	O	1
87	O	1	19	2.4	10	2.3	O	1.4
88	O	1	O	1	O	1	O	1
89	O	1	ND	1	8	1	O	1
90	O	1	16	2.4	10	1	O	1
91	O	1	ND	3.6	8	4.3	O	1
92	O	1	15	2	O	2.3	O	1.6
93	O	1	ND	1.3	7	2	O	1
94	O	1	10	13.6	8	1.3	O	1
Number of calves reacting positively	0/14	0/14	7/10	9/14	12/14	8/14	0/14	0/14

J : day of sampling (inoculation at JO)

I : stimulation index $\dfrac{\text{mean of CPM } (H^3Thy \text{ incorporation}) \text{ in the 6 wells with killed IBR}}{\text{mean of CPM in the six control wells (without killed IBR)}}$

R : percentage of thermostable rosettes forming cells, after three days
    culture with killed IBR.

cells, in unstimulated animals or in stimulated calves at
other times. The booster response is exactly the same: the
lymphocyte population contain about 10% of thermostable rosette
forming cells between the seventh and the fourteenth day after
reinoculation.

Lymphoid organs. We have prepared lymphocyte suspensions
from spleen, thymus, tracheobronchic lymph node, bronchial
washing cells and blood at necropsy of the animals 2, 8 and 14
days after the last virus reinoculation.

On the second day there was no reactivity of lymphocytes
to inactivated IBR virus.

On the eighth day one spleen gave thermostable rosette
forming cells (7 of 10 calves had PBL able to form this
kind of rosette).

On the fourteenth day one spleen and two bronchial
washings gave positive results (5 of 6 calves had PBL
able to form such rosettes).

3. Discussion. We will not discuss the non-specific
activity of lymphocytes on IBR virus, despite the importance
of these reactions during *in vivo* infection, because it does
not depend on previous contact with virus.

We have used transformation tests, which reveal sensitised
lymphocytes which will react specifically to a contact with
the antigen *in vitro*.

Rosette E formation (Photo 1) is a property of certain T
lymphocytes: it is dependent on immunisation status.

Thermostable rosette formation is the property of lymphocyte populations in which a blastic transformation process
occurs, induced by a polyclonal mitogen (PHA or Con A) (Photo 2)
or by the specific antigen which has sensitised re-stimulation
of the lymphocyte *in vitro*. This test is specific (controls were

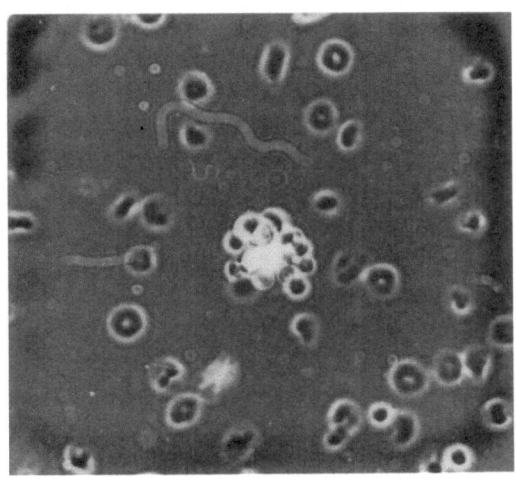

Photo 1. E Rosette, formed at + 4°c between a bovine T lymphocyte and sheep red blood cells. The rosette is thermolabile.

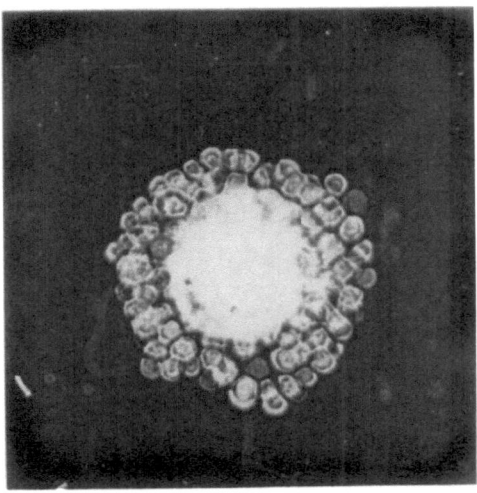

Photo 2. Rosette formed by a bovine lymphocyte incubated three days with PHA. The rosette is thermostable.

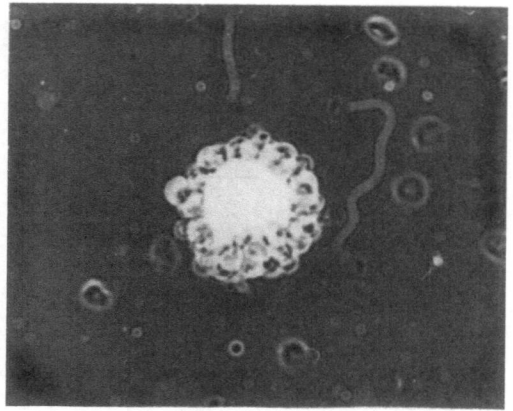

Photo 3. Rosette formed by a bovine lymphocyte incubated three days with
          inactivated IBR virus. The donor had been infected ten days
          earlier by nasal route with IBR virus. The rosette is
          thermostable.

N.B. These two thermostable rosettes are formed by lymphoblasts; in
stimulated cultures, we found also small lymphocytes forming thermostable
rosettes.

kept by immunisation of calves with IBR virus, Hog cholera
virus or Bovine viral diarrhoea virus, and trying to stimulate
lymphocytes *in vitro*).

After three days' incubation with inactivated IBR virus,
we find between 10 and 25% of lymphocytes forming E rosettes;
after thermic treatment, a certain percentage of rosettes
remains only in positively reacting cultures. Are the
thermostable rosette-forming lymphocytes the cells which form
also E rosettes? Are they transformed lymphocytes, or cells
which have adsorbed soluble factor produced by lymphoblasts?
We have not yet elucidated these points.

These two tests are commonly related to thymus-dependent
lymphocytes. The intranasal inoculation stimulates the
appearance of lymphocytes with special properties in the blood
stream and perhaps in spleen and bronchial washings. The
response at the cellular level is of short duration even with
booster inoculations, but this may be only a preliminary and
transient aspect of cellular immunity. The two blastogenic
reactions (thymidine incorporation, thermostable rosette
formation) do not take place always in the same animal at the
same time. This may be because they need different populations
of lymphocytes to support them.

The fact that we found cells able to form thermostable
rosettes in bronchial washings as well as in spleen, does not
indicate the origin of these cells: they can be of local or
systemic origin, or they can be a product of local stimulation.

GENERAL DISCUSSION

We observed reproducible results after inoculation by the
nasal route of IBR virus at the local humoral and systemic
cellular level. The variability of the systemic humoral response
can be linked to the presence of maternal antibodies but also
to the properties of the strain of virus we used, for example,
the capacity to spread from cell to cell, pulmonary tropism,

interferon susceptibility. There is a correlation in the time
of appearance of local antibodies and of cellular reactivity
to the virus inoculated; the two types of response were evident
one week after every virus administration, but the duration of
antibody response increases to more than 30 days with the number
of antigenic stimulations; in contrast, the cellular response
never persists for more than eight days.

The cells which determine the two types of reaction might
have the same origin: the bronchus-associated lymphoid tissue
(BALT) populates the lamina propria with plasmocytes responsible
for immunoglobulin synthesis and the blood stream with migrating
cells. One unique site will be sufficient to initiate the
local humoral and systemic cellular response.

If the two types of response come from cells of different
origins, we have to accept wider spread of the antigen, which
does not seem compatible with the absence of serum antibody
response.

These results have clinical significance.

It is possible to find, after each spontaneous as well as
experimental infection, antibodies in the nasal mucus and
specifically sensitised lymphocytes in the blood. Positive
nasal swabs and reactive cultures of lymphocytes are the direct
consequence of the virus infection. Sometimes it was possible
to isolate virus at the same time. Sometimes it was possible
to isolate at the same time virus and neutralising antibodies
from nasal swabs and to cultivate positive cells from recently
infected calves. We wonder what could be the significance
of the measurement of serum antibodies in establishing a
diagnosis, if pathogenic strains have the same immunological
behaviour. These facts are a good support for the use of local
immunisation with live virus strains which are able to evoke
local antibodies, interferon and very often no reaction in the
serum, to protect specifically the animals in infected herds.

The killed vaccines, given systematically give rise to serum antibodies which are devoid of activity against local infection by the virus.

REFERENCES

Le Jan, C. 1977. Bull. Acad. Vet. Fr. 50, p. 147.

Le Jan, C. and Salmon, H. 1977. Bull. Acad. Vet. Fr. 50, p. 287.

Rouse, B.T. and Babiuk, L.A. 1974. Infect. Immun. 10, No. 4, p. 681.

DISCUSSION

K. Petzoldt *(West Germany)*

Dr. Morein, I have a question concerning your electron micrographs. Have you seen any other effects of IgA antibodies besides the aggregation on the surface of the particle?

B. Morein *(Sweden)*

I have not been looking for any length of time, but we have not. We have not seen any lysis or things like that, in the preparations.

F.J. Bourne *(UK)*

I think you should be content with what you have. Anyone with an interest in IgA realises that the number of functions which this immunoglobulin carries out in a protective sense are very limited. It is very encouraging that here we have another function which IgA antibody can mediate in a protective sense.

Could you clarify one point for me: you have two phases in your mucus - a liquid phase and a gel phase. Are these the products of the same cell?

B. Morein

What I can say is that, physically and chemically they are quite different, but I am not able to tell exactly which cells they are coming from. I have not been looking into that.

F.J. Bourne

In her paper, Dr. Allan mentioned two distinct types of mucus. Do you know if these are products of different cells?

E. Allan *(UK)*

There is some evidence that the gel phase is produced from the epithelial goblet cells, and the serous cells produce the liquid phase.

F.J. Bourne

    So this is equivalent to the human situation?

E. Allan

    Yes.

F.J. Bourne

    My point is that if we could determine that these cells are producing a different type of mucus in relation to the gel and liquid phases, this would have some significance in the protection of these membranes. For instance, if you have a situation where you eliminate the gel phase, your membrane is immediately exposed to virus.

B. Morein

    The tips of the cilia are exposed to virus directly because the cilia grow up into the gel phase. Then again, I do not know how the liquid phase is reacting.

H.M. Pirie *(UK)*

    I think that is an interesting point, because Dr. Allan demonstrated yesterday that in the bronchioles there are normally no mucous cells. Presumably there are no ciliomucins right down in the bottom of the lung, so if the virus is in a very fine aerosol it can get right into the lung, and is more liable to cause infection.

B. Morein

    An infection is quite dependent upon the size of the droplets coming in. It is a very definite size, I think it is 0.2μ, although I might be wrong on that. The virus is actually landing in the respiratory tract at the first infection. It is multiplying in the upper respiratory tract after infection, and then virus is going up and down the tract with the air.

J.M. Sharp *(UK)*

    I would like to make some comments on our experience in SPF lambs with PI3 virus. Our ability to produce disease is

dependent upon the route of inoculation. If we give the virus
in an aerosol, or instil it intranasally, we get virus replication
but no clinical disease, whereas if we inoculate the virus
intratracheally, we obtain very marked clinical disease. We
cannot explain this at the moment and I wondered if perhaps by
putting it intratracheally we were washing the mucus away, dis-
rupting the gel phase so that the virus is getting down to the
cell surface very rapidly in large numbers.

B. Morein

This viral clearance system is working in the nose. In
the trachea, everything is going to the lungs. In order to
introduce particles in the respiratory tract I think you have to
define your droplets and your aerosols very well in order to
know where they are going. I think the people doing that can
place their particles in different levels of the respiratory
tract quite well, but these people are perhaps not pharmacological
people.

J.M. Sharp

The aerosol which we have produced goes right down to the
alveolar level, so we are getting virus deep down into the lungs
but we are not getting evidence of the clinical disease.

C. Howard (UK)

You said that if you give IgA to calves it then gets transported back through the nasal epithelial. Is that through the
epithelial cells?

F.J. Bourne

No, it is through gland cells.

C. Howard

So it is not the same mechanism as you would use to get the
transport of IgA.

F.J. Bourne

    The same cells which transport colostral IgA appear to be transporting IgA in the adult.

C. Howard

    That is supposed to be mediated by the secretion of secretory piece outside the cell.

F.J. Bourne

    Inside the cell.

C. Howard

    And the IgA becomes attached to the secretory piece?

F.J. Bourne

    The secretory piece operates inside the epithelial cell, not outside.

C. Howard

    Yes, but I thought that was how the IgA went on to the epithelial cells.

F.J. Bourne

    As it goes in, yes. But it could be a confusing issue, because when you think of intracellular secretion of IgG, for instance, and IgM, a secretory component is not involved.

    The idea proposed by Brandtzaeg is simply that here you have the epithelial cell's secretory component in the cell. The immunoglobulin comes along to the cell surface, is picked up at this point by secretory component and this is transported across the cell. At this point Dr. Brandtzaeg suggests that the IgA is secreted with secretory component intact so you have no 9S molecule, but this is probably not true for every situation, because we know that in the pig, for instance, 60% of the IgA can be a 9S molecule without the secretory component. We have looked at human colostrum and a similar sort of situation very often exists there. It could be that the secretory

component perhaps detaches itself at this point and is then
re-used for further transport within the cell. What are you
suggesting?

C. Howard

I am saying that if the passively-given IgA already has
secretory piece, how does it get into the cell?

F.J. Bourne

Yes, I see your point. We wondered about that and I do
not know. We carried out some work using human 11S IgA, and
we found that the transport of the 11S IgA was exactly the
same as the 9S IgA.

H.M. Pirie

You may have mentioned it, but I wonder if you could
clarify a point for me. Regarding the cells which secrete the
IgA, particularly in the lung, you mentioned the lung but in
fact it is secreted in the cells in the bronchii or bronchioles
and if it is in the bronchii, is it epithelial cells or the
glands which secrete it?

F.J. Bourne

The evidence of Pat Bradley's work was that it was the gland
cells which secreted IgA, but we do find intracellular IgA
on epithelial cells. You may have seen it on one of the slides.
We have evidence from the gut, from EM studies, that IgA is
in fact intracellular, it is not just sticking on the top. I do
not know how it gets there in the case of these ductal cells.
It could be that it has an intracellular secretory route. We
are not going any further than saying that the duct cells certainly do secrete IgA. The possibility exists that other cells
also secrete IgA. It is very much easier to define this situation in the gut. There we find that only cells at the base of
the villi or in the crypts of Lieberkühn secrete immunoglobulin
molecules; cells further up the villi do not.

H.M. Pirie

I think it is interesting that bronchioles do not have ducts, so that they may be more susceptible to infection.

F.J. Bourne

I do not know. I am not familiar with the histology.

D.R. Snodgrass (UK)

If you stimulate the gut, and the lymphoid system, you said the effect on the CMI becomes systemic. What effect do you have in the respiratory tract after the stimulation of the gut?

F.J. Bourne

As far as I know we have only looked at lymphoid tissue in the lung. You can certainly demonstrate a CMI response in lymphoid tissue in the lung following oral stimulation. This stimulation is very often obtained by presenting antigen in the drinking water, so you cannot rule out the possibility of getting a similar stimulation in the respiratory tract as well.

P.W. Wells (UK)

Professor Petzoldt, when you tried to sensitise lambs with serum containing antibodies to your antigen, produced in calves, were you successful on only one occasion, or were you not successful at all?

K. Petzoldt (West Germany)

We tried passive sensitisation by the inhalation of the positive serum, but we were unsuccessful in these lambs. We repeated the experiment three times. I believe that perhaps the condition of mast cells in lambs is age-dependent. We have seen in other experiments that we cannot use lambs for PCA when we use the lambs before the third day. It may also be a question of dosage.

P.W. Wells

This was bovine serum, though. In experiments we did a few years ago, we showed that we were able to sensitise certain sheep with bovine sera. Do you think this may have been the problem in your case?

K. Petzoldt

This may be the reason.

P. Eyre

I think this is a major problem, because you have a hetero-logous situation, trying to transfer reaginic antibodies from one species to another, and there is a tremendous difference in the ability of the reagins of one species to sensitise another. You cannot assume that this will happen - it may. We showed that you could sometimes get sheep to take bovine reagins but not always. I think that is a major flaw in that argument. I am also a little anxious about your PCA technique because, if you are using relatively crude extracts of vaccines, or what-ever you are using, and using them directly into skin you will, if you are not careful, get direct effects of these substances, whether or not the animal has been previously hypersensitised, either actively or passively, because there are vaso-active substances such as toxins, in these products. I would there-fore suggest that you should do some sort of reverse situation. Buxton and Thomlinson, working in Liverpool about fifteen years ago, did this kind of work with pigs, when they were looking at the gut oedema disease syndrome. You reverse the order of in-jection to prove whether or not the antigen is itself directly vaso-active because it may be. Your tests do not eliminate the possibility that you may have direct vaso-activity.

K. Petzoldt

We tried to exclude this by controls, in the same animals as well as other animals. Up to a certain level we tried to exclude this.

F.J. Bourne

You could also use an anti-IgE presumably.

P. Eyre

Yes, if you can get it.

K. Petzoldt

It is very difficult to get an anti-bovine IgE. That is the problem.

F.J. Bourne

You will have to work in the pig!

H. Ernø (Denmark)

Could you tell me the histology of the positive passive cutaneous anaphylaxis reaction in the bovine: did you look into it or do you know how it looks from other experiments in the bovine species?

K. Petzoldt

No, we did not look at it. I am sorry.

P. Eyre

I could make a very brief contribution to that. It is mainly a vascular reaction. There is very little cellular response because it is a very early vascular lesion.

SESSION 6A

VACCINATION

Chairman:

J.T. Stamp

Co-ordinator:

P.W. Wells

BOVINE RESPIRATORY SYNCYTIAL (RS) VIRUS INFECTION
AND VACCINATION EXPERIMENTS

A. van Nieuwstadt

Centraal Diergeneeskundig Instituut, AFD Virologie,
Houtribweg 39, Lelystad, The Netherlands.

ABSTRACT

Epidemiological studies in the Netherlands have given ample evidence that bovine RS virus is an important and frequently occurring respiratory pathogen of young animals. Hence efforts to develop a vaccine for it are fully justified.

In 27 calves experimentally infected with a wild strain of RS virus in our own isolation units, we have seen only once the serious symptoms that resembled those seen in the field. Thus the protective value of a vaccine must finally be tested in the field because serious respiratory symptoms of the disease, as observed in the field, cannot be reproduced under experimental conditions.

An RS vaccine of the tissue culture adapted strain of Dr. Wellemans of the 'Institut National de Récherches Vétérinaires' in Brussels was tested in experiments in the field. In the autumn of 1976 we did a trial of the vaccine in nine herds and half of the animals of the critical age were vaccinated twice intramuscularly. The other half of the animals were controls. Altogether about 500 calves were vaccinated and only 50% showed a serological response. The vaccine did not have any harmful side effects. In four of these herds there were respiratory troubles in connection with RS virus infections, but in no case was a difference observed in the gravity of the disease symptoms between vaccinated and control animals.

Investigations were started to develop criteria for the evaluation of a vaccine under laboratory conditions. The antibody titre, the number of days·virus was excreted after challenge, and the method of challenge (contact infection or spraying the virus intranasally), were under consideration. Following intranasal infection by aerosol, the wild strain of RS virus could be isolated from nasal swabs up to ten days after infection. However there was no unequivocal reduction in the duration of virus excretion in vaccinated animals, despite a serological response. We tried to challenge the animals by contact infection. It was shown that vaccinated animals were no more protected against infection by contact than by intranasal exposure.

Animals that had experienced an infection with the wild strain of virus could be infected by an intranasal spray of RS virus: at least there was a booster reaction of serum antibodies, but no virus excretion could be demonstrated in nasal swabs in this case.

So far this vaccine does not seem to protect against the infection with the wild strain. Nevertheless some people have found a good protection against the natural disease in the field with this vaccine.

In the autumn of 1976 we carried out some field trials with a bovine respiratory syncytial (RS) virus vaccine. An experimental batch of a modified live virus vaccine, from a tissue culture adapted strain of Dr. Wellemans (Institut National de Récherches Vétérinaires in Brussels), was obtained from a commercial producer.

In 9 herds animals of less than one year old were vaccinated, altogether about 500 calves. On each farm 50% of the calves at the critical age were vaccinated twice intramuscularly, the other half were controls. The vaccine did not have any harmful side effects. We found a significant increase of bovine RS virus antibodies in only 50% of 144 animals serologically investigated, while at the same time none of the control animals showed an increase of antibodies. Serological examination was by virus-neutralisation reaction in a micro-titre system and serum dilutions were tested against 10 $TCID_{50}$ of bovine RS virus.

In 4 of the 9 herds vaccinated, there was an outbreak of respiratory disease later in the autumn. The outbreak co-incided with an infection by bovine RS virus, as judged from serological data. No differences were observed in seriousness of symptoms between vaccinated and unvaccinated animals. We had not specified criteria to compare seriousness of disease symptoms in vaccinated animals and controls. Nowhere in the literature could we find a detailed system to evaluate respiratory disease symptoms. In 4 out of 9 herds in this experiment there were infections with bovine RS virus, but these passed unnoticed and we could trace the infection only by an increase of antibodies, in both vaccinated and unvaccinated animals.

Perhaps vaccination of half of the calves in the critical age prevented a serious outbreak. So far the results of our field trials with modified live virus vaccine of bovine RS virus have not been favourable in every respect. In the case of a bovine RS virus vaccine, protection should be evaluated in a field trial. As with other respiratory viruses, experimental infections under controlled conditions never cause serious respiratory symptoms as observed in the field. Of 27, nearly all, specific pathogen free (SPF) calves which we infected with a wild strain of bovine RS virus, only one had symptoms like those seen in the field, namely: on four successive days a temperature higher than 40°C, reduced appetite, and on auscultation a shrill vesicular respiration. While symptoms cannot be reproduced under experimental conditions and the protective value of a vaccine cannot be tested in this way, we tried to develop other criteria for a good vaccine. Consideration was given to:

The antibody titre induced by the vaccine.

The possibility of infecting vaccinated animals with the wild strain, either by intranasal spray or by contact.

A comparison of the duration of virus excretion by vaccinated animals and controls after challenge with the wild strain.

Some of the results will be presented.

In Figure 1, virus excretion and antibody response of SPF calves is shown after infection by an intranasal spray of a wild strain of bovine RS virus (calf A and B) and after infection by contact (calf C). For infection or challenge of vaccinated animals by an intranasal spray, we always used $10^{5.5}$ PFU of a field strain, isolated in tissue culture. We always used 4 - 6 months old SPF calves in our experiments, unless stated otherwise. Virus isolations were carried out on nasal secretion and sputum samples. Neutralising antibody in blood was measured either by a plaque-reduction test, in which a serum dilution is determined giving 50% survival of the virus, or in the microtitre system, in which a 50% endpoint is determined in a series of serum dilutions against 10 $TCID_{50}$ of the virus. This latter technique gives lower titres, however their exact relations to the titres in a plaque reduction test is not known at this moment. Titres of neutralising antibody are measured in 2 log units. Antibody titres measured in a plaque reduction test are indicated in the tables with a circle around the figure of the titre.

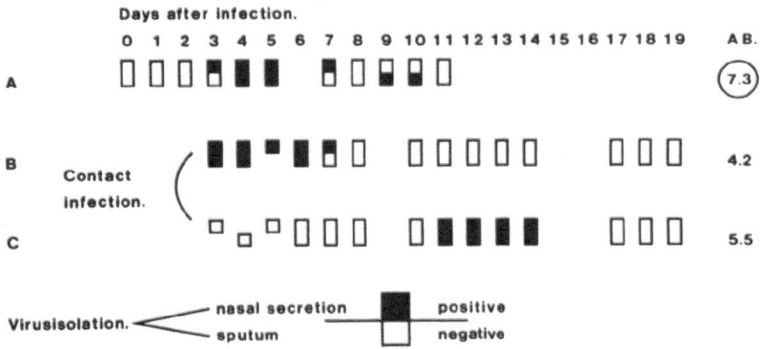

Fig. 1. Virus excretion and antibody responses of SPF calves after infection by an intranasal spray of wild strain bovine RS virus (calf A and B) and after infection by contact (calf C).

In all experimental infections the earliest day on which virus could be isolated was the first day after intranasal infection and the latest was the tenth day. Neutralising antibody in blood was found at the earliest on the ninth day after infection. Three days after intranasal infection with bovine RS virus calf B (Figure 1) was housed together with calf C and infection was transmitted as demonstrated by virus isolation and seroconversion of calf C.

We expected to find very little or no virus excretion at all in vaccinated animals after challenge with the wild strain. Figure 2 gives the results from 4 animals that were vaccinated. Vaccination was carried out with modified live virus of Wellemans and animals were vaccinated once intramuscularly or twice with an interval of three weeks. There was a good serological response: neutralising antibody could already be demonstrated on the seventh day after the initial vaccination. Nevertheless animals could be infected one month after vaccination by an intranasal spray of $10^{5.5}$ PFU of the field strain, despite the presence of neutralising antibody: virus could be isolated on 5, 3, 2 and 5 days after challenge respectively and there was a booster response of antibody. There was no evident reduction in the number of days that the virus could be isolated from airways as compared with non-vaccinated controls.

The question arises as to whether the challenge had been too heavy and should be substituted by contact infection. Two SPF calves were vaccinated with the bovine RS vaccine strain of Wellemans, obtained from industry. Animals were vaccinated twice intramuscularly with $10^{4.35}$ PFU of virus. The antibody response was comparatively low, with titres of 4.1 and 3.4 in 2 log units, but it should be noticed that these titres were obtained by virus neutralisation in the microtitre system. Challenge was by contact infection. Calf B (Figure 3) was infected 3 days earlier by an intranasal spray of wild virus and was housed together with the two vaccinated animals (H,J) and a non-vaccinated control (C). Virus was excreted by the intranasally infected donor calf and transmitted to the un-vaccinated control calf. Virus could be isolated from nasal secretion and sputum of the control calf from the ninth day until the twelfth day after contact and this was followed by a seroconversion. The two vaccinated calves were infected too: both had a booster reaction of antibody and virus was excreted by calf J on the 15th, 16th and 17th day after animals were brought into contact. Vaccination did not appear to have given protection against infection by contact.

Another experiment was performed with 6 calves that had been brought from a local dairy farm. They were housed in our isolation units when two days old. Animals were not colostrum-free and had antibody for bovine RS virus at the age of 4 months, when they were intramuscularly vaccinated with the modified live virus vaccine. It is possible that the vaccine was not effective since antibody titres were not elevated. When 6 months old these animals had relatively low

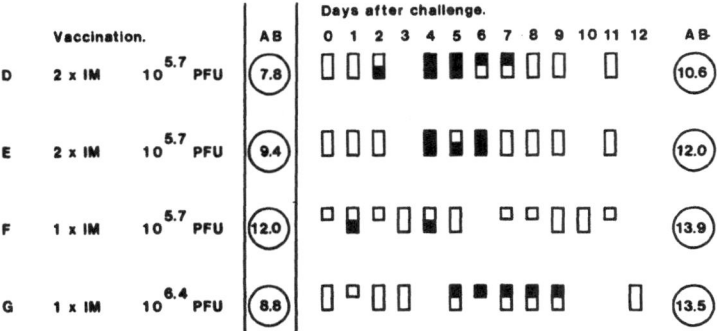

Fig. 2. Virus excretion and antibody responses of SPF calves vaccinated
with modified live bovine RS virus and infected one month later
by an intranasal spray of wild strain bovine RS virus.

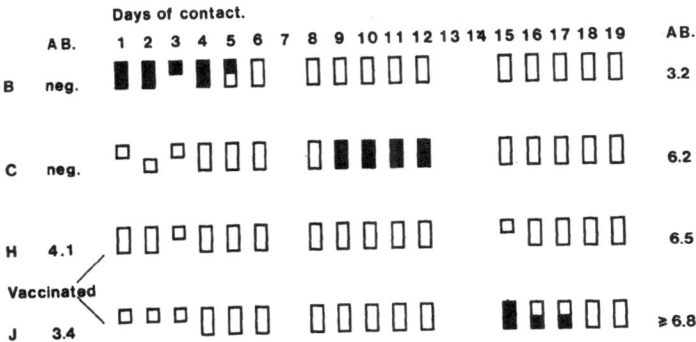

Fig. 3. Virus excretion and antibody responses of SPF calves vaccinated
with modified live bovine RS virus and challenged by contact
infection.

antibody titres, probably from vaccination. One of these
calves 'Q' (Figure 4) was infected by an intranasal spray of
$10^{5\cdot5}$ PFU of a wild strain of bovine RS virus and 3 days later
housed together with the other 5 animals. The virus was

excreted by the infected animal and transmitted to the others, although antibodies were present in the blood. Three calves (R, S, T) excreted the virus from the ninth day after contact and from the other two the virus could be isolated from the twelfth (P) and fifteenth (O) days respectively. Typical symptoms of bovine RS virus infection were observed in one animal only. Calf 'T' was sick and had fever from day 18 until day 21, after the time when virus could be isolated from the airways and by which time antibody production had started. Again no protection against infection by contact was found in this experiment, although the animals had antibodies either passively acquired or actively formed by vaccination.

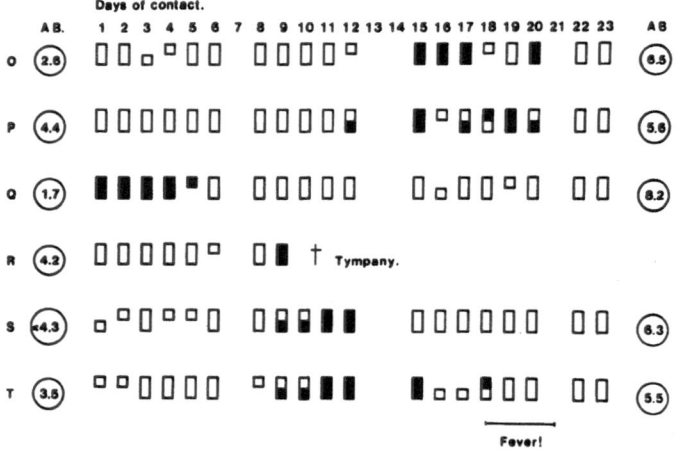

Fig. 4.   Virus excretion and antibody responses of conventionally reared calves vaccinated intramuscularly with modified live bovine RS virus at 4 months of age and exposed to contact infection by the infection of and introduction of calf Q to the group two months later.

The question arose whether or not an animal that has experienced the infection with the wild virus, is protected against a second exposure. Two animals from a group of 5 yearlings which had experienced an experimental infection with the wild strain of bovine RS virus 5 months before and which were still serologically positive, were separated and sprayed again intranasally with $10^{5.5}$ PFU of the wild strain. After three days they were housed with the remaining three. The virus could not be isolated from any of the animals and a secondary serological response was observed only in the intranasally infected animals. Thus virus infection had occurred in these latter animals, although virus was not excreted or transmitted.

In another experiment, 4 colostrum deprived SPF animals, which had experienced a subclinical infection with bovine RS virus in the first month of life, were reinfected 1½ years later. Of these animals, two had a comparatively high anti-body titre (K, L) and two had a low antibody titre (M, N). Animals were infected by an intranasal spray of $10^{5.9}$ PFU of a field strain. In this experiment virus could be isolated from nasal secretions and sputum and there was a secondary antibody response in the blood of all 4 animals (Figure 5).

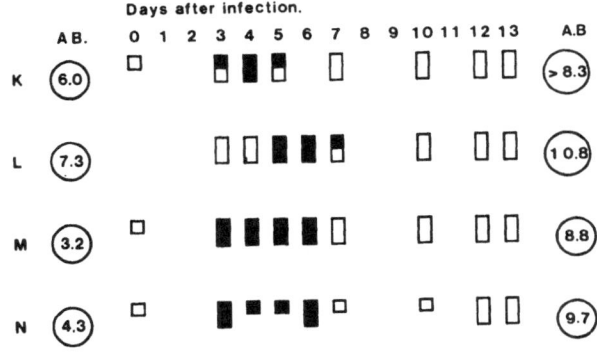

Fig. 5. Virus excretion and antibody responses of colostrum deprived SPF calves infected with bovine RS virus in the first month of life and reinfected 1½ years later.

We may conclude that reinfection is possible after a previous infection with the wild strain of bovine RS virus, at least if the virus is applied by an intranasal spray. Whether or not this is also possible in the case of contact infection should be investigated. We think it is possible, if sufficient time elapses between the first infection and a second exposure. In the field we found that some animals experiencing an infection in the spring as judged from a seroconversion, had a second increase of antibody titre in the following autumn. We wonder if it is possible by vaccination to get a degree of immunity high enough to prevent an infection with the wild virus, for even in the field an infection by the wild strain can be followed by another one some time later. However, perhaps we should be content with a vaccine giving an antibody response and protection from the clinical symptoms and disease caused by infection with virulent virus.

In conclusion we may state:

In field experiments we were not successful in preventing respiratory symptoms due to bovine RS virus infection by vaccination with the Wellemans strain of RS vaccine.

The modified live virus strain of Wellemans induces a good serological response in the SPF animals after intramuscular injection.

It was possible to infect vaccinated animals with a wild strain of bovine RS virus both by an intranasal spray and by contact with a virus-excretor.

In view of our experience that even the natural infection does not give life-long immunity for a second infection, we wonder if prevention of the infection or reduction of virus-excretion is a good criterion for judging protective value of a RS vaccine.

We consider that while vaccination may not result in an immune response of sufficient magnitude to prevent infection by the wild virus, perhaps we should be content if we obtain protection against the symptoms resulting from infection.

RESULTS OF A SMALL FIELD TRIAL WITH A MULTICOMPONENT INACTIVATED RESPIRATORY VIRAL VACCINE.

S.P. Morzaria, B.A. Maund, M.S. Richards and J.W. Harkness
Central Veterinary Laboratory, New Haw, Weybridge, Surrey, England.

ABSTRACT

An inactivated virus vaccine containing strains of Parainfluenza 3, Adenovirus 3, Reovirus 1, Bovine virus diarrhoea and Infectious bovine rhinotracheitis viruses was tested in a group of 60 calves reared in a semi-intensive management system. Both vaccinated and control calves were subjected to prevaccination and postvaccination serological, bacteriological and clinical examinations on a regular basis. Before vaccination, all calves in the test group had antibodies to PI3 and Reovirus 1, and 15/30, 20/30 and 8/30 had antibody to Adenovirus 3, BVD and IBR respectively. In the control group, all calves had antibody to PI3 virus, and 15/28, 26/28, 18/28 and 2/28 had antibody to Adenovirus 3, Reovirus 1, BVD and IBR viruses respectively at the time they arrived on the farm. Following vaccination, only one animal showed a significant rise in antibody titre to Reovirus 1, and none to PI3. Of the calves without serum antibody at vaccination, none subsequently developed antibody to BVD, but 14/15 and 17/22 became seropositive to Adenovirus 3, and IBR respectively. However, in the control group 2/2 developed antibody to Reovirus 1, and 1/10, 6/13 and 3/26 became positive to BVD, Adenovirus 3, and IBR respectively. Bacteriology revealed the presence of a wide variety of commensal bacterial and Mycoplasma bovirhinis in both groups. Analysis of the records of clinical examinations indicated respiratory tract infections occurred among the calves at between 50 and 80 days after arrival, and that there was no significant difference between the test and the control groups. The presence of maternal antibodies appeared to interfere with the response to the antigens present in the vaccine, and the vaccination schedule recommended by the manufacturer does not entirely circumvent this problem.

In the United Kingdom respiratory disease in young
calves can no longer be regarded as occurring sporadically as
reported by Lamont and Kerr (1939); Tutt (1941); Barr et al.
(1951) and Watt (1952). With the increase in intensive
systems of management there has been an increase in the number
of outbreaks of so-called 'virus pneumonia' (Harbourne, 1966)
and the clinical disease can be regarded as endemic in this
country. It is difficult to assess accurately the losses
associated with the condition, but indications from early
surveys in the UK (Leech et al., 1968; Curtis, 1970) are that
the disease is of major economic importance for calf rearers
and beef producers. Recent estimates by Thomas (personal
communication) indicate that the direct losses to the UK beef
industry due to respiratory disease in calves could be as much
as £5.7 million per annum.

In many intensive and semi-intensive systems of calf
management, the prevention of respiratory disease is associated
principally with the use of a combination of chemoprophylaxis
with broad-spectrum antibiotics and the administration of a
viral vaccine. The benefits of such practices have not been
evaluated experimentally in this country. In this paper, we
report a field trial with a commercially manufactured viral
vaccine (Pneumovac Plus; C-Vet Ltd.) currently available in
the UK.

The trial was carried out at the Drayton Experimental
Husbandry farm, Stratford-upon-Avon, Warwickshire, and
employed 60 Friesian calves, 7-14 days old and weighing
between 45-50 kg. Calves were purchased from a calf marketing
group. All were vaccinated against salmonellosis on arrival
using Mellavax vaccine (Burroughs Wellcome & Co). For the
first eight weeks they were reared in a purpose-built calf
house, penned individually in solid-sided pens and bedded on
straw, which was allowed to build-up during the calf rearing
stage. After this they were housed in loose boxes until turn-
out which was 24 weeks after arrival. All calves were fed on
warm milk substitute once daily, and 28 - 30 days after arrival

provided they had eaten at least 700 g concentrates on three consecutive days. Concentrates and water were provided ad lib but hay was restricted to 230 g per calf per day.

The calves for this trial were divided randomly into two equal groups of thirty and one group was vaccinated against respiratory disease while the other was injected with pyrogen-free distilled water as control. The vaccinated and the control calves were distributed alternately in the individual pens.

The vaccine used was Pneumovac-Plus which is a virus vaccine containing inactivated components of parainfluenza virus 3 (PI3), adenovirus 3, reovirus 1, bovine virus diarrhoea (BVD) and infectious bovine rhinotracheitis virus (IBR). The antigens were adsorbed on to aluminium hydroxide (Alhydrogel, Superfos Export, AS., 15, Analiegade, Copenhagen, Denmark). The vaccine was administered intramuscularly according to the manufacturer's recommendations at approximately 2, 5 and 10 weeks of age.

The vaccinated and control calves were subjected to pre- and post-vaccination serology, bacteriology and clinical examinations. For serology, 15 ml of blood was collected from the jugular vein of each of the calves before vaccination and then at fortnightly intervals for 6 months; thereafter samples were taken once a month for a further 3 months. The serum was separated from the clot and stored at -20°C. Sera was subsequently tested for presence of antibodies to the 5 virus antigens present in the vaccine. The following serological tests were employed:

1) PI3: The Haemagglutination-inhibition (HI) test conducted on microtitre plates against 4 haemagglutinating (HA) units of PI3 virus (Strain SF4) and described by Dawson (1964).

2) Adenovirus 3: The Agar-gel precipitation test using the WBRI Weybridge strain of bovine adenovirus type 3 (Darbyshire and Pereira, 1964).

3) Reovirus 1: A micro-HI test using 4HA units of reovirus 1 (Lang strain) as described by Rosen and Abinanti (1960).

4) BVD: A serum-neutralisation test (SN) test (Coggins, 1964) using the NADL strain of the BVD virus,

5) IBR: The SN test (Dawson and Darbyshire, 1964) using the Oxford strain of IBR.

A four-fold rise in antibody titre to any of the above viruses was considered to be a significant serological response.

For bacteriology, the nasal and pharyngeal mucosa of the calves were swabbed with flexible guarded brush swabs as described by Thomas and Stott (1975) and modified by Pritchard and Macleod (1977). The swabs were immediately plated out on to sheep blood agar plates and then transferred into 2 - 3 ml of Eaton's mycoplasma medium (Roberts and Pijoan, 1971) containing 100 µg/ml of ampicillin. Serial dilutions (up to 10^{-6}) of each of the samples were made and one drop of each dilution was placed onto Eaton's agar plates. The plates were incubated at $37^{\circ}C$ in an atmosphere of 7% CO_2 in air and were examined daily for 7 days for mycoplasmas. As far as possible single colonies from the plates were cloned 3 times and identified using the growth inhibition test (Hayflick and Stanbridge, 1967). The swabs were taken at the same time as the bloods.

All calves were examined clinically 3 times a week for 6 months. The examination was limited to the recording of nasal discharge, coughing and respiration rates. Respiration rate was measured for 30 seconds for each calf and the nasal discharge and cough were recorded according to an arbitrary recording system ranging from 0 - 3. For nasal discharge 0 was regarded as no discharge, 1 as slight mucous discharge, 2 as severe catarrhal discharge and 3 as severe muco-purulent discharge. For cough, 0 represented no coughing, 1 as occasional or one single cough, 2 as intermittent cough and 3

as continuous cough during the observation period. These
observations were recorded on forms designed for easy
transcription of the information on to a computer file for
future analysis. To minimise subjective bias, the person
recording clinical signs used a separate form for each day's
observations and was not informed of the vaccinated or non-
vaccinated status of the calves.

All calves were weighted individually once a week throughout the experiment.

Table 1 shows the proportions of calves with antibodies
to PI3, adenovirus 3, reovirus 1, BVD and IBR before and
after vaccination. Before vaccination all calves in the test
group had antibodies to PI3 and reovirus 1 and 15/30, 20/30
and 8/30 had antibody to adenovirus 3, BVD and IBR respectively.
Following vaccination only one calf showed a significant rise
(four-fold) in antibody titre to reovirus 1 and none to PI3.
Of the calves without serum antibody before vaccination, none
subsequently developed antibody to BVD but 14/15 and 17/22
became seropositive to adenovirus 3 and IBR respectively.

TABLE 1

PROPORTION OF CALVES WITH SERUM ANTIBODIES TO THE VIRUS ANTIGENS PRESENT
IN THE VACCINE

Virus	% positive before vaccination			% positive after vaccination*	
	Group to be vaccinated	Control	Total	Vaccinated	Control
PI3	100 (30/30)	100 (28/28)	100 (58/58)	– –	– –
Adenovirus 3	50 (15/30)	53.6 (15/28)	57.7(30/58)	93.3 (14/15)	46.2 (6/13)
Reovirus 1	100 (30/30)	92.9 (26/28)	96.6(56/58)	– –	100 (2/2
BVD	66.7(20/30)	64.3 (18/28)	65.5(38/58)	– (0/10)	10 (1/10)
IBR	26.7(8/30)	7.14(2/28)	17.2(10/58)	77.3 (17/22)	11.3 (3/26)

( ) figures in brackets represent actual numbers

* animals which were serologically negative before vaccination.

In the control group, all calves had antibody to PI3 virus, and 15/28, 26/28, 18/28 and 2/28 had antibody to adeno-virus 3, reovirus 1, BVD and IBR respectively at the time of their arrival on the farm. During the experiment, of the control calves with no antibody on arrival at the farm 2/2 subsequently developed antibody to reovirus 1 and 1/10, 6/13 and 3/26 became positive to BVD, adenovirus 3 and IBR respectively.

Between 16 - 20 weeks of age, all animals (vaccinated and controls) with antibodies on arrival at the farm, except the one with a significant rise in reovirus 1 antibody following vaccination, showed declining, and subsequently insignificant, titres to all the antigens present in the vaccine.

Bacteriology revealed the presence of a large number of commensal bacteria in both the vaccinated and control calves. These were *Moraxella spp.*, *Neisseria spp.*, *Staphylococcus spp.*, *Streptococcus spp.*, *Pasteurella haemolytica* and *P. multocida* and a species of *Micrococci*. *Mycoplasma bovirhinis* was isolated from 48.3% of the calves before vaccination and by the fifteenth week of the experiment all calves had *M. bovirhinis*. No other species of mycoplasmas were isolated.

Results of the clinical examinations are presented in Figures 1, 2, 3 and 4. The average respiration rate of both the vaccinated and non-vaccinated calves showed a significant rise (60 and above) between days 50 and 86 after vaccination and it reached its peak on day 74 (Figure 1). No significant differences were detected in the average respiration rates between the vaccinated and control groups at any stage. From day 86 after vaccination the average respiration rates in both the groups dropped within the normal range. Respiration rates were not recorded after day 112.

The percentage of animals in both groups showing abnormal nasal discharge increased as the trial progressed and reached its peak on day 68 which was 6 days prior to the peak of

503

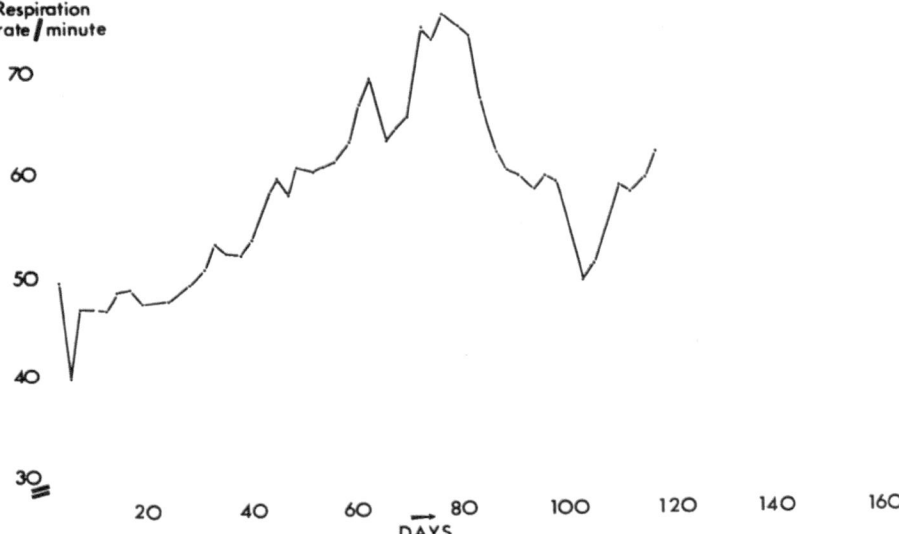

Fig. 1. Average respiration rate.

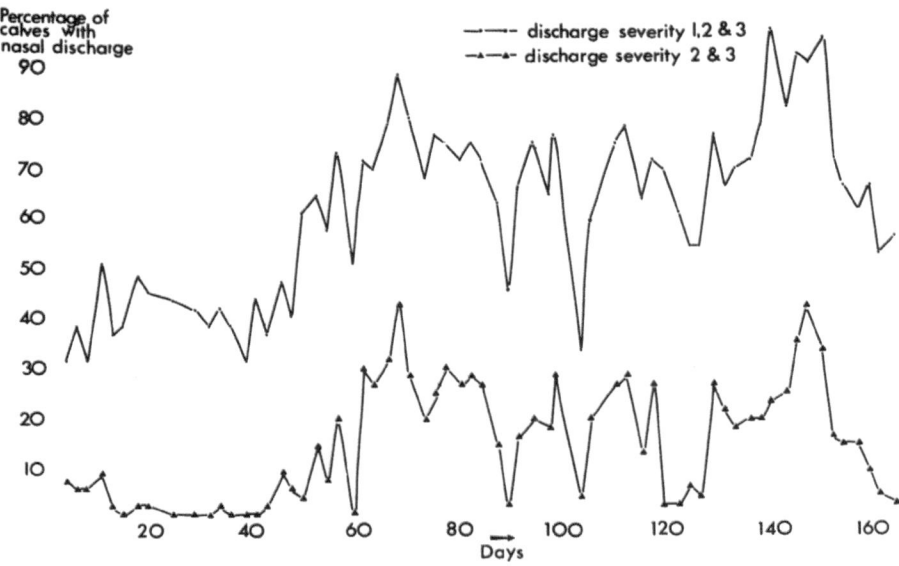

Fig. 2. Proportion of calves with nasal discharge.

504

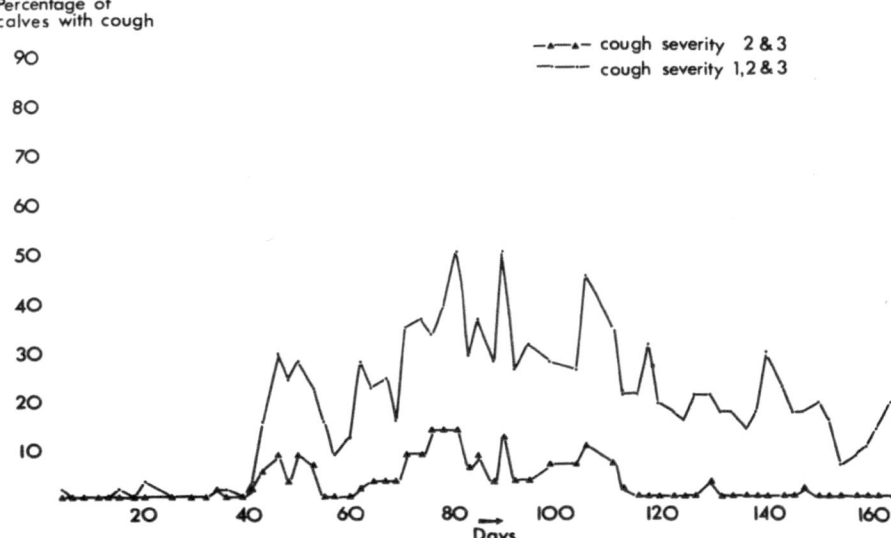

Fig. 3. Proportion of calves with cough.

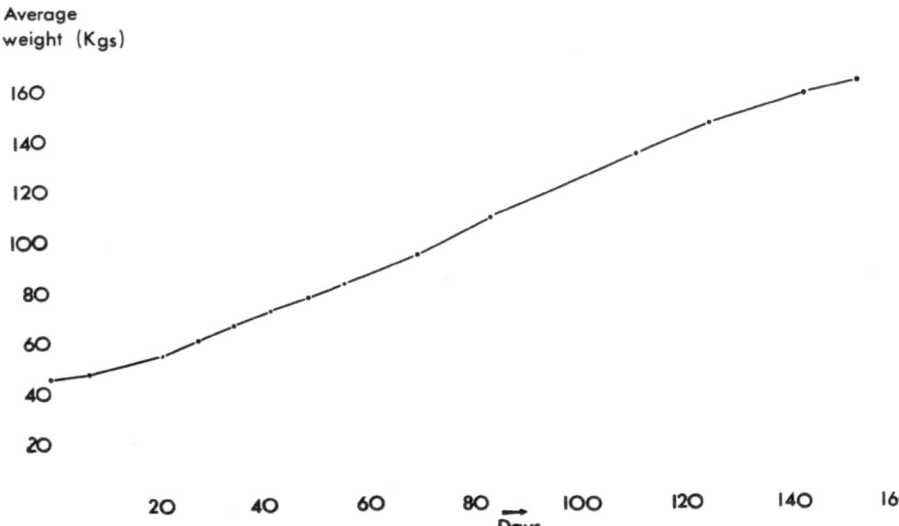

Fig. 4. Average weight of calves.

average respiration rates of both groups (Figure 2). A
second peak of increased nasal discharge was observed on day
137: this peak could not be correlated with respiration rates
since respiration rates were not available for this stage of
the trial. During the period of observations, a nasal discharge
score of 3 (muco-purulent discharge) was recorded only on
one occasion.

On examination of the cough records, it was clear that
the percentage of animals coughing increased from the start
of the trial and between days 70 and 110 more than 30% of the
animals were coughing. An interesting feature of both the
cough and nasal discharge recordings was the fluctuation in
scoring from one set of observations to the next.

DISCUSSION

Serological examination showed that before vaccination,
antibodies to the viral antigens in the vaccine were present
in some of the calves. The proportion of calves carrying
antibody varied with the antigen. The most prevalent were
antibodies to PI3 and reovirus 1 (100% and 96.6% respectively)
followed by BVD and adenovirus 3 (65.5% and 51.7% respectively).
The least common were antibodies to IBR (17.2%) Similar
observations have been made by Harbourne (1966); Thomas (1973);
Thomas and Collins (1974) and Roberts (personal communication).
Following vaccination, of the animals with antibodies only one
animal showed a significant rise in antibody to reovirus 1 while
the rest of the calves showed declining antibody titres to all
the antigens which had reached very low levels or had
disappeared entirely between 16 - 20 weeks of age. The rapid
decline of antibodies was an indication that they were derived
from either selective absorption of high levels of specific
maternal antibody from colostrum or perhaps in utero/trans-
placental infection. The rate of decline appears to closely
parallel that of bovine colostral immunoglobulins (Rossi and
Kiesel, 1972; Logan et al., 1973, Thomas and Collins, 1974).

The inability of the vaccine to boost a serological response
in calves with passive immunity makes it difficult to assess
the antigenicity of the vaccine. Phillip et al. (1973) used
the inability to halt the fall in maternal antibody titre as
a measure of the antigenicity of the vaccine. Considered in
this light, the vaccine we tested was unsatisfactory. But a
better assessment of antigenicity might result from a
consideration of the serological response in antibody-free
calves. In this trial, of the animals with no antibodies on
arrival at the farm, 93.3% and 77.2% of the animals became
positive to adenovirus 3 and IBR respectively following
vaccination but no animal responded to BVD antigen. Further,
only 10% and 46.2% of the susceptible control calves became
positive to adenovirus 3 and IBR respectively. These findings
are essentially in agreement with the results of Phillip et
al. (1973) in that some of the antigens in the vaccine produced
serum antibody in a variable proportion to the test animals.
Throughout the period of this trial, a classical outbreak of
respiratory disease was not observed. But the analysis of the
clinical observation revealed that between days 50 - 86 there
was a significant rise in respiration rates in both the
vaccinated and control groups. Similarly the increase in the
percentage of animals showing nasal discharge and coughing
coincided with this period. While the clinical parameters
recorded, especially nasal discharge and cough, showed large
fluctuations between sets of observations, the subjective bias
was reduced to minimum by the use of a standard and uniform
recording system. Respiration rate was less liable to be
affected by subjective bias and therefore was found to be the
most reliable index, and on the present evidence it appears
that this method of monitoring the disease was sensitive enough
to detect an outbreak of mild respiratory tract illness in both
groups of calves.

It was not possible to correlate the disease outbreak
with either the serological or bacteriological findings.
Bacteria and mycoplasma species isolated from both groups of
calves were identical. The possibility of a challenge due to

micro-organisms not under study in this trial cannot be discounted, but whatever the nature of the challenge there was no evidence that the vaccine provided any protection for the calves. This may have been due to a lack of antigenicity of the vaccine, challenge by a heterologous agent, or the inability of the vaccine to stimulate the appropriate type of antibody at the appropriate site.

In light of the present findings, we cannot but endorse the views of other investigators (Phillip et al., 1973; Thomas and Collins, 1974; Rossi and Kiesel, 1972) that this parenterally administered multicomponent inactivated virus vaccine has little place in the prevention of respiratory disease in calves at the present time. One of the major limiting factors of such a vaccine is its inability to stimulate specific antibody response in calves with passive immunity. Secondly, the recommendations of the vaccine manufacturers are based on the belief that a large proportion of the respiratory disease in calves is caused or initiated by one or a combination of the viruses represented in the vaccine. Recent research (Pirie, 1977) does not support this view and the rationale for the use of such a vaccine has been under attack (Thomas and Collins, 1974). Viruses may or may not be much less important in the aetiology of calf respiratory disease than was believed hitherto, but the use of inadequately proven preparations can only bring viral vaccines of this type into disrepute. This is to be deprecated in view of the fact that some vaccines may have a place in prevention of respiratory disease.

ACKNOWLEDGEMENTS

We thank the Bacteriology Department of the CVL and the Veterinary Investigation Centre, Wolverhampton for carrying out the bacteriology, and Mr. G. Wibberley for his technical assistance.

REFERENCES

Barr, J.M., McMillan, M.M., Jennings, A.R. and Kelly, W.R. 1951. Vet. Rec. 63, p. 652.

Curtis, P.E. 1970. Vet. Rec. 86, p. 454.

Coggins, L. 1964. Am. J. Vet. Res. 25, p. 103.

Darbyshire, J.H. and Pereira, H.G. 1964. Nature, 201, p. 895.

Dawson, P.S. 1964. Res. Vet. Sci. 5, p. 81.

Dawson, P.S. and Darbyshire, J.H. 1964. Vet. Rec. 76, p. 111.

Harbourne, J.F. 1966. Vet. Rec. 78, p. 749.

Hayflick, R. and Stanbridge, E. 1967. Ann. N.T. Acad. Sci. 143, p. 608.

Lamont, H.G. and Kerr, W.R. 1939. Vet. Rec. 51, p. 672.

Leech, F.B., Macrae, W.D. and Menzies, D.W. 1968. MAFF Animal Disease Surveys, report No. 5. HMSO, London.

Logan, E.F., Penhale, W.J. and Jones, R.A. 1973. Res. Vet. Sci. 14, p. 394.

Phillip, J.I.H., Clegg, F.G., Halliday, C.J., Cross, M.H., Hardy, R. and Maund, B.A. 1973. Vet. Rec. 92, p. 420.

Pirie, H.M. 1977. Vet. Rec. 101, p. 255.

Pritchard, D.G. and Macleod, N.S.M. 1977. Vet. Rec. 100, p. 126.

Roberts, D.H. and Pijoan, C. 1971. Br. Vet. J. 127, p. 582.

Rosen, L. and Abinanti, F.R. 1960. Am. J. Hyg. 71, p. 250.

Rossi, C.R. and Kiesel, G.K. 1972. Am. J. Vet. Res. 33, p. 2341.

Thomas, L.H. 1973. Vet. Rec. 93, p. 384.

Thomas, L.H. and Collins, A.P. 1974. Vet. Rec. 94, p. 506.

Thomas, L.H. and Stott, E.J. 1975. Res. Vet. Sci. 18, p. 227.

Tutt, J.B. 1941. Vet. Rec. 53, p. 84.

Watt, J.A.A. 1952. J. comp. Path. Ther. 62, p. 102.

VACCINATION AGAINST BOVINE ENZOOTIC PNEUMONIA

G. Wizigmann

Institute of Medical Microbiology, Infectious and Epidemic
Diseases of Animals, University of Munich, Federal Republic of
Germany.

ABSTRACT

A field trial was carried out with a new vaccine, developed on the
basis of different inactivated virus species (bovine adenoviruses types
1, 3 and 5, reoviruses types 1 and 3, parainfluenza-3 virus).

After 4 consecutive vaccination campaigns (1972-1976) results from
70 043 vaccinated cattle were evaluated.

The vaccine was safe and efficient. A decrease of morbidity from
72% to 6.8% and of mortality from 5.1 to 1% was observed in vaccinated
herds.

Following the results obtained from epidemiologic and pathogenetic investigations carried out by us in the Federal Republic of Germany, we have reached the conclusion that bovine enzootic pneumonia (BEP) is an infectious multifactorial disease. According to present knowledge, its primary cause is a virus infection, but non-microbial, resistance depressing factors are responsible for the conversion of the infection to a clinically manifested disease. The disease is complicated by bacterial infections.

Of particular significance amongst the various types of viruses involved are the adenoviruses (at least 8 serotypes) and the reoviruses (at least 3 serotypes); other viruses that are less involved are the parainfluenza 3 virus, rhinoviruses and the respiratory syncytial virus.

Taking these facts as a basis, we developed a vaccine against BEP. In doing so we took into consideration the fact that, while completely different viruses are responsible for the occurrence of BEP, certain viruses do without doubt dominate in the relation between infection and disease. For this reason the chosen method of vaccination is one using a combined vaccine. Due to immuno-biological as well as economical reasons, it is impossible to produce a combined vaccine that will give protection against all the viruses possibly involved in the BEP. One can, of course, produce a combination of some different immunising antigens without losing effectiveness, but after a certain number has been reached individual antigens begin to lose their effectiveness. One must also keep in mind the economy factor since a vaccine with more than a certain number of antigens would be too expensive.

In view of the above factors and also our epidemiological and pathogenetic investigations during the last few years, we have developed a combined vaccine which has 6 different viruses, namely bovine adenoviruses of the serotypes 1, 3 and 5, reoviruses of the serotypes 1 and 3 as well as parainfluenza 3 virus. We decided to give precedence to a vaccine produced from inactivated viruses which is even more harmless than a living vaccine.

In order to produce the vaccine the viruses were multiplied in tissue cultures, inactivated, mixed and adjuvants were added. The safety and potency of the vaccine were checked in pre-trials. The vaccine proved itself to be safe and effective in regard to the stimulation of formation of specific antibodies.

Furthermore, this combined vaccine has been used in 4 field trials over a period of 4 successive years, in so-called 'problem-herds', which means such farms, in which BEP appeared during the autumn and winter months before the vaccination campaign.

The animals that were inoculated were from 5 weeks to 18 months of age; the average age being 6 months. The inoculation of the animals was carried out during the months of August, September and October; inoculation took place twice with an interval of 4 to 6 weeks. Each time 5 ml of the vaccine was inoculated subcutaneously.

The evaluation of the vaccination results was based on clinical observations made during the time between the second inoculation and the 15th of April in the following year. In addition to this, every veterinary practitioner who took part in the vaccination programme completed a report for each animal involved. As well as questions about the stage of health before and after the vaccination, the report also included questions about the husbandry and management conditions. Moreover the practitioners and the animal owners were asked for their subjective views on the effectiveness of the vaccination.

The number of the practitioner zones included in the 4 vaccination campaigns were 36 (1972/73), 39 (1973/74), 94 (1974/75 and 1975/76) respectively. In all, the results of the vaccination of 70 043 cattle have been evaluated (Table 1).

The number of vaccinated animals and herds was lowest during the first campaign (3 515 animals in 146 herds), and highest during the last campaign (34 328 animals in 1 602 herds).

Fifty five thousand six hundred and thirty six (79.4%) of animals vaccinated during the 4 campaigns stayed completely healthy and 9 648 (13.8%) of the animals developed coughs but showed no signs of feverish illness. Only 4 759 animals (6.8%) developed a typical bovine enzootic pneumonia illness and 1% of the inoculated animals died or had to be slaughtered in emergency.

In order to give critical judgment on the results of the vaccination, the following facts must be taken into consideration:

a) All the vaccinated and evaluated animals came from 'problem-herds'. In such herds the average morbidity rate from BEP is from 50% to 100% (average rate 72%), and the mortality rate is up to 15% (average rate 5.1%).

b) Other than the vaccination no prophylactic measures were taken in these farms.

Following vaccination with our vaccine

the number of farms suffering from BEP decreased from 100% to 32%,

the rate of morbidity from BEP decreased from 72% to 6.8%,

the rate of mortality from BEP decreased from 5.1% to 1.0% which means a reduction of 82% in the number of deaths.

Eighty six per cent to 89% of the farmers were satisfied with the success of the vaccination, and in 89% to 94% of the farms the practitioners evaluated the effectiveness

TABLE 1

VACCINATION AGAINST BOVINE ENZOOTIC PNEUMONIA: RESULTS OF FIELD EXPERIMENTS 1972 - 1976.

Herds and animals	Year of vaccination				Total
	1972/73	1973/74	1974/75	1975/76	
Number of vaccinated herds	146	378	1 110	1 602	
Number of vaccinated animals	3 515 (100.0%)	8 708 (100.0%)	23 492 (100.0%)	34 328 (100.0%)	70 043 (100.0%)
a) healthy	2 806 (79.8%)	7 080 (81.3%)	19 053 (81.1%)	26 697 (77.8%)	55 636 (79.4%)
b) cough only	386 (11.0%)	987 (11.3%)	2 810 (12.0%)	5 465 (15.9%)	9 648 (13.8%)
c) bov. enzoot. pneum.	323 (9.2%)	641 (7.4%)	1 629 (6.9%)	2 166 (6.3%)	4 759 (6.8%)
d) fatal cases	47 (1.3%)	101 (1.2%)	190 (0.8%)	352 (1.0%)	690 (1.0%)

of the vaccine as 'very good' or 'good'.

Our results from the field trials show that, in
principle, it is possible to give prophylactic protection
against bovine enzootic pneumonia using a combined vaccine
based on inactivated 'leading viruses'.

On account of the good results achieved in the field
trials, the vaccine has been commercially produced in the
Federal Republic of Germany since mid 1976.

One should not, however, forget that bovine enzootic
pneumonia is a multi-factorial disease. A significant
prophylaxis should, therefore, not merely be limited to
vaccination. Only an optimal combination of complementary and
mutually supporting measures will lead to an effective, lasting
and complete success.

REFERENCES

Wizigmann, G. 1974. Zbl. Met. Med. B. 21, p. 563.
Wizigmann, G., Dirksen, G., Sandersleben, J.V., Geisel, O., Held, T. and
    Mayr, A. 1976. Tierztl. Umsch. 31, p. 343.

EXPERIMENTAL ASSESSMENT OF PARAINFLUENZA TYPE 3 VIRUS VACCINES

P.W. Wells, J.M. Sharp and W.D. Smith

Animal Disease Research Association, Moredun Institute,
408 Gilmerton Road, Edinburgh, Scotland.

ABSTRACT

In studying the means of assessing efficacy of vaccination against parainfluenza type 3 (PI$_3$) virus infection of the ruminant respiratory tract, experimental models have been developed in specific pathogen free (SPF) lambs. Exposure of SPF lambs to an aerosol of PI$_3$ virus has been shown to result in the mild clinical signs of a transient nasal discharge which was observed in lambs excreting virus. Protection against the clinical signs and virus excretion due to this challenge was obtained by prior intranasal instillation or intramuscular injection of live PI$_3$ virus. Prior administration of inactivated PI$_3$ virus by the same routes was not effective. However, it was shown that if the inactivated PI$_3$ virus antigen was incorporated in adjuvant and given intramuscularly, protection could be achieved.

Clinical illness and histopathological changes in the lungs associated with challenge infection when PI$_3$ virus was given by both the intratracheal and intranasal routes was also prevented by intramuscular vaccination with inactivated PI$_3$ virus in adjuvant. Clinical signs following this challenge in unvaccinated SPF lambs were marked consisting of pyrexia, anorexia, dyspnoea and tachypnoea.

The more recent development of a means of reproducing pneumonic pasteurellosis in SPF lambs by combined infection with PI$_3$ virus and Pasteurella haemolytica has enabled further assessment of the efficacy of intramuscular vaccination with inactivated PI$_3$ virus in adjuvant to be determined. In this challenge system vaccination against PI$_3$ virus prevented the development of clinical signs associated with the PI$_3$ virus infection and significantly reduced the extent and severity of pathological lesions in the lungs due to the super-infection with Paseteurella haemolytica. It is suggested that findings in these experiments may be applied in the assessment and development of effective vaccines of PI$_3$ virus for use in cattle.

In cattle and sheep respiratory infection with para-influenza type 3 (PI3) virus is not usually associated with severe illness and more often is not detected clinically. Consequently experimental assessment of the efficacy of vaccines to PI3 virus infections in these species has depended upon the quantitative assay of virus replication in the nasopharynx (Gilmour et al., 1968; McKercher et al., 1972). However in such experiments as in field trials, conventionally reared animals have been used and the possibility of prior infection during the course of the study could not be excluded. The availability of hysterectomy-derived colostrum-deprived specific pathogen-free (SPF) lambs (Hart et al., 1971) at the Moredun Institute enabled the investigation of immunity to PI3 virus under controlled isolation conditions (Smith, 1975). These experiments were initiated both because of the possible importance of PI3 virus as a pathogen in sheep and since it was thought likely that the results might be applicable to the development of effective vaccines for use in cattle. The purpose of this paper is to review the experimental challenge systems which have been developed for the assessment of in-activated vaccines of PI3 virus in sheep in the hope that these methods may prove to have application in similar studies in cattle.

Vaccination-challenge experiments were carried out in which SPF lambs were inoculated with live or formalin-inactivated PI3 virus by intramuscular injection or intranasal instillation. Intranasal administration of live PI3 virus resulted in a slight transient nasal discharge and stimulated comparable serum but higher nasal secretion antibody titres than did the same concentration of live virus given intramuscularly. There were no obvious clinical signs following the intramuscular injection of the live virus. Inactivated virus given by either route failed to stimulate nasal secretion antibody and resulted in low or undetectable titres of antibody in the serum. Immunity to challenge was assessed by exposure of the lambs to an aerosol of PI3 virus 2 weeks later. Exposure of both the vaccinated and control SPF lambs to an aerosol of PI3 virus failed to result in any distinct signs of clinical disease and the criterion of protection was a reduction of magnitude and duration of virus excretion from the nasopharynx. On this basis, live virus given either intranasally or intramuscularly was protective. Further experiments indicated that the intramuscular injection of inactivated PI3 virus incorporated in Freund's complete adjuvant resulted in an immune response which protected against a similar challenge. The nasal secretion antibody involved in this response was shown to be of the IgG class as compared to IgA antibody which results from intranasal inoculation with live virus (Smith et al., 1975; Smith et al., 1976).

The ovine G2 strain of PI3 virus isolated by Hore (1966) and used in these experiments had been shown to be capable of inducing clinical respiratory disease and pneumonia when given by the combined intratracheal and intranasal routes in newborn lambs (Hore and Stevenson, 1967). A further experimental assessment of an inactivated vaccine of PI3 was carried out using these routes of infection in SPF lambs (Wells et al., 1976). SPF lambs were vaccinated at 10 days of age by intramuscular injection of formalin-inactivated PI3 virus and double-stranded RNA (ds RNA*) emulsified in Bayol F containing 20% Falba (FA). Twenty-five days after vaccination, vaccinated and control SPF lambs were challenged with a total of $10^{8.5}$ TCID 50 of PI3 virus given intratracheally and intranasally. Vaccinated lambs showed a transient febrile response within a few hours of challenge which has been attributed to an immediate-type hypersensitivity reaction associated with some constituent of the tissue culture fluid similar to that observed in previous experiments (Smith, 1975). Apart from some hyperpnoea during this response the lambs were clinically normal and by the third day after challenge when the unvaccinated lambs exhibited marked clinical signs of tachypnoea, dyspnoea, anorexia and dullness, they were completely normal.

* BRL 5907 Beecham Research Laboratories, Brockham Park, Betchworth, Surrey, England.

The clinical signs in the unvaccinated lambs intensified to the sixth day after challenge thereafter regressing. The degree of clinical illness appeared greater than had been described previously (Hore and Stevenson, 1967) and may have been due to the greater concentration of virus or the larger volume of infective tissue culture fluid inoculated. Virus could be isolated from the control group for up to 7 days after infection whereas virus excretion in the vaccinated lambs was restricted almost entirely to the first 2 days after challenge. At necropsy 10 days following infection, no differences were evident between the macroscopic appearance of lungs from vaccinates and controls. It is probable that the bronchiolar and alveolar exudate associated with the clinical signs by Stevenson (1968) had resolved in the control lambs by the time of necropsy.

In these experiments it was established that inactivated PI3 virus vaccines given by intramuscular injection are effective in stimulating serological responses and in conferring protection against challenge infection (Smith, 1975; Wells et al., 1976). With the development of a means of reproducing ovine enzootic pneumonia by combined infection of SPF lambs with PI3 virus and *Pasteurella haemolytica* (Sharp et al., 1978), the opportunity arose to examine the effect of vaccination against the virus component of this combined challenge system (Wells et al., 1978). Infection of SPF lambs by intratracheal and intranasal inoculation with PI3 virus enhances the effect of exposure to an aerosol of *Pasteurella haemolytica* 7 days later. The results of this challenge is marked clinical respiratory illness in over 90% of lambs with pneumonic lesions obvious at necropsy which are typical of natural infection with *Pasteurella haemolytica* (Rushton et al., in preparation).

SPF lambs were vaccinated intramuscularly at 10 days of age with either formalin-inactivated PI3 virus emulsified in IFA or a formalin-inactivated PI3 virus with ds RNA emulsified in IFA. Eight weeks after vaccination lambs were infected by intratracheal and intranasal inoculation with PI3 virus and 7

days later they were exposed to an aerosol of *Pasteurella haemolytica*
biotype A, serotypes 1 and 2 (Gilmour et al., 1975). Lambs
were examined clinically for a period of 2 weeks after inoculation
with PI3 virus and during this time the clinician was unaware
of the identities of the groups. Lambs were awarded a daily
score depending upon their clinical condition. Any lamb
showing severe respiratory disease and considered unlikely to
recover was euthanised. Both groups of vaccinates responded
serologically and were clinically protected against the effects
of infection with PI3 virus. By comparison virus replication
was observed in the nasopharynx of control lambs which exhibited
a febrile response accompanied by tachypnoea, dyspnoea,
anorexia and dullness. After exposure to the aerosol of
Pasteurella haemolytica respiratory illness was observed in
vaccinated and unvaccinated lambs but whereas 9 of 11
unvaccinated lambs died, only 5 of 11 or 2 of 11 died in the
groups vaccinated with either PI3 virus and ds RNA in IFA or
PI3 virus in IFA respectively. As regards clinical assessment,
a statistically significant difference was observed only between
the group given PI3 virus in IFA and the control group.

Examination of lambs at necropsy revealed macroscopic
and microscopic lesions associated with *Pasteurella haemolytica*
infection. The extent of macroscopic lesions estimated by
making lung diagrams and measuring planimetrically the surface
area involved, was significantly less extensive both in the
group receiving IFA vaccine ($p < 0.01$) and in the group receiving
vaccine containing ds RNA in IFA ($p < 0.02$) than in controls.
Clearly, the inactivated vaccines of PI3 virus had prevented
clinical illness attributable to the virus infection and had,
in part, protected against the effects of super-infection with
Pasteurella haemolytica. While this experiment does not suggest
that vaccines of PI3 virus may be of value in the prevention
of naturally occurring pneumonic pasteurellosis in sheep, it
substantiates the previous results which have shown the
efficacy of inactivated vaccines of PI3. It is probably that
a similar vaccine might be useful in cattle and the challenge
methods described could be employed in the investigation of
its worth in preventing bovine respiratory disease associated
with PI3 virus.

520

REFERENCES

Gilmour, N.J.L., Drysdale, A., Stevenson, R.G., Hore, D.E. and Brotherston,
     J.G. 1968. J. Comp. Path. 78, p. 463.
Gilmour, N.J.L., Thompson, D.A., Smith, W.D. and Angus, K. 1975. Res.
     Vet. Sci. 18, p. 340.
Hart, R., Mackay, J.M.K., McVittie, C.R. and Mellor, D.J. 1971. Br. Vet.
     J. 127, p. 419.
Hore, D.E. 1966. Vet. Rec. 79, p. 466.
Hore, D.E. and Stevenson, R.G. 1967. Vet. Rec. 86, p. 26.
McKercher, D.G., Saito, J.F., Franti, C.E., Wada, E.M. and Crenshaw, G.L.
     1972. Am. J. Vet. Res. 33, p. 721.
Rushton, B., Sharp, J.M., Gilmour, N.J.L. and Thompson, D.A. (In preparation).
Sharp, J.M., Gilmour, N.J.L., Thompson, D.A. and Rushton, B. 1978. J.
     Comp. Path. (In press).
Smith, W.D. 1975. Res. Vet. Sci. 19, p. 56.
Smith, W.D., Wells, P.W., Burrells, C. and Dawson, A. McL. 1975. Arch.
     Virol. 49, p. 329.
Smith, W.D., Dawson, A. McL., Wells, P.W. and Burrells, C. 1976. Res. Vet.
     Sci, 21, p. 341.
Stevenson, R.G. 1968. Ph. D. Thesis, University of Edinburgh.
Wells, P.W., Sharp, J.M., Burrells, C., Rushton, B. and Smith, W.D. 1976.
     J. Hyg. Camb. 77, p. 255.
Wells, P.W., Sharp, J.M., Rushton, B., Gilmour, N.J.L., and Thompson, D.A.
     1978. J. comp. Path. (In press).

ENZOOTIC BRONCHOPNEUMONIA IN YOUNG CATTLE, A CONSTANT CHALLENGE TO THE CLINICIAN

H.J. Breukink

Faculteit voor Diergeneeskunde R.U. Vakgroep Inwendige Ziekten Grote Huisdieren, 'De Uithof', Yalelaan 10, Utrecht, Netherlands.

ABSTRACT

A general discussion is given about the problems a clinician is faced with regarding a vaccination programme for enzootic bronchitis and bronchopneumonia. The clinician must make decisions about vaccination while he cannot predict the occurrence of the disease nor the safety or efficacy of the programme. He has difficulties in the clinical diagnosis and it is difficult to obtain undisputed facts. The available information is often confusing not just because it is extensive. There is a need for continous education of the clinician to provide him with the proper knowledge so he can accept the responsibility for vaccination programmes.

INTRODUCTION

Enzootic bronchitis and bronchopneumonia has become a very
important disease among the younger cattle (between 3 and 14
months old) in the Netherlands during the last decade. An
increase in the size of the herds resulting in overcrowding and
inadequate housing, an increase in shipment and an increase in
import from other countries have been important factors in this
respect. Meanwhile we faced all kinds of virus infections, some
of which were completely new to us.

One new type, the so-called 'pinkengriep' seemed to have
started in the eastern parts of the country, while in 1972 the
first case of an infectious bovine rhinotracheitis (IBR)
infection was recognised in the west. Since then apparently
both virus infections have spread over the country causing
serious losses due to death or to a decreased production or
growth rate. Besides IBR and BRS, several other types of virus
have been isolated from cases of enzootic bronchitis. I would
like to discuss the difficulties the clinician is faced with
when a farmer urgently requests preventive measures.

DIAGNOSTIC PROBLEMS

Before one can decide upon the possibility of the use of
certain vaccines one has to consider several facts. Firstly,
as indicated before the enzootic bronchopneumonia is a
polyfactorial disease. Even if we are able to vaccinate against
all the possible types of virus involved, bronchopneumonia could
not be eradicated completely. A very important decrease in the
incidence, however, is possible. Numerous viruses may be
involved but the most important ones seem to be IBR, bovine
virus diarrhoea (BVD), bovine respiratory syncytial virus (BRS),
and parainfluenza type 3 virus (PI3) and fortunately effective
vaccines are available against at least three of them.

Although thorough examination may give some indication one
is never completely sure about the type of virus involved. Only

a few signs of some specific lesions are pathognomonic.

After exclusion of a lungworm infection, especially in younger calves (3 - 5 months), four possible virus infections have to be considered. A lungworm infection, however, can also be complicated by a virus infection.

Signs such as upper respiratory dyspnoea or mouth breathing due to blockage of the upper airways, indicating IBR, severe depression (BVD, BRS), decreased appetite (BVD, IBR), increased respiration rate (highest in BRS), frequent coughing (BRS), abdominal expiration (BRS), excessive salivation (BVD), lesions in the mucous membranes of the mouth (BVD), and the nose (IBR), and pneumonia (BVD, BRS) are important for the clinical differential diagnosis.

The examination of several individuals in a diseased herd is important in order to get a good impression of the clinical picture.

In older calves and yearlings (4 - 14 months) mostly three types of virus can be involved IBR, BRS and PI3 indicating that age differences do exist. Also the season can be of help in the diagnosis, BRS infections occur mostly in the fall and sometimes in the spring, whereas IBR infections occur mainly in the winter. Fatal cases may show characteristic lesions at necropsy especially in infections with IBR, BVD and BRS.

Laboratory confirmation of the suspected infection is very important but the collection of paired serum samples is often difficult and needs adequate registration and planning. This method is time consuming even more so when the laboratories cannot handle large amounts of sera.

VACCINATION PROBLEMS

The clinician faced with the request for preventive measures is provided with a large amount of information about

close contact with pregnant cattle because they may shed vaccine
virus that subsequently can cause abortion in pregnant cattle.
However the duration of the immunity seems to last a lifetime
if the vaccination is administered after colostral immunity
has gone.

Post-vaccination problems other than abortions are rare.
Reactivation of the vaccine virus under stress however may cause
serious problems. The intranasal IBR vaccines, mostly
temperature sensitive (TS) mutants, can be used in the presence
of pregnant cattle and produce a rapid production of interferon.
For the latter reason it has been used as what is called
'treatment' when the first signs of IBR appeared. Vaccination
is a stressor itself and when the diagnosis is not correct
it may aggravate the disease. After vaccination with intranasal IBR vaccines the immunity seems to last only for a short
time. Field experiences indicate that new infections can appear
after a period of not more than 6 months, although manufacturers
recommend only annual vaccination.

Inactivated IBR vaccines should also be repeated annually,
but post-vaccination shed of virus does not occur. There are
reports on fatal hypersensitive reactions or urticaria that
occurred after vaccination with these types of vaccine. If
vaccination of young calves is considered, it is necessary to
know the immunologic status of the animal. Colostral acquired
passive immunity may interfere with successful immunisation but
not all calves get maternal immunity and in individual calves
the duration of this maternal immunity varies.

When calves are vaccinated in the presence of maternal
immunity, a revaccination will be required but the necessary
interval can hardly be predicted.

The advice given by the Dutch National Animal Health
Committee not to vaccinate in closed herds, leaves out the
fact that IBR virus is as ubiquitous as BVD and PI3.

the vaccines provided by the various manufacturers. This
information is often confusing and it is difficult to appreciate
each vaccine objectively. Nevertheless the availability of all
kinds of vaccines, monovalent or polyvalent, stimulates their
use without careful consideration of the circumstances. This
may produce disappointing results endangering a good relationship between clinician and farmer.

The Dutch National Animal Health Committee and research
institutions have warned against the uncontrolled use of
vaccines and have published vaccination programmes adjusted
for each particular form of cattle industry. However, even
these recommendations are sometimes in conflict with the
available information and after all still need adjustment
according to the herd involved.

Regarding the problems with BRS infections, a vaccine is
being tested in the field. This experiment is still in progress
and the results will be available soon.

It has been stated that because of the presence of humoral
antibodies against PI3 in the adult cattle in the Netherlands,
vaccination against this virus seemed useless, but there is no
solid relationship between humoral antibodies and protection.
PI3 vaccines for the same reason give only temporary protection
and one needs regular revaccination.

BVD vaccines are not used regularly in the Netherlands
although they are available. The BVD vaccine is a modified
live virus (MLV) vaccine and may be used in the prevention of
enzootic bronchopneumonia in younger calves. However BVD
vaccines occasionally cause serious troubles especially in combined
vaccines. Such an experience results in a loss of faith in the
use of vaccines.

Now special attention is directed to the use of IBR vaccines
where three types of vaccines are available. The intramuscular
MLV vaccine cannot be used when the vaccinated calves are in

There are certain general considerations that have to be made regarding a vaccination programme. The clinician has to discuss the object of the programme with the owner and has to admit that he cannot predict the safety or efficacy of the programme.

CONCLUSION

In conclusion there is a great need for continous education of the clinician to provide him with the proper knowledge to handle the available vaccines. This should be done by both manufacturers and research workers interested in the control of bovine enzootic bronchopneumonia using vaccination concepts.

DISCUSSION

E. van Opdenbosch *(Belgium)*

I would like to make some comments on the paper by Dr. van Nieuwstadt on behalf of Dr. Wellermans. We agree with some of your results with the RS virus vaccine tests. We have also seen a virus excretion when a natural infection occurred in vaccinated animals and a slight seroconversion after vaccination, so our vaccines do not protect 100% serologically. Nevertheless, up to now our vaccine protected all vaccinated animals against the symptoms of RS virus and this arose under severe field circumstances. We have never seen a case of emphysema nor a case of mortality due to RS virus after vaccination.

As a proof of the effectiveness of our vaccine, we can say this: in an agronomic centre we had 100 animals last year, of which 25 were vaccinated once, 25 were vaccinated twice and 50 were not vaccinated. After the vaccination we had the good fortune to have a natural infection with the following consequences: the animals which were vaccinated twice showed no symptoms. Some of the animals which were vaccinated only once showed slight hypothermia after some time, and one animal died after chronic respiratory troubles. Of the 50 unvaccinated animals, 32 showed the symptoms of RS virus and twelve died, in which RS virus was diagnosed.

In consequence of this outbreak, all the animals on this farm - the vaccinated as well as the unvaccinated - had a positive seroconversion.

It has to be said that our present vaccine contains $10^{5.7}$ infectious doses of tissue culture (IDTC) as compared to $10^{4.35}$ which was used by Dr. van Nieuwstadt. This year we have vaccinated about 50 000 animals from farms which are affected with RS virus yearly. Up until now we have not had one case of mortality or emphysema due to RS virus after vaccination.

The natural RS virus infection in young cattle seems to give protection against the symptoms of RS virus for the rest of their lives. We have never seen RS virus symptoms after the age of 9 months, and in farms where the RS virus occurred every year only the young animals under 9 months showed symptoms, while the older animals reacted only serologically.

We have the following results with the RS virus vaccine. The suppression of clinical symptoms, but not necessarily the absence of seroconversions.

I would like to ask two questions. Are you quite sure that the vaccine you obtained was not contaminated by another agent, or even with the wild RS virus strain, or changed by manipulating in the industry, or in the laboratory, as we know that you have done at least one passage on fibroblast cell culture before using the vaccine in your tests. Furthermore, can you give proof that you are 100% certain that the symptoms which you saw in the vaccinated as well as the unvaccinated animals were really due to RS virus infection? Did you do a direct immunofluorescence test on ultra-thin sections of the lung of animals with symptoms? Did you have one case of mortality of emphysema in the vaccinated as well as the non-vaccinated animals?

We think that our criteria for considering the value of the Wellermans vaccine are more realistic - the prevention, in all the annually-affected farms, of all troubles due to RS virus, as there is 80% of emphysema and 30% mortality in those beef producing farms.

A. van Nieuwstadt (Netherlands)

The vaccine we used came directly from the industrial manufacturers. It was not manipulated in our laboratory. If it was contaminated it was contaminated by the industrial people.

D.R. Snodgrass (UK)

Dr. Harkness, how many doses of the vaccine mentioned in your paper are sold annually in Britain?

J. Harkness *(UK)*

    I cannot give you a figure. It is a substantial number.

J.B. McFerran *(UK)*

    It is generally accepted that this vaccine is not of much value. This is not actually true. If you use it on cattle destined for export it is of considerable value in terms of turning them down on the IBR serology..!

A. Andrews *(UK)*

    I have just been looking at your respiratory data. I notice that your actual increase in respiration rates was at the time you changed the calves' housing. Is that correct? You say that they are in housing for the first 8 weeks. You start your rise round about that time.

J. Harkness

    Yes.

A. Andrews

    Perhaps I am wrong. I was just wondering if there were other factors involved besides an actual agent.

O.C. Straub *(West Germany)*

    We have tested the same vaccine in our country and we have published what we have found as far as IBR is concerned. We found the seroconversion in all of them, but we had to lower the amount of tissue culture effective doses in order even to detect a rise in the antibody titre. We also found that, after the second vaccination, after the 5th week the antibody titres began to go down. Perhaps I should translate the last sentence. We said that it is quite obvious that the vaccine protection does not last for any length of time, because 12 animals which had shown the production of the virus neutralising antibodies had a decrease in titre after the 5th week after the second vaccination. This could only be found because only 10 $TCID_{50}$ were used in neutralisation tests. When these results are compared to other results where 100 $TCID_{50}$ were used, we have to

suppose that animals vaccinated with this vaccine do not become sick when they come into contact with the field virus, but
the virus will be propagated on the mucus membranes of the upper
respiratory tract, and therefore there is a very real danger that
this virus will be spread by animals vaccinated in this way.
Therefore this vaccine should only be used in cattle in feedlot
situations.

H.M. Pirie *(UK)*

You mentioned that *Mycoplasma bovirhinis* started in one calf
and spread. Was there any correlation between the spread of
that organism and the increasing course of virus isolation from
nasal discharges? It seems to go up in about 60 days.

J. Harkness

There is still some work to do. I would have to consult the
other people involved in the trial. I doubt if there was much.

C. Howard

Dr. Wizigmann, did I hear you correctly when you said that
you had no control animals?

G. Wizigmann *(West Germany)*

No, we have not presented any controls. On some farms we
had controls. I should mention that if I make such a field
experiment, at least in our country, it is very difficult to
convince the farmer that it is a good idea to immunise or
vaccinate half of the herd.

The second thing is that, in this special disease called
'pinkengriep', we know that farms which are affected are always
the same every wintertime. This means that the problems are
always on the same farms every year. Therefore I do not think
it is necessary, in this special case, to use some controls as
you mentioned.

The third thing - and I think it is very important - is
that if I have maybe 100 animals and I vaccinate 50 of them

(and there is always some infection present on such farms caused by different viruses) I know that these 50 vaccinated animals, as well as the unvaccinated animals, are in very great danger because every immunity always has an equilibrium point between not only quality but also the quantity of the infectious agents involved, or which are present on the farms.

J.M. Sharp *(UK)*

You presented your data as block figures - 70 000 animals at the end of the day. If you have the figures I wondered whether you could break it down into individual farms. How many farms showed an improvement and how many did not? Was it perhaps 10% which did not?

G. Wizigmann

One hundred percent of the farms were problem farms, with pulmonary bronchopneumonia and on estimation I had only 32% of farms with some cases of bronchopneumonia. This means that 68% of the farms remained completely without bronchopneumonia problems.

J.M. Sharp

That means that 32% continued to have the bronchopneumonia...

G. Wizigmann

Yes, with some animals. In total there were 6.8% of diseased animals.

J.T. Stamp *(UK)*

I think that Dr. Sharp is referring to the percentage on the affected farms.

G. Wizigmann

We know that the number of different viruses possibly involved in the bronchopneumonias is 17 different species and serotypes of viruses. We incorporated 6 of these in our vaccines. With such a vaccine it is logically impossible to protect 100%

of the animals. Although it is theoretically possible to make a vaccine with 15 antigens, I think such a vaccine would be so expensive that no one would use it. Therefore we incorporated 6 antigens which we know would cover the most important and most prevalent viruses involved in the disease.

J.M. Sharp

I think it is rather important, then, in the 32% of farms on which there was no improvement, to know whether you have done any virological or serological studies?

G. Wizigmann

Partially, but not all. That is impossible. I have never found any infection with a virus which was incorporated in the vaccine. I have found, for instance, other adenovirus sero-types, and rhinoviruses as well. I have found respiratory syncytial virus three times.

H. Frerking (West Germany)

I think it is very interesting to hear a little about the situation in Bavaria. Is this only in one district of Bavaria or was it spread all over Bavaria? Was it the typical kind of farming?

G. Wizigmann

All kinds of farms were involved. There were beef fattening farms, calf fattening farms, breeding farms and so on. The vaccine was evaluated over the whole of Bavaria, but we have three regions where the disease mainly occurs. We tested the vaccine especially in these regions.

J.T. Stamp (UK)

My own feeling about Dr. Breukink's paper is that this conference has certainly not been wasted, if for one reason only. For the first time in my life I have heard a clinician say he needed continued education and was asking for proper knowledge! We can all go back to our labs quite content that at least one clinician is going to listen to what we have to say...

G. Wizigmann

You spoke about a type of vaccine. I think the first question should be which viruses are involved in the disease, and which type of virus vaccines can be produced and used. I am convinced that we have great differences in respect of the involvement of the species of viruses between countries. For instance in Belgium we heard that there is a great incidence of respiratory syncytial virus. But in Bavaria it is not often involved in disease. Therefore, if I want to use a vaccine, I have to incorporate the appropriate antigens. I think that is most important.

H.J. Breukink *(Netherlands)*

In Holland we can get, if we wish, any vaccine which is available anywhere. So they pour in vaccines from all possible countries. Any manufacturer who makes vaccines pours them into Holland. The clinician is faced with the problem of what to use, or even whether to use them, and he has to have the right answers. He is faced with what the economical value will be, and if it is worth while using them afterwards. This is where the clinician loses faith in everything - even in Science!

J.T. Stamp

Do you not have a Commission which examines the vaccines coming in, and looks at their credentials before they are marketed, as we have in the UK for instance?

H.J. Breukink

Practically speaking we can use any kind of vaccine we want.

J.T. Stamp

So you have Government permission?

H.J. Breukink

This does not come only from the official sources - it can come from the other way round.

N.J.L. Gilmour (UK)

Could I make a plea for people not to throw out the bacterial component of the multifactorial side completely. I can see the difficulties in the preparation of a suitable virus vaccine for all circumstances, but as the disease is multifactorial, and as one of the components is bacterial, it would seem to be useful to see if you can protect against the bacterial component of the disease as well as the viral. I think that the same applies to mycoplasma and the chlamydia, if these are shown to be important.

SESSION 6B

APPLICATION OF RESEARCH AND FUTURE DEVELOPMENTS

APPLICATION OF RESEARCH AND FUTURE DEVELOPMENTS

J.B. McFerran, D.G. Bryson and M.S. McNulty
Veterinary Research Laboratories, Stormont, Belfast,
Northern Ireland.

ABSTRACT

The parameters associated with rapid and accurate diagnosis of viral infections of the bovine respiratory tract are discussed. It is concluded that immunofluorescent staining of epithelial cells obtained from mucus samples is probably the best diagnostic method.

The viruses associated with respiratory disease are considered. Infectious bovine rhinotracheitis virus, respiratory syncytial virus, parainfluenza virus 3 and adenoviruses are probably the most important aetiologically, but the involvement of other viruses such as bovine viral diarrhoea virus and the picornaviruses cannot be disregarded.

It is suggested that, at present, the use of vaccines provides the only adequate method of controlling respiratory disease. Vaccines must stimulate both local and cell-mediated immunity to be effective. Vaccines based on temperature-sensitive mutants and given intranasally on multiple occasions appear to meet the requirements best.

Over recent years, two trends have become apparent. The first is the increase in the value of cattle and the second is the growth of specialised units, so that the veterinarian is likely to be confronted with outbreaks of respiratory disease involving large numbers of very valuable animals. It is therefore essential that a rapid and correct diagnosis be made. Accurate diagnosis is required on two grounds. Firstly, it may enable rational treatment to be undertaken; the day of the specific viral inhibitor may be approaching. Secondly, it is essential that the current organisms causing disease be identified and the appropriate vaccines used. Current is stressed because in human medicine it is well established that different organisms can cause epidemics in different years and it is unlikely that the bovine field differs. After all the life span of cattle is usually under 3 years and in many cases animals reared in virtual isolation (small or closed herds) are concentrated into feed lots - ie the animal equivalent of army camps or schools.

This communication is limited mainly to virus infections, with special emphasis on the situation experienced in Northern Ireland. Infectious bovine rhinotracheitis does not occur as an important respiratory disease problem. The main respiratory disease problem is pneumonia in housed dairy calves and in intensively reared beef calves in their first period indoors in the autumn or winter. Following a sudden onset, probably due to virus infection, the respiratory signs persist for weeks or months punctuated by periodic exacerbations or 'flare ups'. As well as viruses, Mycoplasma species and Pasteurella species appear to have an important role.

The identification of the micro-organism associated with the acute phase will first be discussed because it is in this area that some of the more important future developments lie. Also from our experience with a very similar situation in poultry, most of the other problems were resolved once the viruses causing the initial infection (eg infectious bronchitis and Newcastle disease) were either eliminated or controlled by

adequate vaccination. Determining the aetiology of
respiratory disease in bovines is not however easy. Often the
acute phase is over before laboratory help is sought. Therefore
as well as those clinically ill, other animals on the farm
(preferably in-contacts) should also be sampled in case they
are in the incubatory stages of the disease.

Many methods have been described for collecting specimens
from living animals. The traditional swab has many disadvantages - it is too short, it is liable to break, it does
not collect enough material and it may be toxic (Hanson and
Schipper, 1976). Various methods have been suggested to overcome these problems. Nasal washings with large volumes of
media are technically difficult; gauze fixed to flexible wire,
tampons (McKercher et al., 1973) and bristle brushes (Thomas
and Stott, 1975) all have their advocates. However large
samples of mucus are advantageous and therefore some form of
mucus sampler is desirable. The mechanical device described
by Baskerville and Lloyd (1977) is satisfactory for this
purpose.

Whilst many viruses, eg adenoviruses, are resistant to
transport and storage, other respiratory viruses, eg respiratory
syncytial, are labile. Because of this it has been advocated
that the specimen should not be frozen (Hambling, 1964) and
some claim it is much better to take the cells to the animal
and inoculate the nasal washings or mucus directly onto the
cells.

The choice of substrate is also important. Primary cells
suffer from the possible presence of latent viruses and variable
sensitivity. Established cell lines, eg MDBK, are in general
not sensitive. Therefore the best choice appears to be diploid
cell lines. These can be prepared from foetal tissue (eg
foetal calf lung) and once established (ie taken to about 14
passes or so), then adequately tested for latent viruses and
sensitivity. The most commonly found latent viruses have
been bovine virus diarrhoea and bovine syncytial viruses. Serum

also can pose difficulties and even foetal calf serum,
supposedly free of globulin, has on occasion been shown to
possess specific antibody to one or more viruses.

Because of the difficulties in isolation and also because
of the long time lag required for isolation, other techniques
have been investigated.

The first is the use of direct electron microscopy.
Whilst we have found EM most useful in identifying viruses once
isolated in cell cultures (McFerran et al., 1971), initial
attempts at direct identification of viruses in nasal swabs
have not been successful although some workers have described
this technique for identifying paramyxoviral (Doane et al.,
1967) influenza and respiratory syncytial viral (Joncas et
al., 1969) infections of man. Recent work on lysis of the
cells deposited from mucus samples, however, appears promising
but must await further evaluation.

The second, and by far the most promising, is the use of
immunofluorescence (IF) on material taken directly from the
animal. Nasopharyngeal secretions removed by suction usually
contain large numbers of respiratory epithelial cells. Other
sources of cells are nasal washings, tampons etc., but in
general they contain much fewer cells. If dead animals are
available for examination then lung impression smears, mucus
scrapings or lung washings may be good sources of potentially
infected cells. However, viral antigen may no longer be
detected when the animal has died. If an animal is slaughtered
in the acute phase, then these techniques are much more
sensitive.

Furthermore the changes in the lungs at this time may be
diagnostic. Thus a productive bronchiolotis with intra
nuclear inclusions and bronchiolar epithelium necrosis suggest
adenovirus infection, whilst alveolar epithelisation, syncytial
formation and intracytoplasmic inclusions suggest PI3 activity.
Tissue from such an animal is ideally suited for virus isolation

and immunofluorescence.

In using the IF technique a number of technical points
must be observed. The respiratory epithelial cells must be
well washed to remove mucus. The antigen must be seen intra-
cellularly and have the appropriate distribution for that
particular antigen. If there is any doubt about specificity,
then duplicate cells should be stained with the appropriate
preimmunisation serum.

In general it is preferable, because of the labour of
conjugation and testing of the large number of antisera
involved, to use the indirect fluorescence technique. This
also allows the use of pools of sera from old animals or from
animals convalescing from respiratory disease to aid in the
diagnosis of new or unexpected micro-organisms.

Immunoperoxidase, especially the indirect test, is
probably an equally sensitive technique to immunofluorescence.
Its advantages are that a fluorescent microscope is not
required, it is less tiring to the eyes and the slides can be
examined when convenient. The disadvantages are that coupling
the antibody to enzyme (usually horse radish peroxidase) is
more difficult. However, the use of the indirect test and
commercially produced coupled antiglobulins overcome this.
The second difficulty is that it may be rather more difficult
to read than immunofluorescence. This difficulty may, in part
at least, be due to the presence of endogenous peroxidases in
leucocytes.

Other techniques are theoretically possible, but have not
to our knowledge been applied to the diagnosis of respiratory
disease. The most promising one is the enzyme-linked immunosorbent assay (ELISA test). This technique could, in theory,
be used to detect either antigen or antibody on the nasal
secretions and again, in theory, there is no reason why 'clini-
sticks' should not become available for diagnosis of specific
virus infections.

Serological methods of diagnosis have in many cases proved disappointing. One reason is by the time help is requested titres are actually already developing and it is therefore difficult to demonstrate rising titres. The second is that with us many calves become infected at 2 - 4 months old when they still have maternal antibody and in spite of virus growth and excretion, show no antibody response. If possible, samples for serological testing should be taken from older animals, which have lost their maternal antibody.

It should be remembered that neither the isolation of organisms nor the development of circulating antibodies are in themselves evidence of the cause of the disease. During a respiratory disease outbreak involving many poultry flocks some years ago, we often isolated as many as 4 viruses and 2 strains of mycoplasma as well as coliforms from broiler chicks at 3 weeks of age. The effective use of attenuated infectious bronchitis vaccine overcame these outbreaks. Although these other organisms (eg adenoviruses and reoviruses) may well have added to the pathological process, their spread was primarily due to the loss of maternal antibody in a population derived from many sources. Similar circumstances apply in many cattle fattening units.

Whilst certain viruses are clearly established as being respiratory pathogens - infectious bovine rhinotracheitis (IBR), parainfluenza 3 (PI3), bovine respiratory syncytial (BRS) and adenoviruses all spring to mind - other viruses are still not fully accepted as respiratory pathogens, eg bovine viral diarrhoea, and yet others have very doubtful claim to importance, eg the reoviruses. Furthermore there may be other viruses to be discovered. There is no reason why influenza, other parainfluenza, other herpes or coronaviruses should not be as important in bovine respiratory disease as they are in other species.

In our situation in which the respiratory form of IBR is virtually absent, the most important viruses appear to be

PI3, BRS and BVD, although we are still not sure whether BVD
is important as a primary respiratory pathogen or if its role
is in modifying the immune response. In a recent survey of 50
outbreaks of respiratory disease in Northern Ireland, antibodies were present in 66%, but active seroconversion could be
demonstrated on only one farm, and the cattle on this farm had
clinical mucosal disease. Adenoviruses are not important with
us, although clearly they can cause major outbreaks of disease
in other areas, often as epidemics. We cannot demonstrate any
role for reoviruses or Chlamydia. One group we do think might
have a role are the picornaviruses - apart from the rhinoviruses. Thus we have on a number of occasions made isolates
of enteroviruses from the nose of ill animals. These isolates
are not faecal contaminants and they often come in epidemics,
eg in 1964 and 1966. In addition enterovirus isolates have been
made from pneumonic lungs. This is not surprising because a
similar picture has been seen in humans. Thus workers in
Manchester (Holzel et al., 1965) isolated Coxsackie B, types
2, 3 and 4, from both upper and lower respiratory tracts and
indeed claimed that respiratory disease was the commonest
manifestation of Coxsackie virus infection in children
admitted to hospital. It should be noted that our commonest
enterovirus isolate, VB/5/27, produces lesions in suckling
mice and, if isolated from humans, would have been classified
as a Coxsackie virus.

Possibly the biggest difficulty in respiratory disease
work has been to reproduce the clinical syndrome. The best
results appear to have been obtained by repeated exposure over
a period of days or by the use of gas powered aerosol
generator (Sinclair and Tamoglia, 1972). But until a standard
method of reproducing disease is recognised and accepted, it
is difficult to establish which organisms are and are not
pathogens and also to formulate realistic control tests for
vaccines. There is also an urgent need for multi-disciplinary
studies on mixed infections by natural routes.

How can respiratory disease and the resulting economic

losses be prevented? Many agree that respiratory disease is
less severe if the environmental conditions are correct and
suggest that the ideal house should be warm, without overheating, with good ventilation but without draughts and that
new arrivals should be quarantined. However, even if someone
could design the perfect house, it would be very many years
before it would be universally adopted. Furthermore the
scientific basis for linking housing recommendations and
standards with control of disease is weak and this is an area
which urgently requires more research.

Therefore to control respiratory disease one must turn
to vaccines. We feel that if the initial virus infection
could be controlled success would be near. This certainly has
been the case in poultry. It is generally recognised that to
produce good protection against respiratory disease it is
necessary to stimulate both general and local immunity with
local immunity the most important. The local immunity in the
respiratory tract is both antibody - IgA mainly, but also IgG,
especially in the anterior part of the nasal cavity (Butler
et al., 1972), and cell-mediated immunity. Interferon probably
only plays a minor role. In poultry we have successfully
controlled infectious bronchitis in our broiler flocks by
vaccination at one day old. These chicks originate from
different parent flocks and thus have different levels of
maternal immunity. Spray vaccination produces a local immunity
in spite of the presence of maternal immunity. There is no
stimulus to the circulatory antibody - which in fact declines -
but these birds are resistant to challenge for at least 8
weeks. A similar managemental situation often exists with
cattle, when calves from many sources are collected together
in one intensive unit, and it appears a similar vaccination
programme would be successful. Thus Mohanty et al (1972)
showed that calves with no detectable circulating antibody to
IBR were immune to challenge 8 weeks later, presumably due to
local immunity. This local immunity can be boosted by a
second intranasal vaccination (Zygraich et al., 1975).
Furthermore, immunity can be stimulated by intranasal vaccination,

even in calves with maternal antibody (Todd, 1973). Therefore
the best method to protect cattle in feed lots might be to
stimulate local immunity by giving 2 or more intranasal
vaccinations during the winter.

Although the most direct method of producing local
immunity is by the use of an attenuated vaccine administered
intranasally, an attenuated vaccine given by a parenteral route
can also stimulate local immunity under certain circumstances
and it is possible also to vaccinate by the use of intranasally
administered inactivated vaccines (Marshall and Frank, 1971;
Frank and Marshall, 1971).

The inactivated vaccine should be free of the defects
usually attributed to an attenuated vaccine. But it must be
remembered it can have its own dangers. The inactivation of
the antigen may not be complete, extraneous micro-organisms may
not be inactivated or it may not provoke the required immune
response. In respiratory syncytial virus infections, there is
a possibility that serum antibody to this virus may play a
part in the pathogenesis of RSV bronchiolitis. Thus 80% of
infants given an inactivated RSV vaccine became seriously ill
after natural exposure, suggesting that serum antibody alone
in this case was not only ineffective but actually dangerous
(Parrott et al., 1975).

Therefore it must be hoped that the use of quick and
accurate diagnostic procedures will allow the use of the
appropriate vaccines. These vaccines must stimulate local
and cell-mediated immunity and it is possible that revaccination
will have to take place at regular intervals to keep this
immunity at optimal levels.

If attenuated vaccines are to be used, ideally they
should fulfil the following criteria; they should not be
excreted, they should be fully attenuated for all ages of
cattle, they should be grown on diploid cells of bovine
origin. If they are excreted, then they must not revert to

virulence after at least 3 back passes. Theoretically the temperature-sensitive mutant vaccine is ideal because the ts mutant should be able to multiply in the upper respiratory tract to give local immunity and yet not be able to invade the lower respiratory tract.

REFERENCES

Baskerville, A. and Lloyd, G. 1977. Vet. Rec. 101, p. 168.

Butler, J.E., Maxwell, C.F., Pierce, C.S., Hylton, M.B., Asofsky, R. and Kiddy, C.A. 1972. J. Immun. 109, p. 38.

Doane, F.W., Anderson, N., Chatiyanonda, K., Bannatyne, R.N., McLean, D.N. and Rhodes, A.J. 1967. Lancet 2, p. 751.

Frank, G.H. and Marshall, R.G. 1971. Am. J. Vet. Res. 32, p. 1707.

Hambling, M.H. 1964. Br. J. exp. Path. 45, p. 647.

Hanson, B.R. and Schipper, I.A. 1976. Am. J. Vet. Res. 37, p. 707.

Holzel, A., Parker, L., Patterson, W.H., Cartmel, D., Wjite, L.R., Purdy, R., Thompson, K.M. and Tobin, J. O'H. 1965. Br. Med. J. 1, p. 614.

Joncas, J.H., Berthiaume, L., Williams, R., Beaudry, P. and Pavilanis, V. 1969. Lancet, 1, p. 956.

McFerran, J.B., Clarke, J.K. and Curran, W.L. 1971. Res. Vet. Sci. 12, p. 253.

McKercher, D.G., Kaneko, J.J., Mills, R.J. and Wada, E.M. 1973. Am. J. Vet. Res. 34, p. 837.

Marshall, R.G. and Frank, G.H. 1971. Am. J. Vet. Res. 32, p. 1699.

Mohanty, S.B., Lillie, M.G., Ingling, A.L., and Hammond, R.C. 1972. J. Am. Vet. Med. Ass. 161, p. 1008.

Parrott, R.H., Kim, H.W., Brandit, C.D. and Chanock, R.M. 1975. Developments in biological standardisation 28, p. 389.

Sinclair, L.R. and Tamoglia, T.W. 1972. Am. J. Vet. Res. 33, p. 2085.

Thomas, L.H. and Stott, E.J. 1975. Res. Vet. Sci. 18, p. 227.

Todd, J.D. 1973. J. Am. Vet. Med. Ass. 163, p. 807.

Zygraich, N., Lobmann, M., Peetermans, J., Vasoboinic, E. and Huygelen, C. 1975. Developments in biological standardisation 28, p. 482.

O.C. Straub *(West Germany)*

    I would like to make a comment on Dr. McFerran's paper. We have clinicians amongst us, and I think it is important to mention the way you take samples of virology and the way you store them until they are placed in tissue culture. I agree that speed is most important. I go to $4^{\circ}C$; I think that $-20^{\circ}C$ is impossible and, if necessary, then $-70^{\circ}C$; but I prefer, if not right away, then $+4^{\circ}C$ until tissue culture.

SUMMARY

D.G. McKercher

Respiratory diseases - and, as I think most of you will
agree, bovine respiratory diseases in particular - are unique
in that the more we learn about them the less we understand them.
In this respect I can well understand Mr. Martin's and Dr.
Breukink's feelings about them in the statements which they have
made.

During this Seminar we have had very excellent presentations
on the aetiology, pathology, epidemiology, diagnosis, prevention
and control of these diseases. However, most of us, I am afraid,
will leave here haunted by the feeling that thus far very little
has been accomplished, and that many problems still remain to be
resolved, despite the diligent efforts of dedicated scientists
in a great many parts of the world.

Apparently the underlying problem is our failure to resolve
the aetiology regarding these respiratory diseases. If we do
not know the cause of a disease, or if we cannot reproduce it,
then it is very difficult to study it under controlled conditions.
That is possibly the main problem which we face now. Take the
IBR virus as an example, and compare the state of our knowledge
of this virus with that of PI3. The difference is that IBR is
reproduceable by experimental means, whereas it is very difficult
to do so with PI3, or the results are very inconsistent. Unless
you can reproduce the condition by experimental means you are
under a great handicap.

With the advent of cell culture 20 to 25 years ago, great
hopes were held for the solution of many viral diseases, by
the isolation of the agent and the development of preventive
measures. This did take place in the case of quite a number of
viral diseases. The virus was isolated, it was modified, vaccines
were produced and the disease was brought under control. But I
think that respiratory viruses were an exception. With the ex-

ception of IBR we are still very much in the situation we were even before cell culture became a reality.

The problem was not that cell culture did not yield the new viruses. In fact many hitherto unknown viruses were recovered by means of cell culture. The big problem was to prove that these viruses were actually pathogens. It is not necessary to name them. They have been discussed today. I agree that some people disagree with others as to the pathogenicity of these viruses. In the hands of some they appear to be more pathogenic than in the hands of others. What is the reason for this? Is it possible that those viruses which exist in the form of serotypes have different pathogenicities associated with these serotypes? It might happen that one man is working with a pathogenic serotype·and the other man is not. Would this account for it? I really do not know. If we refer to the example of PI3 it would not appear to be the case. PI3 will sometimes cause a disease or a clinical infection, and at other times it will not. It is a single serotype as far as we know. Another type of virus which exists in a single serotype, the IBR, consistently produces infection. I do not know whether it is a matter of serotypes, or even a matter of strains.

I think most people believe in synergism. It is believed that many weak viruses do not produce certainly clinical disease unless they are in association with other agents which act as secondaries. The virus is usually regarded as the triggering mechanism and the other agent, usually a bacterium, a chlamydia, or possibly a mycoplasma is regarded as the agent which causes the actual damage. I think that Dr. Allan's paper the other day was interesting in that respect.

What about the environment? We are speaking of respiratory diseases and therefore we are speaking of the lung. At veterinary school we were always taught that the lung is an external organ. If that is the case, and to some extent it is true, it is going to be in direct contact with the environment. As we know, the environment can be very inimical to the lung. Dr. Wiseman brought this out very clearly in his presentation, how such settled things as the amount of rainfall in an area can have an adverse or beneficial effect on the lung.

What about our approach to experimental infection? Are we being too artificial, too experimental, about it? Under field conditions, the animal in any group most susceptible to infection because of stress, or the presence of synergistic flora or other factors is the first one which will become infected. The virus can pick and choose. It can pick up the most susceptible animal. We cannot do this in our experimental infection work. The virus can probably establish itself in a highly susceptible animal even if it is a weak virus; it can set up an infection and then, by contact, the virus goes to the next susceptible animal, and so on. In going through a series of animals it eventually picks up pathogenicity and eventually produces clinical disease. In our experimental inoculations (and possibly I should not indict others by my practices) we tend to use maybe one or two animals in any one experiment. That animal is inoculated and if nothing happens we assume that the virus is not a pathogen, or that the animal is immune, and so on. The point is that the virus has not really had a chance under those conditions to establish it-self and gain pathogenicity. I wonder, therefore, if our ex-perimental methods might not be responsible for many of these failures which are reported. I am only casting these thoughts out. I do not know more than anyone else what the problems are.

The fact that so many people have worked for so many years and yet the aetiology of most of the respiratory infections still remains unresolved is causing people to become impatient and frustrated. Maybe this is a good thing. It probably stimulates us to look into new approaches. This was very well put by Dr. Hall yesterday. He feels that possibly we are emphasising the wrong areas. He was quite interested in the molecular biology approach, and the type of work which Dr. Eyre is doing. I will certainly not try to explain it, but I am sure that it has great merit. I think it is the correct trend. Dr. Straub has talked of interferon therapy. Maybe this is the forerunner of antiviral

therapy. As I mentioned the other day I think that this is
possibly a reality, and we should at least hope so.

Although we must look into these new avenues I do not think
that we should forget the approaches which we are presently
following. Dr. Gilmour is in a very interesting line: apparently
he is able to produce clinical disease in cattle by means of the
parainfluenza 3 virus and the pasteurella organism. Dr. Wells
also has some interesting finds, and although the findings are
in sheep they are possibly applicable to the situation in cattle.
As you well know, some of the reported vaccinations studies were
successful, and others were not. This is not too surprising
when we are dealing with these 'new' viruses - adenoviruses, and
so on. These seem to be very unpredictable viruses and it is
not surprising that the results from vaccines produced from them
would be unpredictable.

Then there is the advance of the immunological knowledge.
A great number of people - Dr. Wells, Dr. Bourne, Dr. Petzoldt -
just to mention some who come to mind, put forward some very
helpful views, and certainly these should be pursued.

Dr. Aalund has mentioned improved management practices in
animal production, based on the anticipated morbidity and mortality, and I think he would have to explain that himself. I do
not pretend to be capable of doing so.

In the same way, Dr. McFerran explained and described new
diagnostic methods.

I think that these are all very hopeful advances and I think
they should be continued, but also in concert with the newer
approaches which have been mentioned. Possibly all of this will
lead to the broader approach which has been talked about by
several investigators, and a co-ordinated multi-disciplinary
effort which has to some degree been lacking in the past, as well
as in the present. I think there is promise of success in the
not too distant future.

I would finally like to acknowledge the thoughtfulness of
the people who invited me here, and I would like to take the
opportunity to thank Dr. L'Hermite and Dr. Martin and Dr. Stamp
and other colleagues here. I am proud to have been associated
with the EEC organisation and I certainly wish you every success.

Thank you very much.

P. L'Hermite *(EEC)*
From what I have heard during the three days of this seminar,
instead of attempting to sum up what has been said I would prefer
to make a proposal that several recommendations should be brought
before the Commission of European Communities that support should
be continued for the work that has already been done in your
various Institutes on respiratory diseases in cattle.

Due to the procedures adopted by the Commission for sub-
mission of research programme proposals, and the ways by which
the decision-making is performed via the Commission and the
Council of Ministers, I propose that these recommendations be
considered under two headings.

A. Fairly long-term research work must be considered on the
mechanisms of the defence reaction, reaction of a particular type
in the case of respiratory diseases.

This can be divided into two main stages:

1) The causal agents, which are tolerated by the bovine
in most cases, become pathogenic under stress conditions
of diverse origin;

2) The second stage originates from the defence reaction,
resulting in a series of distrubances which lead at least
to morbidity and loss of productivity.

Recently, those responsible for agricultural research in
the member States of the Community, who were appointed within the
Standing Committee of Agricultural Research, agreed on a proposal
made by the Commission services for a research programme on protection of cattle and pigs against enteric and respiratory diseases.

In order to set up the programme, scientific experts in this
field of animal pathology will be appointed by each national
authority.

Two topics could be considered for research:

1) Mechanisms of synergenic reactions induced by viruses, bacteria and parasites, as proposed by Professor McKercher in his paper;

2) Study of the defence reaction, both on the basis of a biochemical approach - as already carried out by Professor Eyre - and of an immunological approach.

In addition, a multidisciplinary approach to the different fields - genetic resistance, nutrition/management interactions, physiopathology, environmental factors and clinical research - should be recommended, with a generally improved co-ordination of individual efforts.

B.   Short-term work must also be undertaken to establish at the Community level the criteria for comparing the different serological and immunological tests so that a standardised serological test can be set up for diagnosis which could be systematically applied, with the 'battery' of tests as a reference test.

If possible, a differential serological test could be established.

A further topic might also be dealt with if vaccination proves useful and viable, ie the standardisation of vaccine control at the production and utilisation stages.

I note that I have your agreement on this proposal for a recommendation to the Commission of European Communities.

Now I would like to thank you all for your participation. I would add specific thanks to the local organising committee, to Dr. Stamp and Dr. Martin; and also to all the participants for their attendance and their work - with special mention to Professor McKercher, Professor Eyre and Dr. Morein for having brought to us their knowledge and expertise in this field.

LIST OF PARTICIPANTS

LOCAL ORGANISING COMMITTEE   Animal Diseases Research Association,
Moredun Institute,
408, Gilmerton Road,
GB - Edinburgh EH17 7JH

Dr. W.B. Martin
(Chairman & Local Organiser)

Dr. J.T. Stamp
Dr. N.J.L. Gilmour
Dr. D.R. Snodgrass
Dr. P.W. Wells
Mr. G.E. Jones
Dr. J.M. Sharp
Mrs. Y.M. Morgan
Mrs. P.G. Kenworthy

BELGIUM

Dr. F. Lomba   Faculté Vétérinaire de Liège,
45, rue des Vétérinaires,
1070 - Brussels

Dr. E. van Opdenbosch   Institut National de Recherche
Vétérinaire,
Groeselenberg, 99,
1180 - Brussels

CANADA

Dr. P. Eyre   Professor of Pharmacology,
Department of Biomedical Sciences,
University of Guelph,
Ontario

DENMARK

Professor O. Aalund   (Preventive Medicine)
Royal Veterinary & Agricultural
University,
Bülowsvej, 13,
DK - 1870 - COPENHAGEN V

Dr. V. Bitsch   State Veterinary Serum Laboratory,
Bülowsvej, 27,
DK - 1870 - COPENHAGEN V

Dr. H. Ernø   Aarhus Universitet,
Institut for Medicinsk Mikrobiologi,
Universitets parken,
DK - 8000 - Aarhus

558

FRANCE

Dr. J. Asso

INRA
Station de Recherches de Virologie et
                                d'Immunologie,
Route de Thiverval,
F - 78850 - Thiverval Grignon

Dr. G. Dannacher

Laboratoire de Virologie Animale,
250, rue Marcel Merieux,
F - 69342 - Lyon

Dr. Ch. le Jan

INRA
Station de Recherches de Virologie et
                                d'Immunologie,
Route de Thiverval,
F - 78850 - Thiverval Grignon

IRELAND

Dr. H. Thornberry

Veterinary Research Laboratory,
Abbotstown,
IRL - Castleknock,
Co. Dublin

Dr. E. Weavers

Veterinary Research Laboratory,
Department of Agriculture,
Abbotstown,
IRL - Castleknock,
Co. Dublin

ITALY

Dr. Bergamaschi

Istituto Zoot. Generale,
Facolta di Medicina Veterinaria,
Universita di Milano,
Via Celoria, 10,
I - 20133 - Milan

Dr. P. Pignatelli

Head of Research,
Gruppo Montedison,
Via B. Crespi, 27,
I - 20159 - Milan

Dr. G. Rognoni

Istituto Zootecnia Generale,
Facolta di Medicina Veterinaria,
Universita di Milano,
Via Celoria, 10,
I - 20133 - Milan

NETHERLANDS

Dr. H.J. Breukink,

Faculteit voor Diergeneeskunde R.U.
Vakgroep Inwendige Ziekten Grote Huis-
                    dieren, "De Uithof",
Yalelaan, 10,
NL - Utrecht

Dr. C. Holzhauer,	Prov. Gezondsheidsdienst voor Dieren in Gelderland, "Klein Rosendael" Postbus 10, NL - Rosendael (GLD)
Dr. A. van Nieuwstadt,	Centraal Diergenesskundig Instituut, AFD Virologie, Houtribweg 39 NL - Lelystad

UNITED KINGDOM

Dr. Edna Allan	University of Glasgow Veterinary School Department of Veterinary Pathology Bearsden Road, GB - Glasgow GG1 1QH
Dr. A. Andrews	Meat & Livestock Commission, PO Box 44, Queensway House Bletchley GB - Milton Keynes MK2 2EF
Dr. F.J. Bourne	Department of Animal Husbandry, University of Bristol, Langford House, Langford, GB - Bristol BS18 7DY
Dr. R.N. Gourlay	Agricultural Research Council, Institute for Research on Animal Diseases, GB - Compton, Nr. Newbury, Berks.
Dr. S. Hall	Chief Scientist's Group, Ministry of Agriculture, Fisheries & Food, Great Westminster House, Horseferry Road, GB - London SW1P 2AD
Dr. J. Harkness	Central Veterinary Laboratory, GB - New Haw, Weybridge KT15 3NB
Dr. C. Howard	Agricultural Research Council, Institute for Research on Animal Diseases, GB - Compton, Nr. Newbury, Berks.
Dr. J.B. McFerran	Veterinary Research Laboratories, Stormont, GB - Belfast, Northern Ireland
Mr. B. Martin	21, Hill Street, GB - Kilmarnock, Ayrshire.

Dr. H.M. Pirie	University of Glasgow Veterinary School, Department of Veterinary Pathology Bearsden Road, GB - Glasgow GG1 1QH
Dr. J.M. Rutter	Advisory Board for the Research Councils Department of Education & Science, Elizabeth House, York Road, GB - London, S.E.1.
Dr. I.E. Selman	University of Glasgow Veterinary School, Department of Veterinary Medicine, Bearsden Road, GB - Glasgow GG1 1QH
Dr. E.J. Stott,	Agricultural Research Council, Institute for Research on Animal Diseases, GB - Compton, Nr. Newbury, Berks.
Dr. L.H. Thomas	Agricultural Research Council, Institute for Research on Animal Diseases, GB - Compton, Nr. Newbury, Berks.
Dr. A. Wiseman	University of Glasgow Veterinary School, Department of Veterinary Medicine, Bearsden Road, GB - Glasgow GG1 1QH

UNITED STATES OF AMERICA

Professor D.G. McKercher	School of Veterinary Medicine, University of California, USA - Davis, California

WEST GERMANY

Dr. H.J. Bürger	Institut für Parasitologie, Tierärztliche Hochschule Hannover, Bunteweg, 17, D - 3000 - Hannover 71
Professor Dr. H. Frerking	Rinderklinik, Tierärztliche Hochschule Hannover, Bunteweg, 17, D - 3000 - Hannover 71
Dr. H. Frey	Institut für Virologie der Tierärzt- liche Hochschule, Bunteweg, 17, Kirchrode, D - 3000 - Hannover

Dr. Kunz

Medizinische Tierklinik,
Ludwig-Maximilian Universität,
Veterinärstrasse, 13,
D - 8000 - Munich

Dr. Bror Morein

Temporary Address:

European Molecular Biology Laboratory
(EMBL)

Postfach 10,
D - 2209 - Heidelberg 69

Permanent Address:

The National Veterinary Department of
Biological Products,
S - 104 05 - Stockholm
Sweden

Professor Dr. K. Petzoldt

Institut für Mikrobiologie,
Tierärztliche Hochschule Hannover,
D - 3000 - Hannover 1

Professor Dr. O.C. Straub

Federal Research Institute for Virus
Diseases of Animals,
PO Box 1149,
D - 7400 - Tübingen

PD Dr. G. Wizigmann

Institut für Med. Mikrobiologie,
Infektions und Seuchemedizin,
Ludwig-Maximilians Universität,
Veterinärstrasse, 13,
D - 8000 - Munich

EEC - ADMINISTRATION

Mr. L.D.M. Mackenzie

Commission of the European Communities
DG VI-E-4
Loi 84 - 8/24
200, rue de la Loi
B - 1049 - BRUSSELS
Belgium

Mr. P. L'Hermite

As above

Mr. J. Dehandtschutter

As above

Mr. R. Kuyl

As above

Mr. G.J. Breslin

Commission of the European Communities
DG XIII
Batiment Jean Monnet
Plateau du Kirchberg
LUXEMBOURG
Luxembourg

RECORDING PERSONNEL

Mr. S.E.W. Hallam	Janssen Services 14, The Quay, Lower Thames Street, LONDON EC3R 6BU UK
Mr. R. Rice	Janssen Services 14, The Quay, Lower Thames Street, LONDON, EC3R 6BU UK